Pediatrics
at a GLANCE

editors

Steven M. ALTSCHULER, MD
CHAIRMAN and **ASSOCIATE PROFESSOR**
Department of Pediatrics
University of Pennsylvania;
PHYSICIAN-IN-CHIEF
Children's Hospital of Philadelphia
Philadelphia, Pennsylvania

Stephen LUDWIG, MD
PROFESSOR
Department of Pediatrics
University of Pennsylvania;
ASSOCIATE PHYSICIAN-IN-CHIEF
Children's Hospital of Philadelphia
Philadelphia, Pennsylvania

APPLETON
& LANGE

Developed by Current Medicine, Inc.
Philadelphia

Current Medicine, Inc.

400 Market Street
Suite 700
Philadelphia, PA 19106

Managing Editor:	Lori J. Bainbridge
Developmental Editors:	Scott Thomas Hurd, Elise M. Paxson
Art Director:	Paul Fennessy
Design and Layout:	Jerilyn Bockorick
Illustration Director:	Ann Saydlowski
Typesetting:	Ryan Walsh
Production:	Lori Holland, Sally Nicholson
Indexer:	Maria Coughlin

Library of Congree Cataloging-in-Publication Data

Pediatrics at a glance / editors, Steven Altschuler, Stephen Ludwig.

      p. cm.

      Includes bibliographical references and index.

      ISBN 0-8385-8142-0 (soft bound)

        1. Pediatrics–Handbooks, manuals, etc. I. Altschuler, Steven, 1953– . II. Ludwig, Stephen, 1945– .

        [DNLM: 1. Pediatrics–handbooks. 2. Diagnosis, Differential–in infancy & childhood–handbooks.   WS 39 P3716 1997]

      RJ48.P434 1997

      618.92–dc21

DNLM/DLC

for Library of Congress   97-41516

                                           CIP

Printed in the United States by Edwards Brothers

10 9 8 7 6 5 4 3 2 1

Distributed worldwide by Appleton & Lange.

Section Editors

Allergy, Immunology, and Pulmonary

Nicholas A. Pawlowski, MD
Associate Professor
  Department of Pediatrics
  University of Pennsylvania;
Chief
  Allergy Section
  The Children's Hospital of Philadelphia
  Philadelphia, Pennsylvania

Contributors

Terri F. Brown-Whitehorn, MD
Allergy/Immunology Fellow
  Department of Immunologic and Infectious Diseases
  University of Pennsylvania
  Immunologic and Infectious Diseases
  The Children's Hospital of Philadelphia
  Philadelphia, Pennsylvania

Joel Fiedler, MD
Associate Physician
  Allergy Section
  The Children's Hospital of Philadelphia
  Philadelphia, Pennsylvania

Richard M. Kravitz, MD
Assistant Professor
  Department of Pediatrics
  University of Pennsylvania;
  Division of Pulmonary Medicine
  The Children's Hospital of Philadelphia
  Philadelphia, Pennsylvania

Cardiology

Marie Gleason, MD
Clinical Associate Professor
  Department of Pediatrics
  University of Pennsylvania School of Medicine;
Director
  Outpatient Services
  The Children's Hospital of Philadelphia
  Philadelphia, Pennsylvania

Victoria Vetter, MD
Associate Professor
  Department of Pediatrics
  University of Pennsylvania School of Medicine;
Chief
  Division of Cardiology
  The Children's Hospital of Philadelphia
  Philadelphia, Pennsylvania

Emergency Medicine and Trauma

Kathy Shaw, MD
Associate Professor
  Department of Pediatrics
  University of Pennsylvania School of Medicine;
  Division of Emergency Medicine
  The Children's Hospital of Philadelphia
  Philadelphia, Pennsylvania

Contributors

Evaline A. Allesandrini, MD
  Division of Emergency Medicine
  The Children's Hospital of Philadelphia
  Philadelphia, Pennsylvania

Elizabeth R. Alpern, MD
Instructor
  Department of Pediatrics
  University of Pennsylvania School of Medicine;
Fellow
  Division of Emergency Medicine
  The Children's Hospital of Philadelphia
  Philadelphia, Pennsylvania

M. Douglas Baker, MD
Associate Professor
  Department of Pediatrics
  Yale University;
Chief
  Division of Pediatric Emergency Medicine
  The Children's Hospital at Yale–New Haven
  New Haven, Connecticut

Thomas H. Chun, MD
Instructor
  Department of Pediatrics
  University of Pennsylvania School of Medicine;
  Division of Emergency Medicine
  The Children's Hospital of Philadelphia
  Philadelphia, Pennsylvania

Joel A. Fein, MD
Assistant Professor
  Department of Pediatrics
  University of Pennsylvania School of Medicine;
  Division of Emergency Medicine
  The Children's Hospital of Philadelphia
  Philadelphia, Pennsylvania

Mark D. Joffe, MD
Associate Professor
  Department of Pediatrics
  University of Pennsylvania School of Medicine;
  Division of Emergency Medicine
  The Children's Hospital of Philadelphia
  Philadelphia, Pennsylvania

Jane Lavelle, MD
Assistant Professor
  Department of Pediatrics
  University of Pennsylvania School of Medicine;
  Division of Emergency Medicine
  The Children's Hospital of Philadelphia
  Philadelphia, Pennsylvania

Contributors

Frances Marie Nadel, MD
Instructor
Department of Pediatrics
University of Pennsylvania School of Medicine;
Division of Emergency Medicine
The Children's Hospital of Philadelphia
Philadelphia, Pennsylvania

Kevin C. Osterhoudt, MD
Instructor
Department of Pediatrics
University of Pennsylvania School of Medicine;
Division of Emergency Medicine
Section of Clinical Toxicology
The Children's Hospital of Philadelphia
Delaware Valley Regional Poison Control Center
Philadelphia, Pennsylvania

Barbara Pawel, MD
Clinical Assistant Professor
Department of Pediatrics
University of Pennsylvania School of Medicine;
Division of Emergency Medicine
The Children's Hospital of Philadelphia
Philadelphia, Pennsylvania

Jill C. Posner, MD
Instructor
Department of Pediatrics
University of Pennsylvania School of Medicine;
Division of Emergency Medicine
The Children's Hospital of Philadelphia
Philadelphia, Pennsylvania

Steven M. Selbst, MD
Professor
Department of Pediatrics
University of Pennsylvania School of Medicine;
Division of Emergency Medicine
The Children's Hospital of Philadelphia
Philadelphia, Pennsylvania

Martha W. Stevens, MD
Assistant Professor
Department of Pediatrics
University of Pennsylvania School of Medicine;
Division of Emergency Medicine
The Children's Hospital of Philadelphia
Philadelphia, Pennsylvania

George A. Woodward, MD
Assistant Professor
Department of Pediatrics
University of Pennsylvania School of Medicine;
Division of Emergency Medicine
The Children's Hospital of Philadelphia
Philadelphia, Pennsylvania

Endocrinology

Thomas Moshang, MD
Professor
Department of Pediatrics
University of Pennsylvania School of Medicine;
Division of Endocrinology
The Children's Hospital of Philadelphia
Philadelphia, Pennsylvania

Charles A. Stanley, MD
Professor
Department of Pediatrics
University of Pennsylvania School of Medicine;
Division of Endocrinology
The Children's Hospital of Philadelphia
Philadelphia, Pennsylvania

Gastroenterology

Christopher Liacouras, MD
Assistant Professor
Gastroenterology and Nutrition
University of Pennsylvania;
Director
Endoscopy Suite
Division of Gastroenterology and Hepatology
The Children's Hospital of Philadelphia
Philadelphia, Pennsylvania

General Pediatrics

Stephen Ludwig, MD
Professor
Department of Pediatrics
University of Pennsylvania;
Associate Physician-in-Chief
Children's Hospital of Philadelphia
Philadelphia, Pennsylvania

Hematology and Oncology

Catherine S. Manno, MD
Associate Professor
Division of Pediatrics
University of Pennsylvania;
The Children's Hospital of Philadelphia
Philadelphia, Pennsylvania

Contributors

Michael D. Hogarty, MD
Instructor
Division of Oncology
The Children's Hospital of Philadelphia
Philadelphia, Pennsylvania

Ann Leahy, MD
Assistant Professor of Pediatrics
Division of Oncology
The Children's Hospital of Philadelphia
Philadelphia, Pennsylvania

Michael N. Needle, MD
Assistant Professor of Pediatrics
The Children's Hospital of Philadelphia
Philadelphia, Pennsylvania

Metabolic and Genetic Disorders

Paige Kaplan, MD
Professor of Pediatrics
   Department of Metabolism and Genetics
   University of Witwatersrand
   Johannesburg, South Africa;
   Division of Metabolism and Genetics
   The Children's Hospital of Philadelphia
   Philadelphia, Pennsylvania

Nephrology

Bernard S. Kaplan, MB, BCh
Professor
   Department of Pediatrics
   University of Pennsylvania School of Medicine;
   Division of Nephrology
   The Children's Hospital of Philadelphia
   Philadelphia, Pennsylvania

Seth Schulman, MD
Assistant Professor
   Department of Pediatrics
   University of Pennsylvania School of Medicine;
   Division of Nephrology
   The Children's Hospital of Philadelphia
   Philadelphia, Pennsylvania

Neurology

Stephen G. Ryan, MD
Assistant Professor
   Department of Neurology and Pediatrics
   University of Pennsylvania;
   Division of Neurology
   The Children's Hospital of Philadelphia
   Philadelphia, Pennsylvania

Rheumatology

Gregory F. Keenan, MD
Assistant Professor
   Rheumatology Section
   University of Pennsylvania;
   Wood Center
   The Children's Hospital of Philadelphia
   Philadelphia, Pennsylvania

Preface

The practice of pediatrics is undergoing monumental changes as the result of a rapid evolution in health care delivery and financing and ongoing new developments in clinical diagnosis and therapy. The focus away from specialty-dominated care toward a primary-care model is forcing primary-care providers to assume a greater and more comprehensive role in the care of their patients. In this system of health care, the availability of current, organized, and easily accessible clinical information is critical to the delivery of quality, efficient, and cost-effective care. *Pediatrics at a Glance* has been developed by pediatric faculty at the Children's Hospital of Philadelphia and the University of Pennsylvania School of Medicine to provide the primary-care provider with an easy-to-use and concise reference source to be used while caring for patients.

The section editors and authors are all experienced clinicians and educators who have continually excelled in their interactions with primary-care providers. During the editorial process, care has been taken to ensure that each chapter conforms to a standard format. We hope that the consistent chapter organization that provides a spread of two facing pages (diagnosis on the left and treatment on the right) for each disorder will be a useful aid in determining for an individual patient the most appropriate diagnostic tests and treatment plan.

As editors, we would like to thank all the section editors and authors for their hard work and timely contributions to this project. Their commitment to excellence in patient care and education is readily apparent in the completed text.

Steven M. Altschuler, MD

Stephen Ludwig, MD

Contents

Contents

Contents by specialty

Figure acknowledgments

We gratefully acknowledge the publishers and individuals
who allowed us to use the following illustrations.

Page 280. Adapted with permission from Gay NJ et al.: Age
specific antibody prevalence to parvovirus B19: how many
women are infected in pregnancy? Communicable Diseases
Report 1994, 4:R104–R107.

Page 298. Adapted with permission from Fleisher G, Ludwig
S: Textbook of Pediatric Emergency Medicine, ed 3. New
York: Williams and Wilkins; 1993:1236–1287.

This book provides current expert recommendations on the diagnosis and treatment of all major disorders throughout medicine in the form of tabular summaries. Essential guidelines on each of the topics have been condensed into two pages of vital information, summarizing the main procedures in diagnosis and management of each disorder to provide a quick and easy reference.

Each disorder is presented as a "spread" of two facing pages: the main procedures in diagnosis on the left and treatment options on the right.

Listed in the main column of the Diagnosis page are the common symptoms, signs, and complications of the disorder, with brief notes explaining their significance and probability of occurrence, together with details of investigations that can be used to aid diagnosis.

The left shaded side column contains information to help the reader evaluate the probability that an individual patient has the disorder. It may also include other information that could be useful in making a diagnosis (*e.g.*, classification or grading systems, comparison of different diagnostic methods).

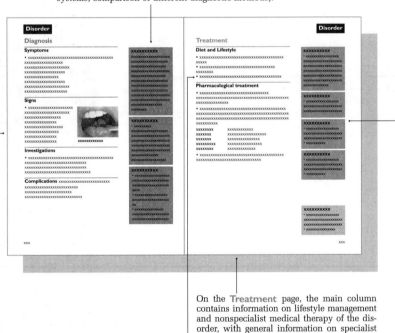

On the Treatment page, the main column contains information on lifestyle management and nonspecialist medical therapy of the disorder, with general information on specialist management when this is the main treatment.

Whenever possible under "Pharmacological treatment," guidelines are given on the standard dosage for commonly used drugs, with details of contraindications and precautions, main drug interactions, and main side effects. In each case, however, the manufacturer's drug data sheet should be consulted before any regimen is prescribed.

The main goals of treatment (*e.g.*, to cure, to palliate, to prevent), prognosis after treatment, precautions that the physician should take during and after treatment, and any other information that could help the clinician to make treatment decisions (*e.g.*, other nonpharmacological treatment options, special situations or groups of patients) are given in the right shaded side column. The key and general references at the end of this column provide the reader with further practical information.

Diagnosis [1]

Symptoms

- History can provide helpful clues to the cause of the abdominal mass.

Infrequent bowel movements: constipation or intussusception.

Abdominal trauma: pancreatic pseudocyst.

Dysuria: renal disease.

Weight loss: malignancy, Crohn's disease, abscess.

Irregular menstrual cycle: pregnancy, ovarian disease.

Signs

Jaundice: liver or biliary disease.

Fever: Crohn's disease, malignancy, or abscess.

Hematuria: renal disease.

Abdominal distension: 30%–40% of patients.

Failure to thrive: malignancy, renal disorders.

Investigations

Physical exam: the abdominal examination should be soft and nontender. In infants, the liver edge and spleen tip may be palpable and a full bladder may be mistaken for a hypogastric abdominal mass. Solid masses will be dull by palpation whereas hollow organs will provide a high pitch. Bruits can be appreciated in vascular tumors.

Rectal exam: to define mass (intestinal or in pelvis) and check for occult bleeding.

Blood tests: complete blood count (malignancy, abscess, anemia, hemolysis); chemistry panel (liver gallbladder and renal disease); amylase and lipase (pancreatic or ovarian disorders). A screen for vanillylmandelic acid (VMA) will identify neuroblastoma.

Abdominal ultrasound: the most useful test for abdominal masses in children. This test is noninvasive and easily performed and can usually identify the involved organ. **Limitations:** operator variability and intestinal gas may obscure findings [2].

Abdominal CT: provides excellent anatomic detail and is very useful after abdominal ultrasound.

Abdominal plain film: can provide information on the presence of constipation, calcifications (gallstones, kidney stones, teratoma, adrenal hemorrhage, neuroblastoma, meconium peritonitis), and chest involvement.

MRI: beneficial when evaluating liver and kidney masses, vascular disorders, and tumors [3].

Intravenous urography: useful in assessing kidney disorders.

Intestinal contrast (upper gastrointestinal, barium enema) and endoscopy studies: when intestinal involvement is suspected (Crohn's disease, abscess).

Laparoscopy or laparotomy: performed when direct visual interpretation and biopsy is required.

Differential diagnosis

Abdominal wall: hernia, omphalocele.

Adrenal: neuroblastoma, hemorrhage, pheochromocytoma.

Bladder: posterior urethral valves, obstruction.

Extraintestinal: mesenteric/omental cyst, teratoma, lymphangioma, ascites, meconium peritonitis.

Gallbladder/biliary tree: choledochal cyst, hydrops, stone.

Gastric: foreign body, bezoar, gastroparesis.

Intestine: constipation, volvulus, duplication, intussusception, abscess, megacolon, lymphoma.

Kidney: hydronephrosis, Wilm's tumor, ureteropelvic junction obstruction, cystic kidney disease, renal vein thrombosis.

Liver: storage disease, infection, congenital hepatic fibrosis, hemangioendothelioma, tumor.

Ovary: torsion, dermoid, tumor.

Pancreas: pseudocyst.

Spleen: leukemia, Gaucher's disease, Niemann-Pick disease, portal hypertension, hemolytic anemia.

Uterus: pregnancy (ectopic), hydrometrocolpos.

Epidemiology

- Neuroblastoma, Wilm's tumor, and teratoma are the most common tumors.

Neonate: most masses are retroperitoneal and benign (>50% from the urinary tract); less than 10% involve the intestine.

Older child: likelihood of malignancy increases (50% retroperitoneal malignancy in children >1 y).

Adolescents: increased chance of ovarian and uterine disease; appendiceal disorder; or liver, gallbladder, biliary abnormalities.

Location of mass

Epigastric: stomach, pancreas.

Right upper quadrant: liver, gallbladder, stomach, adrenal.

Left upper quadrant: spleen, stomach, adrenal.

Flank: kidney, adrenal, intestinal, extraintestinal.

Periumbilical: intestinal, extraintestinal, abdominal wall.

Right/left lower quadrant: ovary, appendix (right), intestinal, extraintestinal.

Hypogastric: bladder, uterus, intestinal.

Treatment

Diet and lifestyle

Depends on the etiology of the mass.

Pharmacologic treatment

Chemotherapy: malignancies.

Enzyme replacement: Gaucher and Niemann-Pick disease.

Laxatives and enemas: constipation.

Diuretics: ascites.

Motility agents (cisapride, metoclopromide): gastroparesis.

Nonpharmacologic treatment

Surgery: indicated for tumors and the majority of ovarian, renal, bladder, and intestinal disorders.

Interventional radiology: drainage of abscess or cyst, intussusception, gallbladder and biliary abnormalities.

Endoscopy: intestinal foreign body

Treatment aims

To treat the etiology of the abdominal mass.

Emergencies

• Patients who present with an abdominal mass and signs and symptoms of intestinal obstruction, a toxic appearance, fever, gastrointestinal bleeding, hematuria, right lower quadrant pain, pancreatitis or toxic megacolon should be immediately evaluated.

Prognosis

• Depends on the etiology of the mass.

• Constipation is successfully treated with medication. Intussusception recurs in 10% of patients. Hernias, benign tumors, bezoars, and cysts are treated definitively with surgery. The prognosis of malignancies varies depending on the etiology.

Follow-up and management

• Malignancies, most renal and liver diseases, and storage diseases (Gaucher and Niemann–Pick) require long-term follow-up.

Key references

1. Healey PJ, Hight DW: Abdominal masses. In *Pediatric Gastrointestinal Disease*. Edited by Wyllie R, Hyams JS. Philadelphia: WB Saunders; 1993:281–292.
2. Teele RL, Henschke CI: Ultrasonography in the evaluation of 482 children with an abdominal mass. *Clin Diagn Ultrasound* 1984, 14:141–165.
3. White KS: Imaging of abdominal masses in children. *Semin Pediatr Surg* 1992, 1:269–276.

Diagnosis

Symptoms

Pain or swelling of the scrotum or testicle.

Bilateral disease: rare in patients with torsion of the testicle or appendix testis.

Nausea or vomiting: common in patients with testicular torsion.

Epididymitis: history of prior urologic instrumentation, painful voiding, or urethral discharge.

History of trauma: testicular hematoma, rupture, or dislocation; can also be seen with testicular torsion.

Signs

Bilateral disease suggests trauma or infection.

Erythema of overlying skin is a non-specific sign.

Testicular torsion: high-riding and transversely located testicle.

Cremasteric reflex: absent in patients with testicular torsion. If present, this strongly suggests another diagnosis [1].

Location of tenderness: posterior in epididymitis; superior–anterior in torsion of the testicular appendage.

Scrotal pain without testicular involvement: vasculitides.

Investigations

• Complete blood count generally unhelpful in differentiating diagnoses.

Epididymitis

• Urinalysis reveals pyuria in only one third of patients with epididymitis, unhelpful in other diagnoses.

• Urethral swab for *Chlamydia* sp. isolation, chocolate agar for isolation of *Neisseria gonorrhea*.

• Serological testing for syphilis should be performed in any patient suspected of having a sexually transmitted disease.

Testicular torsion

• Handheld doppler useful only for testing success of detorsion procedure.

• Color doppler flow study useful in diagnosing testicular torsion in adolescents and adults, less useful in young children.

• Study of choice for children is radionuclide scintography (Technetium-99).

Complications

• Delay in diagnosis of testicular torsion can result in nonviability of the testicle.

• Orchitis can result in impaired sterility, rarely infertility.

• Traumatic rupture or dislocation can result in ischemic compromise and subsequent loss of testicular viability.

• Incarcerated inguinal hernia can result in bowel strangulation, gangrene, and septicemia.

Differential diagnosis [2]

Swollen and painful
Testicular torsion.
Torsion of appendix testis.
Incarcerated hernia.
Epididymitis/orchitis.
Vasculitides.
Henoch–Schönlein purpura.
Kawasaki disease.
Familial Mediterranean fever.
Trauma.
Rare entities.
Bleeding into tumor.
Peritonitis.
Intra-abdominal hemorrhage.
Spermatic vein thrombosis.
Swollen and not painful
Inguinal hernia.
Hydrocele.
Varicocele.
Spermatocele.
Tumor.
Acute idiopathic scrotal edema.

Epidemiology

• Of boys presenting with acute scrotal complaints [3]:
38% had testicular torsion,
31% had epididymitis or orchitis,
24% had torsion of the appendix testis,
7% had idiopathic pathology or normal findings.

Etiology

Torsion
Bell clapper deformity, in which tunica vaginalis completely surrounds testicle rather than allowing for normal posterior fixation within the scrotum.

Epididymitis
Sexually active male children: *Neisseria gonorrhea, Chlamydia trachomatis*.
Prepubertal patients: *Pseudomonas* sp., *Escherichia coli*, or *Enterococcus* sp.

Treatment

Nonpharmacologic treatment

For testicular torsion

Immediate: detorsion procedure. Twist testicle towards ipsilateral thigh and observe for resolution of pain and swelling [4].

Surgical removal of nonviable testicle.

Bilateral orchiopexy.

Pharmacologic treatment

For epididymitis

Sexually active patient and their partners:

Standard dosage   *Gonorrhea:* Ceftriaxone 250 mg intramuscularly.

Cefixime 800 mg orally, single dose.

Chlamydia: Doxycycline 100 mg twice daily for 10 days.

Azithromycin 2 g orally, single dose.

Prepubertal patients: trimethoprim-sulfamethoxazole 2 cm^3/kg divided twice daily for 7–10 d.

Other treatment options

For torsion of appendix testis/orchitis

Rest.

Testicular elevation.

Analgesia.

For vasculitides

See pharmacologic treatments for Kawasaki syndrome, anaphylactoid purpura, familial Mediterranean fever.

• For traumatic injury to testicles, incarcerated hernia, or testicular cancer, refer to appropriate subspecialist (urology, general surgery).

Treatment aims

To manually correct testicular torsion and follow-up with surgical management.

To treat infectious causes with appropriate antibiotic therapy.

To palliate inflammatory lesions.

Prognosis

Testicular torsion

• Testicle viability depends on promptness of treatment.

100% if torsion corrected within 3 h of symptom onset.

50%-75% within 8 h.

20% within 24 h.

0% after 24 h.

Testicular trauma

• Surgical exploration within 3 d of injury can reduce the need for orchiectomy, shorten hospitalization, and relieve disability [5].

Infectious causes and vasculitides

• No threat to testicular viability; possible impaired fertility after acute orchitis.

Key references

1. Zderic SA, Duckett JW: Adolescent urology. *AUA Update Series.* [Houston, TX]:American Urological Association, Inc.; 1994.

2. Fein JA: Pathology in the privates: acute scrotal swelling in children and adolescents. *Pediatric Emergency Medicine Reports* 1997, **2**:47-56.

3. Knight PJ, Vassy LE: The diagnosis and treatment of the acute scrotum in children and adolescents. *Ann Surg* 1984, **200**:664673.

4. Cattolica EV: Preoperative manual detorsion of the torsed spermatic cord. *J Urol* 1985, **133**:803–805.

5. Cass AS, Luxenberg M: Value of early operation in blunt testicular contusion with hematocele. *J Urol* 1988, **139**:746–747.

Diagnosis

Symptoms

• Large left-to-right shunts may occur with ventricular septal defect (VSD), atrioventricular canal defect (AVC), patent ductus arteriosus (PDA), and atrial septal defect (ASD). Age at presentation with symptoms varies according to the size of the cardiac shunt, degree of associated pulmonary hypertension and vascular resistance.

Large shunts with pulmonary hypertension

• Patients present in infancy with poor feeding, poor weight gain, easy fatiguability and a cardiac murmur.

Full-term infant: a VSD is the most likely cause; may be multiple; muscular and perimembranous defects are most common; high rate of spontaneous closure over time; malalignment and canal type defects need surgical closure.

Premature infants: a large PDA may worsen respiratory status.

Patients with genetic syndromes (ie, trisomy 21): VSD or AVC are most likely.

Large shunts without pulmonary hypertension

• ASD is most common cause; approx 75% are secundum type, occurring in the mid-atrial septum; next in frequency is the primum ASD (incomplete AVC) occurring in the lower part of the atrial septum and associated with cleft mitral valve; less common is the sinus venosus type, occurring in the upper septum near the superior caval inflow and associated with partial, anomalous right-pulmonary venous drainage.

• Patients are asymptomatic with a murmur. Growth is usually normal.

• Patients may exhibit dyspnea on exertion and palpitations as older children, teens, and young adults.

Signs

Tachycardia for age, possible gallop rhythm, harsh systolic murmur along the left sternal border that radiates to the back, a loud narrowly split S2, a diastolic rumble over the LV apex (mitral area).

Tachypnea with clear lung fields.

Hepatomegaly.

Equal pulses throughout.

Altered growth parameters: preserved head and length rate of growth, but slowed rate of weight gain.

Investigations

Electrocardiography

VSD, ASD: sinus tachycardia, persistent right axis deviation, RVH or biventricular hypertrophy; in ASD, RAE (peaked P wave in lead II).

Complete AV canal: right superior axis ("northwest axis"= negative QRS deflection in lead I, avF), RVH.

Primum ASD: left superior axis (positive QRS deflection in lead I and negative QRS deflection in lead avF), RAE, RVH (rSR' pattern).

PDA: normal or leftward axis for age, LVH, LAE.

Chest radiography: cardiomegaly, increased pulmonary arterial markings, prominent main pulmonary artery segment, left atrial enlargement on lateral projection, some patients with right aortic arch.

Echocardiography: to delineate the presence of one or more septal defects and other associated cardiac anomalies, such as pulmonary or stenosis and coarctation of the aorta; pulmonary arterial pressure estimate made by measuring the pressure gradient across a VSD or PDA or by measuring the right ventricular pressure using the tricuspid valve regurgitant jet, if present; cardiac chamber dimensions can be measured.

Cardiac catheterization: indicated to document pulmonary artery pressure or Qp:Qs ratio if not able to be determined by echocardiography; assessment of pulmonary vascular reactivity with vasodilators can be done in patients with long-standing pulmonary hypertension.

Differential diagnosis

• In patients presenting with initial findings of cardiomegaly, altered growth parameters, respiratory symptoms, cardiac murmur, or change in activity level, one must differentiate between:
A large left-to-right shunt with CHF.
Cardiomyopathy with CHF.
An untreated cardiac arrhythmia (tachycardia or bradycardia) with CHF.

Etiology

• In general, left-to-right shunt lesions are random birth defects without a specific genetic inheritance pattern, although there are clearly families where multiple affected members have VSD or ASD. Patients with diverse chromosomal anomalies, especially trisomies, have an increased incidence of septal defects, suggesting a genetic role. Environmental factors also are important; fetal exposure to certain viruses (ie, congenital rubella) or other agents (ie, ethanol, anticonvulsants, maternal diabetes with hyperglycemia and fetal hyperinsulinism) result in increased incidence of congenital heart defects, especially left-to-right shunts.

Epidemiology

• VSD accounts for ~20% of congenital heart defects, with an incidence of ~2:1000 live, term births; slight female predominance; most common defect in chromosomal syndromes.
• ASD accounts for 6%–10% of congenital heart defects; incidence, 1:1500 live, term births; slight female predominance.
• PDA (without prematurity history) accounts for 5%–10% of congenital heart defects; incidence, 1:2000 live, term births.
• CAVC: accounts for 3%–5 % of congenital heart defects occurring ~2:10,000 live births but accounts for up to 40% of congenital heart disease in patients with trisomy 21; slight female predominance.

Complications

Congestive heart failure (CHF), endocarditis, pulmonary artery hypertension and pulmonary vascular obstructive disease (Eisenmenger syndrome), cardiac arrhythmias (SVT, atrial flutter, ventricular ectopy), aortic valve regurgitation (aortic cusp prolapse into the VSD), and subaortic stenosis (fibrous) or right ventricular muscle bundle (associated with nature's attempts at spontaneous VSD closure).

Treatment

Diet and lifestyle

• In general, there are no restrictions. Infants may need higher caloric density of formula or breast milk to maintain adequate weight gain with a large shunt and CHF with poor growth.

Pharmacologic treatment

Endocarditis prophylaxis: suggested for all VSD, AV canal, and primum ASD patients; not required for isolated ASD, or 6 months after closure of PDA or pericardial patch repair of ASD.

Anticongestive medications: digoxin, diuretics, and afterload reduction are standard.

Nonpharmacologic treatment

Surgical intervention

Large VSD and CAVC: surgical repair within the first year of life is indicated when there is persistent pulmonary hypertension, cardiomegaly, and/or failure to thrive.

ASD: surgical repair generally performed after 2–3 years of age, if right heart volume overload is present.

PDA: in premature infants, surgical ligation is indicated in ill infants who have failed medical treatment with indomethacin; in term infants and older children, surgical repair of a small ductus arteriosus is elective after 1 year of age or sooner if there is left heart volume overload; this may be performed through a standard left thoracotomy or with video-assisted thoracoscopy.

Digoxin

Standard dosage	Digoxin, (loading dose[TDD]): 30–40 mug/kg i.v. or p.o. in 3 divided 8 h apart (0.50, 0.25, 0.25 of TDD, respectively).
	Digoxin (maintenance dose): 10 mug/kg/d divided every 12 h (12 h after loading is completed).
	Lasix, 1 mg/kg i.v. or p.o. every 12 h, up to 4 mg/kg/d.
	Aldactone, 1–3 mg/kg/d p.o. every 12 h.
	Captopril, 1–3 mg/kg/d p.o. every 8 h.

Catheter intervention

• Nonsurgical coil embolization of small PDAs in the cardiac catheterization lab is an alternative option that has gained increased popularity in the past 5–8 years with 90%–95% complete occlusion rate.

Treatment aims

To recognize and treat heart disease that may result in damage to the heart and lungs, resulting in death from congestive heart failure, pulmonary hypertension, and pulmonary vascular occlusive disease.

Prognosis

Small left-to-right shunts: aside from the risk of endocarditis, long-term prognosis is excellent.

Moderate left-to-right shunts: modest elevation in pulmonary vascular resistance, and volume loaded chambers, often leads to surgical intervention in the older child.

Large left-to-right shunts: if appropriate medical and surgical therapy is done within the first year, long-term prognosis is very good; if unrepaired, leads to Eisenmenger syndrome, in which pulmonary vascular occlusive disease results in shunt reversal, cyanosis, and early death from hypoxia, stroke, arrhythmias, and congestive heart failure.

General references

Brook M, Heymann M: Patent ductus arteriosus. In *Moss and Adams' Heart Disease in Infants, Children and Adolescents*, ed 5. Edited by Emmanouilides G, Allen H, Riemeschneider T, Gutgesell H. Williams and Wilkins: Baltimore; 1995:746–764.

Feldt R, Porter C, Edwards W, *et al.*: Atrioventricular septal defetcs. In *Moss and Adams' Heart Disease in Infants, Children and Adolescents*, ed 5. Edited by Emmanouildes G, Allen H, Riemenschneider T, Gutgesell H. Williams and Wilkins: Baltimore, 1995:704–724.

Kidd L, Driscoll D, Gersony W, *et al*: Second natural history study of congenital heart defects: results of treatment of patients with ventricular septal defects. *Circulation* 1993, **87 (suppl I)**:I38–I51.

Porter C, Feldt R, Edwards W, *et al*.: Atrial septal defects. In *Moss and Adams' Heart Disease in Infants, Children and Adolescents*, ed 5. Edited by Emmanouilides G, Allen H, Riemenschneider T, Gutgesell H. Williams and Wilkins: Baltimore; 1995:687–703.

Diagnosis

Symptoms

- Often a child is unaware of the enlargement of lymph glands and thus will not directly or specifically complain.
- If the node(s) are painful and enlarged, the child will have reason for presenting with a symptom.
- Other symptoms may be of general malaise or fatigue, loss of appetite, weight loss, fevers, night sweats, or change in sleep patterns.
- Children too young to articulate their symptoms may revert to younger behaviors or exhibit behavioral situations that evoke parental attention.

Signs

Localized adenopathy: consider the area of distribution of the node and determine any inciting source of irritation, infection, or mechanical trauma. Some localized nodes are of immediate concern, *eg*, nodes in the supraclavicular area.

Generalized adenopathy: consider systemic infections and neoplastic diagnoses.

- Palpation of the size and texture of the node(s) is important. Many normal children will have nodal enlargement up to 1–1.5 cm. These nodes are usually firm but slightly spongy and nontender. Nodes that are tender, warm, and red suggest enlargement due to infection (adenitis). Nodes that are hard or rubbery suggest tumor. Masses that are fluctuant may be nodes with necrotic centers, but a nonadenopathic mass must also be considered.
- Evaluate the child for any other signs such as other areas of lymphoid hyperplasia (*eg*, tonsil, adenoids) and other findings of a generalized process (*eg*, liver, spleen enlargement).

Investigations

- The need for investigations beyond a thorough history and physical examination will depend on the amount of adenopathy, location, and accompanying signs and symptoms.
- The finding of enlarged lymph nodes on examination prompts consideration of a large differential diagnosis that contains many common benign entities as well as other diagnoses with serious, long-term, life-threatening implications.

Complete blood count: will be helpful in most cases. Look for abnormalities in all three cell lines: erythrocytes, leukocytes, and platelets. A sedimentation rate will help to identify chronic inflammatory conditions.

Other tests: PPD (purified protein derivative), monospot test or Epstein-Barr virus (EBV) titers (particularly in preadolescents), HIV testing if there are risk factors, and chest radiography.

Node biopsy: for tissue diagnosis in nodes that are chronic, unresponsive to therapy, rapidly advancing, and defying identification. A CT scan of the area prior to the biopsy will help to define the anatomy and guide the procedure.

Needle aspiration: for nodes that are fluctuant, this may yield an offending organism and guide antibiotic therapy.

Complications

- Complications result when a diagnosis is missed that requires special therapy, *eg*, tuberculosis or malignancy.
- Other complications are caused by needle aspiration that is performed in a way that leads to a chronic draining sinus.

Differential diagnosis

Generalized nodes: infections, eg, non-specific viruses, EBV, cytomegalovirus (CMV), sarcoid, or HIV; tumors, eg, leukemia, lymphoma (both Hodgkin's and non-Hodgkin's types), histiocytosis or neuroblastoma; inflammatory disorder, eg, juvenile rheumatoid arthritis (JRA), Kawasaki disease, systemic lupus erythematosus (SLE); medications, eg, phenytoin, isoniazid.

Localized nodes: infection, primarily bacterial (*Staphylococcus* and *Streptococcus*), tuberculosis, atypical tuberculosis, cat-scratch disease, or EBV; other sources of inflammation, eg, dental abscesses, chronic eczema, cellulitis, scalp irritants.

Etiology

- The most common cause for diffuse adenopathy is nonspecific viral infection. Usually there will be a mild prodromal illness and not many signs or symptoms. Adenopathy will be generalized and the size of the nodes less than 1–1.5 cm.
- Localized adenopathy usually stems from an infective process originating in the nose or throat or soft tissues and has accompanying signs of redness, tenderness, and warmth. The usual cause is bacterial: *Staphylococcus aureus* or *Streptococcus*.
- Other causes are more rare.

Treatment

General treatment

• The initial approach to the child with localized adenopathy and the findings of adenitis is to carefully measure the size, location, and consistency and begin antibiotic therapy. Use of an agent that will be effective against *Staphylococcus* and *Streptococcus* is advised, *eg*, cephalexin, 50 mg/kg/d for 10 days. Amoxicillin/clavulinic acid is an acceptable agent as well. If the adenitis is in response to a dental infection, clindamycin, 30 mg/kg/d, may be preferred to cover anaerobic organisms.

• The patient may apply warm compresses if symptomatic relief is achieved by doing so.

• Adenitis should respond over a 2-week period with less inflammatory signs and perhaps some decrease in node size.

• For children with more generalized adenopathy, initial laboratory assessment is indicated. A normal CBC and sedimentation rate is generally reassuring that no serious condition exists, although this is not absolute. A PPD should be added to this initial screen.

• If history and physical examination suggest other diagnoses, *eg*, mononucleosis, then appropriate laboratory confirmation should be sought.

• If no clear cause is apparent and the adenopathy has persisted for 3–4 weeks, then further testing should be undertaken.

• The patient should be allowed to resume their own level of activity and a balanced diet should be encouraged.

Treatment aims

To establish a working diagnosis based on history, physical examination, and limited laboratory studies.

To apply a therapy.

To evaluate for expected response or resolution.

• If response does not occur, widen the differential diagnosis.

Other treatments

• If the child is showing generalized signs and if there are abnormalities on the CBC or sedimentation rate, then direct referral to a pediatric center is indicated to confirm the suspected diagnosis of malignancy.

• Presumed infected nodes that do not respond to oral antibiotics may also require admission to the hospital for treatment with intravenous antibiotics.

Prognosis

• For adenopathy with infectious causes, the prognosis is excellent.

• For adenopathy with neoplastic causes, prognosis will depend on the kind of tumor and its stage of progression.

Follow-up and management

• Children with adenopathy must be followed carefully and reexamined frequently to make sure that they are following an expected course for their condition.

General references

Chesney J: Cervical adenopathy. *Pediatr Rev* 1994, **15**:276–284.

Mazur P, Kornberg AE: Lymphadenopathy. In *Textbook of Pediatric Emergency Medicine*, ed 3. Edited by Fleisher G, Ludwig S. Baltimore: Williams & Wilkins; 1993: 310–317.

Putnam T: Lumps and bumps in children. *Pediatr Rev* 1992, **13**:371–378.

Adrenal hyperplasia, congenital

Diagnosis

Symptoms

Lethargy, vomiting, or poor feeding: in newborns.

Oligomenorrhea: in adolescent females.

Signs

In newborn or infant: ambiguous genitalia; hypotension, tachycardia, hypothermia, shock; hyponatremia, hyperkalemia, acidosis.

In older child: premature pubic hair, clitoral enlargement in female or enlargement of penis.

In adolescent: hirsutism and pustular, cystic acne.

Investigations

Ambiguous genitals: *see* Ambiguous genitalia.

Plasma corticotropin concentration: will be elevated.

Serum 17-hydroxyprogesterone, 17-hydroxypregnenolone, and 11-deoxycortisol concentrations: will be elevated as will the serum androgens.

Cortrosyn stimulation testing using 250 μg dose of cortrosyn: useful to categorize the child with nonclassic congenital adrenal hyperplasia (CAH).

Bone age: assess advancement due to androgens in older child.

Complications

Death or brain injury: in newborns.

Development of true central precocious puberty: in older children.

Infertility: in adolescents.

Differential diagnosis

In newborn: ambiguous genitalia (see Ambiguous Genitalia); shock (sepsis, hyponatremic dehydration, pyloric stenosis).

Older child: premature adrenarche, true precocious puberty, exogenous anabolic steroid ingestion, and virilizing tumors.

Adolescent: polycystic ovary disease, virilizing tumors, infertility.

Etiology

Inherited autosomal recessive disorder with the genetic mutations described for the following conditions:

21-hydroxylase (cytochrome $P450_{21}$) deficiency: chromosome 6.

3-β hydroxylase (cytochrome $P450_{21}$) deficiency: chromosome 1.

Cholesterol desmolase deficiency: StAR (steroidogenic acute regulatory protein).

17,20 lyase deficiency (cytochrome $P450_{c17}$).

Epidemiology

• 21-Hydroxylase deficiency is the most common disorder, estimated 1:10,000 to 1:20,000; higher incidence in Yupik Eskimos because of consanguinity.

• Nonclassic CAH is estimated to be very common in Ashkenazi Jews.

Treatment

Lifestyle

- Compliance in taking medication is very important.
- An increasing dose of glucocorticoids should be taken during physical stress.
- A warning bracelet, necklace, or other medical alert aid should be worn at all times to inform others that the patient is taking glucocorticoids and is glucocorticoid dependent.
- Parents should be taught to administer hydrocortisone parenterally during severe illness.

Pharmacologic treatment

For newborn or infant in shock

- Administer hydrocortisone (25–50 mg i.v. every 4–6 h). The most important aspect of resuscitation is replacement of fluids and sodium. Often the infant will need 2–3 times the usual maintenance of normal saline during the first 24 h. Occasionally, the patient may require hypertonic saline. Generally no treatment is required for the hyperkalemia.

Standard dosage	*For pharmacologic maintenance treatment:* hydrocortisone, 10–15 mg/m^2 divided in three doses daily.
	9-α fludohydrocortisone, 0.05 to 0.30 mg as necessary based on renin level.
	Late-onset or nonclassic CAH in adolescents: 0.5 mg dexamethasone or 5 mg prednisone each night.
Contraindications	None. Important to recognize that the usual practice of discontinuing glucocorticoids with varicella and other such illnesses does not pertain to the adrenal insufficient patient.
Special points	During acute illness: 50 mg/m^2 divided in three doses for several days as necessary.
Major drug interactions	None.
Side effects	Chronic overtreatment will retard growth and result in short stature.

Treatment aims

To provide sufficient glucocorticoid and mineralocorticoid to maintain normal metabolic status and suppress abnormal androgen secretion.

Prognosis

- The children with severe salt-loss are at risk for sudden death during illness.
- Normal life span and fertility is anticipated with compliant pharmacologic treatment.

Follow-up and management

- Serum concentrations of adrenal steroids and renin activity should be monitored every 6 months.
- Height and weight measurements should be maintained in appropriate channels.
- Radiologic determination of bone age should be monitored every 1–2 y.

Other treatments

Classic CAH: none.
Nonclassic CAH: patients may elect no treatment if hirsutism and infertility are not concerning.

General references

Bose HS, Sugawara T, Strauss JF III: The pathophysiology and genetics of congenital lipoid hyperplasia. *N Engl J Med* 1996, **335:**1870–1878.

Miller WL, Levine LS: Molecular and clinical advances in congenital adrenal hyperplasia. *J Pediatr* 1987, **111:**1–17.

Donohoue PA, Parker K, Migeon CJ: Congenital Adrenal Hyperplasia. In *The Metabolic and Molecular Bases of Inherited Disease.* Edited by Schriver CR, Beaudef AL, Sly WS *et al.* New York: McGraw Hill, 1995:2929–2966.

Diagnosis

Symptoms

Onset is often insidious.

Weight loss, fatigue, and anorexia.

Syncope.

Hyperpigmentation, darkening of moles and scars.

Polyria, enuresis, vomiting, and diarrhea.

Neurologic complaints: memory loss, decreased capabilities in school work.

Pubertal delay, poor linear growth, amenorrhea in girls.

Signs

Hyperpigmentation.

Hypotension, tachycardia.

Cachexic and chronically ill appearance.

Investigations

Electrolytes: hyponatremia, hyperkalemia, and acidosis; hypoglycemia; hypercalcemia.

Plasma corticotropin concentration: markedly elevated in primary adrenal insufficiency.

Plasma renin activity: markedly elevated and serum aldosterone concentration is low (except in the syndrome of corticotropin unresponsiveness).

Serum cortisol concentration: is extraordinarily low.

Long-chain fatty acids: are elevated in adrenoleukodystrophy and should be evaluated in all children with Addison's disease because of the poor neurologic prognosis.

Cortrosyn stimulation testing: cortisol unresponsiveness to 1 µg of synthetic corticotropin indicates adrenal insufficiency. Elevated corticotropin levels indicate primary adrenal insufficiency.

Complications

Death from adrenal crisis.

Severe brain damage from hypoglycemia in infants (corticotropin unresponsiveness).

Neurologic deficits, leading to death, in adrenoleukodystrophy.

Other associated autoimmune disorders in Addison's disease: including mucocutaneous candidiasis, chronic active hepatitis, and other endocrine disorders.

Differential diagnosis

Other causes of hypoglycemia (see Hypoglycemia).

Anorexia nervosa.

Sepsis in infants.

Renal disease.

Etiology

Addison's disease, autoimmune adrenalitis.

Familial polyglandular autoimmune disease.

Corticotropin deficiency (genetic panhypopituitarism or isolated corticotropin deficiency, septo-optic dysplasia, brain tumor, or brain tumor treatment).

Familial corticotropin unresponsiveness.

Adrenoleukodystrophy.

Congenital adrenal hyperplasia.

Adrenal hemorrhage, adrenal infection (tuberculosis, HIV adrenalitis).

Epidemiology

• More common in girls, even in the familial polyglandular autoimmune disorder.

• Adrenoleukodystrophy is X-linked and more common in males.

Treatment

Lifestyle

• Compliance in taking medication is of major importance.

• Increasing dose of glucocorticoids during physical stress.

•A warning bracelet, necklace, or other medical alert aid should be worn at all times to inform others that the patient is taking glucocorticoids and is glucocorticoid dependent.

•Parents should be taught to administer hydrocortisone parenterally during severe illness.

Pharmacologic treatment

For shock

Standard dosage   Hydrocortisone, 50–100 mg i.v. every 4–6 h.

Special points   Most important aspect of resuscitation is replacement of fluids and sodium. Often the child will need 2–3 times the usual maintenance of normal saline during the first 24 h. Occasionally, the patient may require hypertonic saline. Generally no treatment is required for the hyperkalemia.

For maintenance treatment

Standard dosage   Hydrocortisone, 10–15 mg/m^2 divided in three doses daily.

9-α fludohydrocortisone, 0.05–0.30 mg as necessary based on renin level.

For acute illness

50 mg/m^2/d during acute illnesses.

Treatment aims

To provide sufficient glucocorticoid and mineralocorticoid to maintain normal metabolic status.

Prognosis

Good if patient is compliant in taking glucocorticoid replacement; there is a risk for adrenal crisis and sudden death.

Follow-up and management

• Serum concentrations of adrenal corticotropin and renin activity should be monitored every 6 mo.

• Height and weight measurements should be maintained in appropriate channels.

• Radiologic determination of bone age should be monitored every 1–2 y.

General references

Grinspoon SK, Biller BMK: Clinical review: laboratory assessment of adrenal insufficiency. *J Clin Endocrinol Metab* 1994, **79**:923–931.

Moser HW, Moser AE, Singh I, O'Neill B: Adrenoleukodystrophy: survey of 303 cases. Biochemistry, diagnosis, and therapy. *Ann Neurol* 1984, **16**:628–641.

Oelkers W: Adrenal insufficiency. *N Engl J Med* 1996, **335**:1206–1211.

Diagnosis

Symptoms
- Symptoms depend on the underlying malformation and its location.
- Patients may be asymptomatic.

Cough.

Wheeze.

Dyspnea.

Stridor.

Hoarseness.

Dysphagia.

Signs
- Physical findings depend on the underlying malformation and its location.

Examination may be normal.

Decreased breath sounds, rhonchi, rales or dullness to percussion over the area of the malformation.

Fixed or unilateral wheezing.

Stridor.

Hoarseness.

Respiratory distress.

Investigations
Chest radiograph: useful for localizing the malformation; frequently obtained for other reasons, with a congenital lung malformation being an incidental finding. Both posteroanterior and lateral views are needed to localize the malformation.

Chest computed tomography scan: also useful for further delineating the malformation and for viewing its internal structures and its relationship to neighboring organs.

Barium swallow: useful for determining if the malformation is compressing nearby gastrointestinal structures.

Airway films: to asses airway caliber.

Chest magnetic resonance imaging scan: useful in cases of pulmonary sequestration to identify the arterial feeding vessel or to identify and better define cases of arteriovenous malformations or anomalous vascular structures.

Angiography: useful in cases of pulmonary sequestration to identify the arterial feeding vessel or to better identify arteriovenous malformations or anomalous vascular structures.

Bronchoscopy: useful for assessing airway patency and dynamics, for identifying intraluminal lesions or extrinsic airway compression, and for removing foreign bodies.

Complications
Bronchial compression: with secondary atelectasis or recurrent or chronic pneumonia.

Respiratory distress: can be due to compression of the airways or surrounding lung tissue or from a hypoplastic lung.

Hemoptysis.

Esophageal compression with resultant dysphagia.

- *Note*: many congenital malformations of the airway have accompanying congenital malformations of other organs.

Differential diagnosis

Extrathoracic malformations

Laryngomalacia.

Subglottic stenosis.

Laryngeal web.

Laryngotracheoesophageal cleft.

Subglottic hemangioma.

Tracheomalacia.

Tracheal stenosis.

Tracheal compression secondary to a vascular malformation (ie, vascular ring or sling).

Tracheoesophageal fistula.

Intrathoracic malformations

Tracheobronchomalacia.

Aberrant right upper lobe bronchus ("pig bronchus").

Arteriovenous malformation.

Bronchogenic cyst.

Pulmonary cyst.

Cystic adenomatoid malformation.

Pulmonary sequestration.

Congenital lobar emphysema.

Hypoplastic lung.

Congenital diaphragmatic hernia.

Miscellaneous

Laryngeal papillomas.

Mediastinal masses (see Mediastinal masses).

Pneumonia.

Tuberculosis with a cavitating granuloma.

Secondary bronchial compression and resultant atelectasis caused by foreign body, hilar adenopathy, cardiomegaly, bronchiectasis, cystic fibrosis, lung abscess, pneumothorax.

Etiology

Dependent on the underlying malformation.

Epidemiology

Dependent on the underlying malformation; however, in general, most of these congenital lesions are rare.

Treatment

Diet and lifestyle
• No specific dietary or lifestyle changes are required.

Pharmacologic treatment
Dependent on the underlying malformation.

Antibiotics: if infection is present (*ie*, pneumonia, tuberculosis, lung abscess).

Steroids or interferon: can be useful aids in treating airway hemangiomas.

Nonpharmacologic treatment
Dependent on the underlying malformation.

Surgery: to correct any vascular anomaly or to remove the malformation (*ie*, bronchogenic cyst or pulmonary sequestration).

Tracheostomy: to maintain the patency of the patient's airway.

Embolization of isolated arteriovenous malformations: an option in select cases.

Observation: sometimes an option if the malformation is benign and delay in treatment will not adversely effect the outcome (*ie*, select cases of congenital lobar emphysema or smaller airway hemangiomas).

Treatment aims
To alleviate symptoms.
To maintain a patent airway.
To treat underlying pathology.
To prevent reoccurrence of lesion.
To prevent recurrent infections secondary to bronchial obstruction.

Prognosis
• Depends on underlying malformation.
• In laryngotracheomalacia, the prognosis is excellent, with most patients outgrowing their problem by 2–3 years of age.
• In airway hemangiomas, most spontaneously involute by 3 years of age.
• In most congenital lung malformations, the prognosis is excellent if the lesions are removed before recurrent infection becomes an issue.
• In congenital lung malformations, which have a propensity to expand (congenital lobar emphysema, cystic adenomatoid malformations), if expansion is occurring and causing respiratory distress, delay in surgical removal is associated with a poor prognosis.

Follow-up and management
• In isolated malformations, follow-up is short term. Chest radiographs and pulmonary function tests can prove useful for following pulmonary involvement.

General references
Haddon MJ, Bowen A: Bronchopulmonary and neurenteric forms of foregut anomalies: imaging for diagnosis and management. *Radiol Clin North Am* 1991, **29**:241–254.

Hudak BB: *Respiratory Diseases in Children: Diagnosis and Management.* Williams and Wilkins: Baltimore; 1994:501–532.

Keslar P, Newman B, Oh KS: Radiographic manifestations of anomalies of the lung. *Radiol Clin North Am* 1991, **29**:255–270.

Kravitz RM: Congenital Malformations of the Lung. *Pediatr Clin North Am* 1994, **41**:453–472.

Lierl M: *Pediatric Respiratory Disease: Diagnosis and Treatment.* WB Saunders: Philadelphia; 1993:457–498.

Mancuso RF: Stridor in neonates. *Pediatr Clin North Am* 1996, **43**:1339–1356.

Salzberg AM, Krummel TM: *Kendig's Disorders of the Respiratory Tract in Children.* WB Saunders: Philadelphia; 1990:227–26.

Allergic rhinoconjunctivitis

Diagnosis

Symptoms

Ocular pruritus.
Ocular discharge and tearing.
Photophobia.
Above with sneezing.
Nasal itching and/or congestion.
Rhinitis.

Signs

Eyelid edema: as lacrimation.
Chemosensitivity: with injection with nasal edema and secretions.

Investigations

Allergy skin testing.
Radioallergosorbent testing.
Nasal smears: for eosinophils (not diagnostic).

Complications

Sinusitis.

• Otherwise exceedingly rare.

Differential diagnosis

Vernal conjunctivitis.
Bacterial or viral conjunctivitis.
Upper respiratory infection.
Nonallergic rhinitis.
Nasal polyps.
Toxic exposure.

Etiology

Allergic sensitization with exposure.

Epidemiology

Commonly spring and early fall.
Pollen counts usually highest in early morning.
Strong family history usually present, though not necessary for diagnosis.

Treatment

Pharmacologic treatment

General guidelines
- Nasal steroids are used in patients with moderate-to-severe allergic symptoms.
- Antihistamines should be used as necessary.

Over-the-counter ocular antihistamine/decongestants
Naphazoline 0.025% and pheniramine (Naphcon A).
Naphazoline 0.027% and pheniramine (Opcon A).
Naphazoline 0.05% and antazoline (Vasocon A).

IX
Standard dosage   Cromolyn, iodoxamide, 1–2 up to 4 times per day.

Levocabastine 1 three times per day.

Olopatadine 1 twice per day (ages 3 and up).

Ketorolac 1 four times per day (age 12 and up).

First-generation principle classes of antihistamines
Alkylamines (chlorpheniramine, brompheniramine).

Ethanolamines (clemastine, diphenhydramine).

Phenothinazines (promethazine).

Second-generation principle classes of antihistamines
Standard dosage   Loratadine, 5 mg/5 cm^3 and cetirizine, 5 mg/5 cm^3.

Astemizole, 10 mg once per day.

Terfenadine, 60 mg twice per day (ages 12 and up).

Fexofenadine, 60 mg twice per day (ages 12 and up).

Nasal steroids
Beclomethasone: (ages 6 and up) triamcinolone, fluticasone, flunisolide, available as aqueous.

Budesonide: nonaqueous.

Special points   Ocular drops sting less if kept refrigerated.

Many antihistamines are combined with decongestants.

Second-generation antihistamines (with the exception of cetirizine) are nonsedating.

All other nasal steroids have approval for age 12 and up.

Main drug interactions   Macrolide antibiotics and terfenadine PNO astemizole.

Main side effects   First generation antihistamines: drowsiness.

Paradoxical hyperactivity.

Nasal steroids: burning, epistaxis.

Other treatment options   Immunotherapy, if patient fails to respond to medical therapy.

Treatment aims
To improve symptoms.

Prognosis
Excellent; allergies will usually "burn out" in sixth decade of life.

Follow-up and management
- Patients should begin therapy prior to allergy season yearly.

Other information
- Patients can develop tolerance to specific antihistamines.
- It may be necessary to switch antihistamines yearly.

General references

Friedlander MH: Management of ocular allergy. Ann All Asthma Imm 1995, **75**:212–222.

Juniper EF. Aqueous beclomethasone in treatment of ragweed pollen induced rhinitis: further exploration of "as needed" use. J All Asthma Imm 1993, **92**:66–72.

Naclerio RM: Allergic rhinitis. N Eng J Med 1991, **325**:860–869.

Diagnosis

Symptoms

None: may have lethargy, vomiting, or poor feeding in congenital adrenal hyperplasia

Signs

Penile–phallic structure: small, underdeveloped with hypospadius or very enlarged clitoral-appearing structure.

Scrotum–labia: scrotalized, ruggated, fused labia or cleft scrotum.

Testicular or gonadal structure in scrotal sac or cryptorchid.

Investigations

Ultrasound imaging of internal genital ducts: the absence of uterus indicates the presence of testicular tissue and mullerian inhibiting hormone.

Chromosome analysis to document genotype.

Serum concentrations to document genotype.

Serum concentrations of corticotropin, 17-OH progesterone, testosterone, androstenedione: to evaluate for the various forms of congenital adrenal hyperplasia.

Vaginogram-contrast radiographic study of urethra–vaginal vault.

Complications

Shock or death in patients with congenital adrenal hyperplasia.

Poor phallic growth at puberty in patients with partial androgen insensitivity.

Infertility.

Differential diagnosis

Virilization of female.

Undervirilization of male.

True hermaphroditism (gonadal combination of testicular and ovarian elements).

Chromosomal aberrations.

Etiology

Virilization of female

Congenital adrenal hyperplasia.

Virilization due to maternal androgens.

Virilization due to maternal exposure to androgens.

True hermaphroditism.

Idiopathic.

Undervirilization of males

Congenital adrenal hyperplasia.

Partial androgen insensitivity.

5-α Reductase deficiency

True hermaphroditism.

Hypospadius with or without cryptorchidism.

True hermaphroditism

Translocation of *SRY* gene.

Chromosomal aberrations

Mosaicism of sex chromosomes (eg, 45XO/46XY).

Epidemiology

Virilization of female: most frequent is congenital adrenal hyperplasia.

Undervirilization of male: most frequent cause is hypospadius.

Treatment

Lifestyle
Psychological counseling for parents for reassurance of gender of child.

Pharmacologic treatment
• Pharmacology treatment is only necessary for infants with ambiguous genitalia with congenital adrenal hyperplasia. (*See* Adrenal hyperplasia, congenital.) The impotant treatment for children with ambiguous genitals is appropriate surgical correction, *ie*, fixing the genitals for appropriate gender.

For newborn or infant in shock
• Administer hydrocortisone, 25–50 mg i.v. every 4–6 h. The most important aspect of resuscitation is replacement of fluids and sodium. Often the infant will need 2–3 times the usual maintenance of normal saline during the first 24 h. Occasionally, the patient may require hypertonic saline. Generally no treatment is required for the hyperkalemia.

Standard dosage	*For pharmacologic maintenance treatment:* hydrocortisone, 10–15 mg/m^2 divided in three doses daily.
	9-α fludohydrocortisone: 0.05–0.3 mg as necessary based on renin level.
	Late-onset or nonclassic congenital adrenal hyperplasia in adolescents: 0.5 mg dexamethasone or 5 mg prednisone each night.
Contraindications	None, but it is important to recognize that the usual practice of discontinuing glucocorticoids with varicella and other such illnesses does not pertain to the adrenal insufficient patient.
Special points	During acute illness: 50 mg/m^2 divided in three doses for several days as necessary.
Major drug interactions	None.
Side effects	Chronic overtreatment will retard growth and result in short stature.

Treatment aims
To correct ambiguous genitals to best support sexual function as adult.
To maintain ability for fertility if possible.

Prognosis
Excellent in general.
Children with congenital adrenal hyperplasia: risk for adrenal crisis.
Cases of gender reversal: risk for psychosocial maladjustment.

Follow-up and management
See Adrenal hyperplasia, congenital.
Evaluate psychosocial adjustment.
Evaluate gonadal function as child approaches teenage years.
Evaluate genital surgical correction for sufficiency for sexual function.

Other treatments
Surgical correction needed (genitoplasty).

General references
Migeon CJ, Berkowitz GD, Brown TR: Sexual differentiation and ambiguity. In *The Diagnosis and Treatment of Endocrine Disorders in Childhood and Adolescence.* Edited by Kappy MS, Blizzard RM, Migeon CJ. Springfield, IL: Charles C. Thomas; 1994:573–716.

Moshang T, Jr., Thornton PW: Endocrine disorders in newborn. In *Neonatology.* Edited by Avery G, Fletcher MA, MacDonald MG. Philadelphia: JB Lippincott Co.; 1993:764–791.

Diagnosis

Symptoms
Malaise, weakness, sense of "doom" (prodromal).

Itching, swelling, and/or flushing of skin.

Nasal itch, congestion, sneeze.

Hoarseness, dyspnea, wheeze, chest tightness, cough.

Palpitations, headache.

Nausea, dysphagia, abdominal pain (cramping), bloating.

Anxiety, mental status changes.

Signs
Urticaria: red, elevated, non-pitting papules or plaques; individual lesions are transient (2 hours or less) and resolve without residuum.

Erythema and angioedema.

Pallor and cyanosis possible.

Diaphoresis.

Nasal mucosal edema, rhinorrhea.

Edema of tongue, pharynx, larynx.

Stridor.

Tachypnea, chest wall retraction, wheeze, hyperinflation, pulmonary edema, bronchorrhea, pulsus paradoxicus.

Hypotension, tachycardia, arrhythmias, cardiac arrest, coronary insufficiency with ST–T wave changes in electrocardiogram, cardiac enzyme abnormality.

Vomiting, diarrhea, increased peristalsis, fecal and urinary incontinence.

Syncope and seizures.

Investigations

Immediate management period
• Initial investigations aimed at management of acute system dysfunction but should not delay treatment.

• Search for causative factors (eg, sting sites) in unconscious patients.

• Focused history to identify causative trigger and complicating conditions.

• Measurement of serum tryptase (mast cell protease; half-life about 2 hours in circulation); rise in histamine more transient and not helpful.

• Secondary laboratory abnormalities may be present (hemoconcentration, thrombocythemia, chest hyperinflation, elevated cardiac enzymes, ECG evidence for infarction, ischemia or rhythm disturbances).

Later diagnostic interventions
Allergy evaluation: correlation of exposure with presence of allergen-specific immunoglobulin E; skin testing and RAST methods; assess 14 or more days later to allow for regeneration of antibody.

Challenge procedures: selected circumstances, under controlled conditions.

Urinary catecholamines and plasma histamine: when recovered, to investigate carcinoid syndrome and mastocytosis.

Skin or bone biopsy: to confirm mastocytosis.

Complications
• Failure to reverse progression may lead to severe consequences for major organ system function.

• High risk factors for mortality include cardiovascular collapse and asphyxiation.

• Prior β-blocker use complicates resuscitation.

Differential diagnosis
Vasovagal reaction (pallor and diaphoresis common; no tachycardia with hypotension).

Hereditary angioneurotic edema.

Cardiac: infarction, arrest, dysrhythmia, hypovolemic shock.

Pulmonary: foreign body, aspiration, embolus, pneumothorax, epiglottis, severe asthma.

Neurologic: head injury, epilepsy, cerebrovascular accident.

Endocrine: hypoglycemia, carcinoid, pheochromocytoma.

Mast cell disorders: systemic cold-induced urticaria, systemic heat-induced (cholinergic) urticaria, systemic mastocytosis.

Drug reaction (idiosyncratic, pharmacologic, toxic).

Miscellaneous: anxiety/hyperventilation, factitious stridor, Munchausen syndrome.

Etiology
• Anaphylaxis is an acute, life-threatening syndrome consistent with sudden release of mediators from mast and other cells. Anaphylactoid reactions resemble IgE-mediated anaphylaxis but are induced by other mechanisms resulting in mediator release.

• Most stringent definition of anaphylaxis includes 1) systemic rather than localized manifestations, 2) dysfunctions in at least one major target organ (eg, cardiovascular, larynx, lung), 3) distinct signs of mast cell activation (urticaria, itch, flush), 4) appropriate history of exposure, 5) detection of antigen-specific IgE (or direct release trigger), and 6) elimination of conditions that may mimic anaphylaxis.

Epidemiology
• U.S. mortality from anaphylaxis/anaphylactoid reactions ranges from 700 to 1800 per year. β-Lactam antibiotics cause 400 to 800 deaths per year and hymenoptera stings cause about 40 deaths per year.

• Allergen immunotherapy injections cause anaphylaxis in ~2.5 out of 1000 injections but only about 3 deaths per year.

• Newer, nonionic, low-osmolar radiocontrast media rarely cause anaphylaxis.

• Prior exposure and sensitization are prerequisites for IgE-mediated anaphylaxis.

Treatment

Lifestyle management

• Patients should avoid proven and suspected triggers, have easy access to auto-injectable epinephrine, consider use of medic alert bracelet, and avoid β-blocker drugs if possible. Education of patient and responsible caregivers about trigger avoidance and emergency treatment is advised. Any chronic illness, especially pulmonary and cardiovascular, should be optimally managed.

Pharmacologic treatment

Immediate measures

Standard dosage   Aqueous epinephrine, 1:1000, 0.01 mL/kg subcutaneously, upper extremity; repeat up to twice at 20-minute intervals (maximum dose, 0.4 mL).

For laryngospasm

• Consider nebulization of aqueous epinephrine (0.5 mL/kg of 1:1000 diluted in 3 mL of normal saline; maximum dose, 5 mL [2.5 mL in patients ≤ 4 y]) or racemic epinephrine (2.25% solution, 0.05 mL/kg/dose, diluted in normal saline; maximum dose, 0.5 mL).

• Place patient Trendelenburg position.

• Establish and maintain airway, giving oxygen as needed.

• Start intravenous line with normal saline.

Standard dosage   Diphenhydramine, 1 to 2 mg/kg i.v., i.m., or orally (if appropriate) to a maximum dose of 50 mg; repeat up to every 6 h as indicated (2 mg/kg/24 h; maximum dose, 300 mg/24 h).

Ranitidine, 1 mg/kg/dose i.v., i.m., or orally (if appropriate) to maximum dose of 50 mg; repeat up to every 6 h as indicated (5 mg/kg/24 h; maximum dose, 400 mg/24 h).

Methylprednisolone, 1 mg/kg/dose i.v., i.m. (or prednisone orally if appropriate) to a maximum dose of 100 mg (yields no immediate benefit, but reduces risk of recurrence or protracted anaphylaxis); repeat up to every 6 h (maximum dose 2 mg/kg/24 h).

For acute bronchospasm

• Administer standard doses of β-$_2$-agonists via aerosol delivery
• Consider intravenous theophylline.

Treatment of hypotension

Aqueous epinephrine: 1:10,000, 0.1 mL/kg i.v. every 3–5 min for 2–3 doses; maximum dose, 5 mL; consider i.v. infusion of 0.01–1.0 µg/kg/min, titrated to effect.

• Consider dopamine infusion (inotropic effect) if fluid status corrected and epinephrine ineffective.

• Consider norepinephrine (potent vasopressor) if unresponsive to fluid correction, epinephrine, and dopamine.

• Treat ventricular arrhythmias as appropriate.

Treatment of hypotension in patients using β-blockers

• Administer isoproterenol (no α-agonist activity) via continuous infusion if unresponsive to epinephrine. Consider glucason in refractory cases.

Treatment aims

To manage acute emergency, to identify trigger and initiate avoidance measures, and to monitor for protracted and recurring anaphylaxis (at least 12 hours).

Prognosis

Excellent, if trigger avoidance successful.

Follow-up and management

• Encourage avoidance measures.
• Maintain emergency medication supply.
• Consult subspecialist as indicated.

General principles

• Assess rapidly and establish close monitoring of vital signs and cardio-pulmonary status.
• Maintain oxygenation, perfusion, cardiac output.
• Prepare for intubation or tracheostomy.
• Take clinical history to identify trigger.
• If possible, stop absorption of trigger with a venous tourniquet above reaction site (sting, injection), and administer local subcutaneous epinephrine (dose below) to delay absorption.

General references

Atkinson TP, Kaliner MA: Anaphylaxis. *Med Clin North Am* 1992, **76**:841–853.

Bochner BS, Lichtenstein LM: Anaphylaxis. *N Engl J Med* 1991, **324**:1785–1790.

Lawlor GJ, Rosenblatt HM: Anaphylaxis. In *Manual of Allergy and Immunology: Diagnosis and Therapy.* Edited by Lawlor GJ, Fischer TJ. Boston: Little, Brown and Co; 1988:??–??.

Middleton E, Reed CE, Ellis EF, *et al* (eds.): *Allergy Principles and Practice*, ed. 4. Philadelphia: CV Mosby; 1993:??–??.

Anemia, aplastic

Diagnosis

Symptoms

• Symptoms and signs are due to and relate to the severity of the peripheral blood pancytopenia.

Fatigue, shortness of breath on exertion, headache, palpitation: symptoms of anemia.

Easy bruising and petechiae, gum bleeding, buccal hemorrhage, visual disturbance due to retinal hemorrhage: symptoms of thrombocytopenia.

Mouth and tongue ulcers: symptoms of infection due to leukopenia.

History of jaundice: may indicate postherpetic aplasia or associated paroxysmal nocturnal hemoglobinuria.

Signs

Pallor.

Ecchymoses, petechiae of skin and mouth, retinal hemorrhage: bleeding manifestations are usually more common than infection.

Fever.

Mouth and tongue ulceration.

Pharyngitis, pneumonia.

Skin and perianal abscess.

Skeletal, skin, and nail anomalies; short stature: may occur in congenital aplastic anemia.

• Spleen, liver, and lymph nodes are not enlarged.

Investigations

Full blood count and examination of blood film: shows pancytopenia (isolated cytopenias may occur in early stages), macrocytosis (mean corpuscular volume >100 fL).

Reticulocyte count: shows absolute reticulocytopenia.

Bone-marrow aspiration and biopsy: shows hypocellular bone marrow, no tumor infiltration, no increase in reticulin, colony-forming cells low or absent; cytogenetic studies exclude preleukemia; in Fanconi's anemia, cultured peripheral blood lymphocytes show increased chromosomal breaks with DNA cross-linking agent (eg, diepoxybutane).

Investigations

Vitamin B$_{12}$ and folate levels: should be normal.

Ham's test: classically negative in aplastic anemia and positive in paroxysmal nocturnal hemoglobulin (PNH).

Liver function tests and viral studies: to detect antecedent hepatitis; test for hepatitis A, B, and hepatitis C, Epstein–Barr virus; cytomegalovirus; and parvovirus B19 (parovirus classically causes pure erythrocyte aplasia).

Chest and sinus radiography.

Hand and forearm radiography: may be abnormal in congenital aplastic anemia.

Abdominal ultrasonography: to exclude splenomegaly; anatomically displaced or abnormal kidneys in Fanconi anemia.

Complications

Bleeding due to thrombocytopenia, infection due to neutropenia.

Failure of random donor platelet transfusions to increase recipient's platelet count: due to sensitization to HLA antigens from blood transfusions.

Late clonal evolution to myelodysplastic syndrome or acute myeloid leukemia in 10%.

Differential diagnosis

Myelodysplastic syndrome (with hypoplasia).

Hypoplastic acute lymphoblastic leukemia.

Other bone marrow infiltration: eg, lymphoma.

Severe infection: eg, tuberculosis, overwhelming gram-negative or gram-positive sepsis may cause pancytopenia.

Etiology

Congenital causes:
eg, Fanconi's anemia, dyskeratosis congenital

Aquired causes:
Idiopathic: in majority of patients.

Drugs: eg, nonsteroid anti-inflammatory drugs, gold, chloramphenicol, sulfanomide.

Chemicals: benzene, organic solvents, aniline dyes.

Viruses: hepatitis A, B (hepatitis C) and other as yet unidentified viruses; Epstein–Barr virus.

Paroxysmal nocturnal hemoglobinuria: 25% of patients later develop aplastic anemia.

Thymoma.

Rare causes:
Systemic lupus erythematosus, pregnancy.

Epidemiology

• The annual incidence in the US is 2–8 : 1,000,000.

• The male:female ratio is equal.

Treatment

Diet and lifestyle

• Patients with thrombocytopenia should restrict their activities to avoid trauma and resultant serious bleeding. There are no specific dietary recommendations.

Pharmacologic treatment

• Definitive treatment is reserved for patients with diagnosis of severe aplastic anemia (two of three peripheral blood counts: absolute neutrophil count <500/μL, platelets <20 000/μL, corrected reticulocyte count <1%) with bone marrow cellularity <30%.

Allogeneic bone marrow transplantation

For HLA-identical siblings.

Immunotherapy

Standard dosage	Antithymocyte globulin (ATG), 160 mg/kg total dose given over 4–8 days.
	Cyclosporin, 5–10 mg/kg/day divided twice daily given to ATG-treated patients for 3–6 months (or until time of response).
	Granulocyte colony-stimulating factor (G-CSF), 5 μg/kg/day subcutaneously for patients on cyclosporin, until neutrophil count improves.
Special points	ATG: Patients require hospitalization and monitoring during infusion of ATG for possible anaphylaxis, serum sickness. Prophylactic corticosteroids, acetaminophen, diphenhydramine may help prevent untoward side effects.
	Cyclosporine:blood levels must be monitored.
	G-CSF: Growth factors should not be given alone for treatment of aplastic anemia.
Main side effects	Anaphylaxis, serum sickness (see Special Points).

Treatment aims

Transfusion independence, normal blood counts, normal bone marrow cellularity.

Other treatments

Blood transfusions: erythrocyte transfusions to maintain hemoglobin >10–12 gm/dL. Platelet transfusions during ATG therapy to maintain count >20,000/μL. When ATG treatment is ended, platelet transfusions are given to maintain platelet count >10,000/μL or to treat bleeding episodes.

Androgens: eg, decaburabolan, oxymethalone; not first-line therapy.

High-dose corticosteroid: not first-line therapy.

Prognosis

• There is a complete or partial response to immunotherapy in 75%–80% of patients.

• Late relapses of aplastic anemia following immunotherapy have been reported.

• Very young patients with very severe aplastic anemia have poor response to immunotherapy.

• Disease may evolve to myelodysplasia and leukemia, particularly after G-CSF treatment.

Follow-up and management

• Patients require follow-up until counts have been normal for 3–5 y.

General references

Brown KE, Tisdale J, Barrett J, et al.: Hepatitis-associated aplastic anemia. *N Engl J Med* 1997, **336**:1059–1064.

Hows JM: Severe aplastic anemia: the patient without a HLA-identical sibling. *Br J Haematol* 1991, **77**:1–4.

Young NS, Alter BP: *Aplastic Anemia: Acquired and Inherited.* Philadelphia: WB Saunders Co.; 1994.

Anemia, autoimmune hemolytic

Diagnosis

Symptoms
Jaundice.

Dark urine.

Paleness (may precede jaundice).

Fatigue.

Abdominal pain.

Signs
Jaundice.

Pallor.

Splenomegaly.

Fever.

Investigations
Complete blood count: The hemoglobin is moderately to markedly decreased; the total leukocyte count may be moderately elevated with a shift to the left; the platelet count is normal; the mean cell volume is normal.

Reticulocyte count: increased with erythrocyte destruction; may be low at onset of disease.

Peripheral blood smear: erythrocyte morphology significant for microspherocytes, polychromasia, nucleated erythrocytes. There are no erythrocyte fragments.

Direct antiglobulin test (direct Coombs test): positive usually for IgG. Most autoimmune hemolytic anemia of childhood is warm reacting.

Indirect antiglobulin test (indirect Coombs test): positive for antibody in the serum.

Special: Bone marrow aspiration; performed if there is a suspicion of concomitant malignancy.

Complications
Severe, rapidly developing anemia may lead to heart failure, shock.

Erythrocyte incompatibility and *in vivo* erythrocyte destruction: causing difficulty in treating severe anemia with transfusion.

Differential diagnosis
Evan's syndrome autoimmune hemolytic anemia with immune thrombocytopenia, immune neutropenia, or both.

Secondary to an underlying malignant disorder: Hodgkin's lymphoma, non-Hodgkin's lymphoma.

Drug-induced hemolytic anemia.

Hemolysis associated with antibody-producing diseases: systemic lupus erythematosus, juvenile rheumatoid arthritis, chronic active hepatitis.

Paroxysmal nocturnal hemoglobinuria: rare.

Etiology
May occur 1–3 weeks after a viral infection, usually respiratory.

Cold agglutinin disease (IgM-mediated hemolysis may follow infection with Epstein-Barr virus or *Mycoplasma*).

Epidemiology
Peak incidence 3–6 y, slightly more common in males.

Treatment

Diet and lifestyle
• No specific dietary recommendations are necessary. Acutely anemic require hospitalization and bed rest with careful monitoring of vital signs and evidence of ongoing hemolysis. Once discharged from hospital, activity as tolerated is recommended.

Pharmacologic treatment

Standard dosage   Methylprednisone, 0.5–1.0 mg/kg/day in four divided doses in the acute phase of hemolysis.

Prednisone, maintenance dose of 2 mg/kg until hemoglobin approaches normal.

Special points   *Methylprednisolone*: when stable may change to oral corticosteroid.

Anemia, constitutional aplastic (Fanconi anemia)

Diagnosis

• Bone marrow failure presents with an insidious onset in children who may or may not have phenotypic abnormalities. Children with Fanconi anemia have often been recognized prior to the development of bone marrow failure.

Symptoms

Easy bruising.

Petechial rash.

Gum bleeding.

Nose bleeding.

Paleness, fatigue.

Fevers, unusual infections.

Signs

Bruises, petechiae, mucosal bleeding.

Pallor.

Flow murmur.

Short stature.

Micrognathia, microphthalmia.

Upper limb abnormalities (absent or hypoplastic thumbs with or without absent or hypoplastic radii).

Cafe-au-lait spots.

Investigations

General investigations

Complete blood count: the hemoglobin, erythrocyte count, and platelet count are variably decreased. The mean cell volume is increased to > 100 fL. Neutropenia may by present. In Fanconi anemia, thrombocytopenia or leukopenia precede pancytopenia.

Peripheral blood smear: the erythrocytes are large. The leukocyte morphology is normal. Platelets appear decreased and may be smaller than normal.

Reticulocyte count: normal or decreased.

Hb F quantitation: increased.

Bone marrow aspiration: bone marrow cellularity is moderately to severely decreased depending on when in course of disease bone marrow is obtained.

Special investigations

Ham test: positive in paroxysmal nocturnal hemoglobinuria.

Chromosomal fragility testing with diepoxybutane: increased fragility diagnostic of Fanconi anemia.

Renal ultrasound: horseshoe kidney, other anatomical abnormalities.

Plain films of upper extremities.

MRI of spine: increased fat in spinous processes associated with decrease in hematopoietic elements.

Complications

• 10% develop leukemia, 5% other cancers, 4% liver disease (hepatic tumors, pelias hepatis).

Differential diagnosis

Acquired aplastic anemia.

Leukemia.

Myelofibrosis.

Other causes of constitutional aplastic anemia:

Dyskeratosis congenital (very rare).

Schwachman-Diamond syndrome (can progress from neutropenia to pancytopenia).

Amegakaryocytic anemia (very rare; can progress from thrombocytopenia to pancytopenia).

Etiology

The genetic defects responsible for Fanconi anemia are currently being defined. The first gene described in association with Fanconi anemia has been designated *FAC*.

Epidemiology

Fanconi anemia is a rare autosomal recessive disorder. Male:female ratio is 1.3.

Treatment

Diet and lifestyle

• A varied, healthy diet is encouraged. There are no specific restrictions. When peripheral blood counts are normal, the patient is encouraged to participate fully in normal activities. Thrombocytopenic patients must avoid activities that place them at risk for head injury and the potential for intracranial bleeding. Neutropenic patients are required to seek medical attention with the development of significant fever.

Pharmacologic treatment

Standard dosage	Androgens alone: Oxymetholone (United Pharmaceuticals, Inc., Buffalo Grove, IL), 2–5 mg/day orally.
	Nandrolone decanoate, 1–2/kg/wk.
	Androgens with corticosteroids: above doses of androgens with prednisone, 5–10 mg every other day.
Special points	*Oxymetholone*: associated with hepatic toxicity.
	Nandrolone decanoate: when given i.m., associated with pain and bleeding at injection site.

Other treatments: supportive care

Transfusions

• Erythrocytes and platelets should come from non-family members.

• Cellular blood products should be irradiated and leukoreduced.

• Transfuse erythrocytes with posttransfusion hemoglobin (goal, 10–13 g/dL); platelet transfusions as needed to prevent spontaneous bleeding episodes.

Hematopoietic growth factors

• Concern about leukemogenic effects of cytokines.

Bone marrow transplantation

• Offers cure for aplastic anemia and prevention of possible development of leukemia.

• Preparative regimens are difficult for Fanconi's anemia patients to tolerate.

• Decision for bone marrow transplantation in Fanconi's anemia patient requires discussion with experienced pediatric hematologist and pediatric bone marrow transplantation physician.

Treatment aims

To improve peripheral blood counts, approximately 50% of patients will respond to corticosteroids; response in erythrocytes first, followed by leukocytes.
• Platelet rise may not be observed for months. Some patients lose their response.

Prognosis

Median survival, 16 y.
Twenty-five percent live beyond age 26 y.
Prognosis improves as more is known about the disease.

Follow-up and management

As with other rare hematological disorders of childhood, patients with Fanconi anemia should be primarily treated by physicians familiar with this rare disease. Surveillance for liver disease, progression of bone marrow failure, and leukemic transformation is necessary.

General references

Alter BP: Fanconi's anemia: current concepts. *Am J Pediatr Hematol Oncol* 1992, **14**:17–76.

Gluckman E, Auerbach AD, Horowitz MM, et al.: Bone marrow transplantation for Fanconi anemia. *Blood* 1995, **86**:2856–2862.

Young NS, Alter BP: Aplastic anemia: acquired and inherited. Philadelphia: WB Saunders Co.; 1994.

Anemia: iron deficiency

Diagnosis

Definition
• Iron-deficiency anemia is due to inadequate intake that develops slowly. Symptoms may not be noticed by family members.

Symptoms
Crankiness.

Lethargy.

Pale appearance.

Signs
Pallor.

Tachycardia.

Tachypnea.

Investigations
Complete blood count: Hemoglobin is mildly to severely decreased. The mean cell volume and mean corpuscular hemoglobin are decreased. Leukocytes are normal in number and appearance. Platelets are normal or increased.

Peripheral blood smear: erythrocytes are hypochromic and microcytic; erythrocytes vary in size and shape.

Reticulocyte count: decreased.

Serum iron: decreased.

Total iron-binding capacity: increased.

Serum ferritin: decreased.

Complications
• Predisposition to infection is due to neutrophil dysfunction.

• Impaired absorption of fat, vitamin A, and xylose may occur.

Differential diagnosis

Etiology

Inadequate iron intake in face of rapid growth.

Inadequate iron absorption.

Occult gastrointestinal bleeding (less common in children).

Epidemiology

Peak ages: second year of life and in rapid growth phase of adolescence.

Infants at risk have a history of prematurity, formula without iron, or early introduction of cow's milk.

Treatment

Diet and lifestyle

• Nutritional iron deficiency can be avoided by consuming a diet with iron-containing foods.

Infants and toddlers should not drink excessive amounts of cow's milk.

In those with cow's milk protein allergy, cow's milk should be avoided altogether.

Pharmacologic treatment

Standard dosage   Iron supplementation: ferrous sulphate, 6 mg/kg/day of elemental iron.

Special points   Best absorbed if given on an empty stomach; may be divided into two or three daily doses.

Treatment aims
To raise hemoglobin to normal range.
To replenish total body iron stores.
To avoid recurrence of iron deficiency anemia through dietary counseling and proper foods.

Other treatments
Parenteral iron (iron dextran): rarely indicated.
Erythrocyte transfusion: can usually be avoided by treating with oral iron and observing carefully. Transfusions are necessary only if heart failure is imminent.

Prognosis
Excellent for cure of anemia.
Psychomotor developmental delay may result despite adequate treatment of anemia with iron.

Follow-up and management
Initial response to iron (reticulocytosis) is observed within days of the institution of therapy; with adequate iron supplements, iron deficiency anemia is corrected.

General references
Bessmar JD, McClure S: Detection of iron deficiency anemia. *JAMA* 1991, **266**:1649–1653.

Dallman PR, Yip R, Oski FA: Iron deficiency and related nutritional anemias. In *Hematology of Infancy and Childhood*, edn 4. Edited by Nathan DG, Oski FA. Philadelphia: WB Saunders Co.; 1993.

Walter T, deAndraca I, *et al.*: Iron deficiency anemia: adverse effects on infant psychomotor development. *Pediatrics* 1989, **84**:7–10.

Diagnosis

Symptoms

Many patients have no symptoms; the disease is suspected on routine blood count.

Dyspnea on exertion, tiredness, headache.

Painful tongue.

Paraesthesias in feet, difficulty walking: vitamin B_{12} deficiency only.

Infertility.

Signs

Pallor of mucous membranes: if hemoglobin concentration <9 g/dL.

Mild jaundice.

"Beefy red" glossitis.

Signs of vitamin B_{12} neuropathy: if present.

Investigations

General investigations

Complete blood count: raised mean cell volume (>100 fL), reduced erythrocyte count, hemoglobin, and hematocrit, low reticulocyte count, reduced leukocyte and platelet counts (in severely anemic patients). Red cell distribution width very high.

Peripheral blood smear: shows macroovalocytes, hypersegmented neutrophils (>five nuclear lobes).

Bone marrow analysis: in severely anemic patients, the bone marrow is very hypercellular with increased proportion of early cells, many dying cells, megaloblastic erythroblasts, giant and abnormally shaped metamyelocytes, and hypersegmented megakaryocytes.

Serum indirect bilirubin and lactic dehydrogenase measurement: raised concentrations demonstrate ineffective erythropoiesis.

Direct Coombs test: usually negative, although positive for complement in some patients.

Tests for vitamin B_{12} or folate deficiency: serum B_{12} low in B_{12} deficiency, normal or slightly low in folate deficiency; serum folate normal or raised in B_{12} deficiency, low in folate deficiency; erythrocyte folate normal or low in B_{12} deficiency, low in folate deficiency.

Deoxyuridine suppression, serum homocysteine, and methylmalonic acid measurement: additional tests performed in some laboratories to demonstrate lack of B_{12} or folate.

Special investigations

Diet history: to exclude veganism, low folate intake.

Surgical history: surgical removal of terminal ileum.

Schilling test: for B_{12} absorption; abnormal in pernicious anemia.

Endoscopy and jejunal biopsy: if gluten-induced enteropathy is suspected in patients with folate deficiency.

Complications

Neuropathy: due to B_{12} deficiency.

Neural tube defects in fetus: risk reduced by folate treatment.

Differential diagnosis

Other causes of macrocytosis: liver disease, hypothyroidism, aplastic anemia, myelodysplasia, acute myeloid leukemia, reticulocytosis.

Causes of megaloblastic anemia: Transcobalamin II deficiency.

Antifolate drugs: methotrexate, pyrimethamine (reverse by folinic acid), cotrimoxazole.

Drugs inhibiting DNA synthesis: cytosine, arabinoside, hydroxyurea, 6-mercaptopurine, azathioprine, 5-fluorouracil.

Congenital abnormalities of vitamin B_{12} or folate metabolism.

Congenital abnormalities of DNA synthesis: eg, orotic aciduria.

Etiology

Causes of vitamin B_{12} deficiency

Diet deficiency: eg, in vegans or in infants born to mothers with pernicious anemia who are vegans.

Pernicious anemia.

Congenital intrinsic factor deficiency.

Total or subtotal gastrectomy.

Chronic gastritis.

Blind loop syndrome.

Ileal resection or abnormality, eg, Crohn's disease.

HIV infection.

Specific malabsorption with proteinuria.

Fish tapeworm.

Causes of folate deficiency

Dietary deficiency: poor-quality diet, goat's milk, specialized diets.

Malabsorption: gluten-induced enteropathy, tropical sprue, congenital.

Increased turnover: pregnancy, prematurity, hemolytic anemias, myelofibrosis, widespread inflammatory or malignant diseases.

Increased losses: congestive heart failure, hemodialysis or peritoneal dialysis.

Alcohol abuse: anticonvulsant treatment.

Epidemiology

Megaloblastic anemias related to diet (occurs in communities where veganism is common or in people for whom dietary folate intake is reduced).

Pernicious anemia unusual in children <10 g.

Occurs in whites and nonwhites.

Treatment

Diet and lifestyle

• The quality of the diet must be increased in patients with dietary folate deficiency.

For vitamin B_{12} deficiency

Standard dosage	**(for patients who cannot absorb B_{12})** Cyanocobalamin, 0.2 μgm/kg/day for 7 d s.c. or i.m. Maintenance: 1 mg s.c. or i.m. per month.
Contraindications	Rare hypersensitivity.
Special points	No evidence suggests that more frequent doses are needed for B_{12} neuropathy.
Main drug interactions	None.
Main side effects	None.

For folate deficiency

Standard dosage	Folic acid, 1 mg orally daily for 4 months, then 5 mg daily or weekly as needed.
Contraindications	B_{12} deficiency, malignancy (unless deficiency is clinically important).
Special points	B_{12} deficiency must be excluded because B_{12} neuropathy could be precipitated or aggravated.
Main drug interactions	None.
Main side effects	None.

• Folic acid should be used as prophylaxis.

• For premature babies (birth weight <1500 g), folic acid, 1 mg daily, is indicated.

For patients with congenital hemolytic anemia (eg, sickle cell disease), folic acid, 1 mg daily, is indicated.

Treatment aims

To correct anemia by replenishing body stores of vitamin.

To correct underlying disease.

To restore normal neurological status (vitamin B_{12} deficiency).

Other treatments

Packed erythrocyte transfusion should be used only if essential: removal of equivalent volume of plasma in patients with congestive heart failure.

Prognosis

Prognosis depends mainly on the underlying cause.

Life expectancy is reduced slightly in patients with pernicious anemia because of the risk of carcinoma of the stomach.

Follow-up and management

Patients with pernicious anemia should have annual clinical review and blood counts.

Routine endoscopy is not recommended.

Patients having total gastrectomy or ileal resection need prophylactic hydroxocobalamin, 1 mg every 3 mo, from the time of surgery for life.

General references

Cooper BA, Roseblatt DS, Whitehead VM: Megaloblastic anemia. In *Hematology of Infancy and Childhood*, edn 4. Edited by Nathan DG, Oski FA. Philadelphia: WB Saunders Co.; 1993:354–390.

Hoffbrand AV, Jackson BFA: The deoxyuridine suppression test and cobalamin-folate interrelations. *Br J Haematol* 1993, **85**:232–237.

Savage DG, Lindenbaum J: Folate-cobalamin interactions. In *Folate in Health & Disease*. Edited by Bailey L. New York: Marcel Dekker; 1994:237–285.

Appendicitis

Diagnosis

Symptoms

• The classic triad is pain, vomiting, and fever.

Abdominal pain: begins in the midabdomen or periumbilical area. Pain most often localizes to the right lower quadrant after 4–6 hours, but this is variable depending on the anatomical location of the appendix.

Vomiting: usually follows rather than precedes abdominal pain. This may be less consistent in young children [4]. Vomiting occurs in about 80% of patients, and generally occurs only once or twice.

Low-grade fever: usually develops after the onset of abdominal pain.

Anorexia: is quite common and is seen even in young children who cannot verbalize feelings of nausea. Some say the diagnosis of appendicitis should be questioned if anorexia is not reported.

• Most patients report obstipation before the onset of abdominal pain, but 5%–10% report loose stools.

Signs

• Guarding and focal peritoneal signs are expected.

Pain in the right lower abdominal quadrant (McBurney point): in two thirds of patients; this finding is not present when the child has an appendix in the pelvis or retroperitoneal area; suprapubic or flank pain may be present in those cases; shaking the child, precipitating a cough, or asking the child to hop on the right foot may help to localize the pain [6]; patients usually prefer to lie quietly as movement increases the pain [6].

Rectal examination that elicits sudden pain: (as opposed to discomfort from the examiner's finger) confirms the presence of inflammation and is found in 50%–80% of cases; a boggy mass suggesting an abscess may also be palpable in 25% [4]; rectal examination is especially helpful if the appendix lies in the pelvis.

Psoas sign: with the patient lying on his or her left side, the examiner should slowly extend the right thigh; this stretches the psoas muscle and produces pain if the appendix is inflamed.

Obturator sign: passively rotate the flexed right thigh internally with the patient supine; irritation indicates a positive obturator sign.

Peritoneal signs: inconsistent.

Investigations

Complete blood count: generally reveals an elevated white blood cell count early in the course; a left shift is noted later in the course; the white blood count will be markedly elevated with a left shift if perforation has occurred.

Urinalysis: shows ketosis and, sometimes, a few white blood cells if the appendix lies over the ureter or adjacent to the bladder.

Abdominal radiographs: often normal, but they reveal a fecalith in 8%–10% of cases; many consider radiographs to be unnecessary in making the diagnosis [6]; most radiographs show diminished air in the gastrointestinal tract (from anorexia, nausea), an ileus, air–fluid levels, and indistinct psoas margins with scoliosis concave toward the right; air in the appendix is also noted in some cases; free air in the abdomen may be seen if perforation has occurred.

Abdominal ultrasound: helpful if there are equivocal signs and symptoms; this study is sensitive in 85% of cases with a specificity of 94% [2]; the probability of appendicitis after a normal ultrasound is 6% [2].

Surgical consultation: indicated when the diagnosis is clear or when appendicitis can not be safely ruled out [6].

Differential diagnosis

Gastroenteritis: expect nausea, vomiting, and diarrhea [5].

Urinary tract infection: expect more white blood cells and bacteria in the urinalysis.

Constipation: fever is unusual.

Lower lobe pneumonia: usually associated with cough, fever, and tachypnea.

Pelvic inflammatory disease: surgical consultation may be warranted.

Renal colic: expect more red blood cells in the urinalysis.

Etiology

• The condition is usually caused by obstruction of the lumen of the appendix by inspissated fecal material or by hyperplastic lymphoid tissue. Bacteria invade the wall of the appendix at sites of inflammation leading to infarction. Infections with inflammation such as those caused by *Yersinia* sp., *Salmonella* sp., *Shigella* sp., and some parasites play a role.

Epidemiology

• Appendicitis is one of the most common abdominal surgical conditions in childhood.

• There are about 80,000 cases per year in the United States.

• Appendicitis occurs in patients of all ages.

• It is rare in children <2 y old; the peak age is 12 y.

Complications

• The condition is misdiagnosed in 7%–12% of patients aged less than 15 years, and in 57% of those aged less than 6 years.

• Perforation occurs in 25%–30% of cases. In preschool children, perforation is noted in 50%–70%. Once perforated, there are usually signs of generalized peritonitis with a rigid, tender abdomen. The child will appear quite ill, with pallor, dyspnea, and grunting. Radiographs may reveal free abdominal air in these cases.

Treatment

Pharmacologic treatment
• Antibiotics are recommended.

Standard Dosage   Ampicillin 200 mg/kg/d.
Gentamicin 7.5 mg/kg/d.
Possibly clindamycin 25 mg/kg/d.

Nonpharmacologic treatment
• Surgery is required after appropriate intravenous hydration and stabilization.
• Management of pain and fever are also important.
• Placement of a nasogastric tube may provide comfort preoperatively.

Important information
• Do not ignore the findings of abdominal tenderness, especially in the lower right quadrant [3–5].

• Since the diagnosis is often difficult, it may be wise to admit some children with abdominal pain to the hospital for close observation, even if their initial presentation is not classic for appendicitis.

• Admit the child who has any two of the following three indicators: classic history, impressive physical examination, abnormal laboratory studies. This will allow for reexamination every 1–2 hours [6].

• Reexamination of the child at several points in time is crucial, because the findings will change as the condition evolves.

• Remember that tenderness may be lessened temporarily if the appendix has recently perforated.

• Radiographs, if obtained, should be carefully reviewed and acted on when abnormal.

• Consider evaluation of the abdomen with ultrasound if the diagnosis is not obvious.

• Document the findings of abdominal and rectal examination carefully.

Treatment aims
To correct metabolic acidosis and electrolyte abnormalities.
To restore hydration.
To remove the inflamed appendix.

Prognosis
• Prognosis is quite good after surgery.
• In cases of perforation, prognosis is also favorable, although the hospital course may be prolonged by several days.
• Mortality is ~1%–3%, and death usually occurs in misdiagnosed patients [5].

Follow-up and management
• If the diagnosis is suspected but is not confirmed and the child is discharged, follow-up within 12–24 h is suggested [5].

Key references
1. Brender JD, Marcuse EK, et al.: Childhood appendicitis: factors associated with perforation. J Pediatr 1986, **76:**301–306.
2. Crady SK, Jones JS, Wyn T, et al.: Clinical validity of ultrasound in children with suspected appendicitis. Ann Emerg Med 1993, **22:**1125–1129.
3. Reynolds SL, Jaffe DM: Diagnosing abdominal pain in a pediatric emergency department. Pediatr Emerg Care 1992, **8:**126–128.
4. Rothrock SG, Skeoch G, Rush JJ, et al.: Clinical features of misdiagnosed appendicitis in children. Ann Emerg Med 1991, **20:**45–50.
5. Rusnak RA, Borer JM, Fastow JS: Misdiagnosis of acute appendicitis: common features discovered in cases after litigation. Am J Emerg Med 1994;12:397–402.
6. Schnaufer L, Mahboubi S: Abdominal Emergencies. In Textbook of Pediatric Emergency Medicine, ed 3. Edited by Fleisher G, Ludwig S. Baltimore: Williams and Wilkins; 1993:1309–1314.

Diagnosis

Symptoms

Painful, swollen, warm joints, with morning stiffness and impaired function: onset usually insidious, sometimes rapid; characteristically in hands or feet, occasionally monoarticular (most often in a knee); often accompanied by tiredness; pauciarticular usually involves the knee; polyarticular affects large and small joints; systemic desease may result in fever, rash, severe malaise, as well as joint pain.

Signs

Articular

Warm, tender, swollen joints: decreased range of movement; peripheral joints most often affected; characteristic symmetry of involvement; proximal interphalangeal, metacarpophalangeal, wrist, and metatarsophalangeal joints usually affected.

Extra-articular signs of juvenile rheumatoid arthritis

	Pauciarticular (1–4 joints)	Polyarticular (4 or more joints)	Systemic (any number, may be absent initially)
Fever	absent	absent	common
Rash	absent	absent	common
Uveitis	common	common	absent
Nodules	absent	rare	absent
Serositis, pericarditis	absent	rare	common

Investigations

• No single diagnostic test is available; the diagnosis relies on some or all of the following:

ESR, ANA, RF, Lyme titer (in endemic areas): for evidence of inflammation.

Immunology: rheumatoid factor positivity (not essential for diagnosis).

Radiography: initially shows soft tissue swelling periarticular osteoporosis, later and finally erosions around affected joint.

Blood count: for anemia of chronic disease, thrombocytosis.

Serum immunoglobulin measurement: for polyclonal gammopathy and to identify immunoglobulin A–deficient patients.

• In addition, the duration of morning stiffness, level of functional impairment, and number of inflamed joints must be monitored in established disease.

Complications

• The following occur in patients with established disease and global decline in function or severe systemic malaise.

Widespread active synovitis.

Septic arthritis.

Systemic rheumatoid disease.

Iatrogenic problems: *eg*, NSAIDs and anemia, methotrexate, and white cell count suppression and infection.

Atlantoaxial subluxation.

Non-Hodgkin's lymphoma: possible.

Amyloidosis.

Osteoporosis and fracture.

Differential diagnosis

Seronegative spondylarthritis.

Reactive arthritis: gastrointestinal or sexually acquired.

Viral arthritis: *eg*, rubella, hepatitis B virus infection.

Septic polyarthritis: *eg*, staphylococcal or gonococcal infections.

SLE.

Lyme disease.

Hypermobility.

Etiology

• The cause of juvenile rheumatoid arthritis is unknown, but the following have a role:

Genetic factors: subtypes of HLA DR4 in polyarticular disease.

Hormonal factors: remission during pregnancy; contraceptive pill protects from disease.

Epidemiology

• Juvenile rheumatoid arthritis is a significant disease that affects up to 110 per 100,000 children.

• It is a chronic disease, with high prevalence and low incidence.

Pauciarticular: affects ages 1–6 and many more girls than boys.

Polyarticular: affects ages 8–16 and more girls than boys.

Systemic: affects ages 1–16 and approximately the same number of girls as boys.

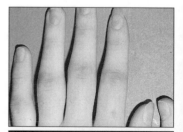

Polyarthritis of the proximal interphalangeal joints in a 15 year-old girl with RF+ juvenile rheumatoid arthritis.

Treatment

Diet and lifestyle
• Activity should be encouraged, but high-impact activity intensifies joint inflammation.
• Physical therapy, taught exercise, and "joint protection" are helpful to maintain strength and function.
• Omega-3 fatty acids may reduce inflammation.

Pharmacologic treatment

NSAIDs
• The response is variable and idiosyncratic; if one drug fails, another from a different group may be worth trying.
• The most commonly used drugs are diclofenac, ibuprofen, indomethacin, naproxen, and salicylate.

Standard dosage	Naprosyn: 1–20 mg/kg/day divided in 2 doses. Ibuprofen: 30–40 mg/kg/day divided in 4 doses. Indomethacin: 2–3 mg/kg/day divided in 3 doses.
Contraindications	Caution in peptic ulceration, asthma, renal impairment, pregnancy, and elderly patients.
Main drug interactions	Diuretics, warfarin.
Main side effects	Dyspepsia, altered bowel habit, renal impairment, fluid retention.

Second-line agents
• These are increasingly started early in the disease process, particularly in patients who do not respond to NSAIDs or who respond partially [2–4].

Standard dosage	Sulfasalazine, 50 mg/kg/day divided in 2 doses. Methotrexate, 0.3–0.5 mg/kg orally once weekly. Plaquenil: 4–7 mg/kg/day in one dose.
Contraindications	*Sulfasalazine:* sulfonamide and salicylate hypersensitivity. *Methotrexate:* pregnancy, liver disease. *Plaquenil:* visual impairment, pregnancy.
Special points	*Sulfasalazine:* full blood count and liver function tests every 4 wk for 2 mo, monthly for 2–3 mo, then 2-monthly. *Methotrexate:* full blood count monthly, liver function test every 2 wk for 2 mo, then every month for 2 mo, and then every 2 mo. alcohol use should be avoided. *Plaquenil:* need visual-field testing every 6 mo.
Main drug interactions	*Sulfasalazine:* warfarin, co-trimoxazole. *Methotrexate:* co-trimoxazole, trimethoprim, phenytoin.
Main side effects	*Sulfasalazine:* nausea, rashes, hepatitis. *Methotrexate:* nausea, diarrhea, rash, pulmonary hypersensitivity, blood dyscrasias, infection. *Plaquenil:* nausea, visual acuity loss (rare).

Other options
Gold (i.m.); cycolsporin; penicillamine; local steroids; systemic steroids: either induction before or adjunctive to second-line agents in poorly controlled disease; immunosuppressants: for severe articular or extra-articular disease.

Nonpharmacological treatment
Physical therapy: during active disease.
Occupational therapy, including nightime splints.
Surgery: synovectomies, arthroplasty, arthrodesis, tendon repair; for painful joints (particularly at night), functionally restricted joints, and joints that do not respond to other treatments.

Treatment aims
To decrease pain and symptoms and signs of inflammation.
To prevent progression of irreversible joint damage.
To monitor for and treat extra-articular manifestations.
To reduce disability.

Prognosis
• The prognosis is very variable.
• Poor prognostic markers include polyarticular disease, high-titer rheumatoid factor, persistently raised ESR.

Follow-up and management
• Second-line treatment must be monitored regularly.
• Stable disease needs occasional assessment for progressive functional decline.
• Active disease needs regular follow-up so that modifying the various treatment options can be considered.
• Care should be shared between primary care and rheumatologic consultants.

General references

Cassidy JT, Levinson JE, Brewer EJ Jr: The development of classification criteria for children with juvenile rheumatoid arthritis. In *Bulletin on the Rheumatic Diseases,* vol. 38, no. 6. Edited by Hess EV. Arthritis Foundation: Atlanta; 1989:1–7.

Gäre BA, Fasth A: Epedimiology of juvenile chronic artheritis in Southwestern Sweden: a 5-year prospective study. *Pediatrics* 1992, **90**:950–958.

Giannini EH, Brewer EJ, Kuzmina N, *et al.*: Methotrexate in resistant juvenile rheumatoid arthritis. *N Eng J Med* 1992; **326**:1043–1049.

McCarthy PL, Wasserman D, Spiesel SZ, *et al.*: Evaluation of arthritis and arthralgia in the pediatric patient. *Clin Pediatr* 1980, **19**:183–190.

Arthritis, septic

Diagnosis

Symptoms

• Symptoms and signs are more difficult to interpret in the presence of preexisting joint disease and may be muted in immunosuppressed.

• Polyarticular infection is rare [1,2].

Pain: most consistent feature; typically progressive; may be worse at night; with pre-existing joint disease, change or exacerbation of pain is an important warning sign.

Loss of function, limp: possibly presenting feature in children [2].

Fever: possibly only manifestation.

Signs

Swelling and local tenderness, pain and restriction of movement.

Heat: common.

Local erythema: possible.

Fever: although temperature normal in up to one-third of patients.

Monoarticular presentation: typical [1].

Location: a large joint: knee, hip, elbow, or ankle; other joints; including small joints, are rarely affected [1].

Investigations

• Most investigations are nonspecific, and results may be normal; a high index of suspicion is necessary to make the diagnosis [4].

• Adequate specimens must be obtained for microbiological examination before antimicrobial treatment is started.

Synovial fluid analysis: Gram stain positive in >50% of patients; culture positive in up to 80%; presence of leukocytes <50,000 helpful but not diagnostic.

Glucose and protein: do not aid in diagnosis.

Blood cultures: positive in 50% (may be presenting feature of subacute bacterial endocarditis and may be positive when synovial fluid is negative).

Pharyngeal and urogenital swabs: should be obtained if gonococcal infection suspected.

Plain radiography: usually unhelpful in early stages of infection [2].

Complications

Death: rare in children.

Loss of function of joint.

Loss of prosthesis.

Osteomyelitis: from direct spread.

Bacterial endocarditis, disseminated intravascular coagulation.

Differential diagnosis

Toxic synovitis.

Osteomyelitis.

Serum sickness.

Acute flare of inflammatory joint disease.

Avascular necrosis.

Slipped capital femoral epiphysis.

Hemarthrosis.

Lyme disease.

Henoch–Schönlein purpura.

Trauma.

Etiology

• Pathogens depend on age and predisposing factors; most infections are due to *Staphylococcus aureus* and streptococci; in children aged <5 y, *Haemophilus influenzae* type b has been an important pathogen, but now less so since vaccination has been made available. Gonococcal infection appears to be in decline but should be considered in sexually active patients.

• Spread is usually hematogenous; joint disease or blunt trauma may act to localize blood-borne pathogens.

• Direct inoculation during surgery, injection, or trauma occurs but is unusual.

• Risk factors include extremes of age, previous joint disease, diabetes mellitus, immunosuppression (iatrogenic or congenital) and corticosteroids.

Epidemiology

• Septic arthritis is the cause of about 5% of all childhood arthritides.

Treatment

Diet and lifestyle

• Weight bearing should be avoided until patient has impoved symptomatically.

Pharmacologic treatment

General principles

• A possible septic arthritis is a medical emergency and should be urgently referred to a specialist (rheumatologist or orthopedic surgeon).

• High-dose antibiotics are given i.v. for at least 2 weeks, then orally for at least a further 2–4 weeks, depending on the clinical response and presence of prosthesis.

• Antibiotics should be started only after appropriate specimens for culture have been obtained.

• Initially, a "best guess" choice of antibiotics is used, based on the most probable pathogen, patient's age, and sensitivies of pathogen; treatment is later tailored by the results of the Gram stain and culture.

Possible "best-guess" regimen

Child aged <5 years: an i.v. antistaphlococcal penicillin and ceftriaxone.

Child aged >5 years: an i.v. staphylococcal with ceftriaxone if gonococcal infection likely.

Vancomycin i.v. for methicillin-resistant *Staphylococcus aureus*.

Specific drugs

Standard dosage	Oxacillin, 150 mg/kg/d i.v. divided in 4 doses, maximum 3 g i.v. every 6 h. Ceftriaxone, 100 mg/kg/d i.v., maximum 1 g per d. Vancomycin, 40 mg/kg/d i.v. 4 doses, maximum dose 1 g i.v. every 6–12 h.
Contraindications	Hypersensitivity.
Special points	Complete blood count needed twice weekly.
Main drug interactions	None.
Main side effects	Rash, hypersensitivity reaction (rare), neutropenia (after prolonged treatment), diarrhea.

Nonpharmacologic treatment

Repeated medical aspiration or surgical drainage [3].

• Surgery is indicated for the following:

Hip involvement

Inability to drain medically.

Failure to improve on antibiotic or medical management.

Osteomyelitis.

Prosthetic joints (surgical drainage, debridement, or removal).

Treatment aims

To prevent septicemia or osteomyelitis.
To preserve joint function.
To resolve infection.

Prognosis

• Excellent in cases treated within 4 d of onset [3,4].
• The prognosis is worse if treatment is delayed in patients with predisposing joint or systemic disease.
• Infection of prosthetic material carries a particularly poor prognosis; revision or removal of the prosthesis is a common outcome.

Follow-up and management

• The ESR and the synovial fluid WBC count should fall as the patient responds to therapy.
• Prompt physical and/or occupational therapy is important in order to maximize range of motion.

Key references

1. Fink CW, Nelson JD: Septic arthritis and osteomyelities in children. *Clin Rheumatic Dis*1986, **12**:423–435.

2. Shaw BA, Kasser JL: Acute septic arthritis in infancy and childhood. Clin Orthop 1990, **257**:212–225.

3. Wilson NIL, DiPaola M: Acute septic arthritis in infancy and childhood: 10 years' experience. *J Bone Joint Surg* 1986, **68-B**: 584–587.

4. Weldon CJ, Long SS, Fisher MC, *et al.* Pyogenic arthritis in infants and children: a review of 95 cases. *Pediatr Infect Dis J* 1986, **5**:669–676.

Asthma

Diagnosis

Symptoms

Cough: with or without sputum production; night cough is usually more pronounced than day cough; may be easily inducible by physical triggers during and after an exacerbation.

Sputum production: distinguish airway secretions originating from chest versus the upper airways by nature of cough, the presence of cough upon arising, and mobilization of secretions after inhaling.

Breathlessness: with acute exacerbations; patients with chronic dyspnea may have become accommodated and show a decreased sense of breathlessness.

Chest tightness: may be perceived as "pain," but it is qualitatively different.

Wheeze: absence of wheeze does not eliminate the diagnosis of asthma.

Signs

Tachypnea

Tachycardia

Accessory muscles of respiration use.

Retractions: supraclavicular, intercostal, subcostal.

Auscultation of the lungs

Decreased air entry into lungs, rhonchi and/or rales, increased expiratory phase: altered inspiratory:expiratory ratio, **asymmetric breath sounds:** possible due to atelectasis or airway plugging; **pulsus paradoxicus,** and anxiety or agitation.

Life-threatening features

Cyanosis, confusion, fatigue, exhaustion, reduced consciousness, bradycardia, silent chest, and paradoxical thoracoabdominal movement.

Retractions cease without clinical improvement.

Investigations

Acute episode

Peak flow rate and/or spirometry: assess severity; **oximetry in room air; arterial blood gas:** especially if patient shows features of impending respiratory arrest; **chest radiography:** if physical examination suggests abnormality such as pneumonia, barotrauma, or cardiac condition; **electrocardiography:** if cardiac dysfunction suspected; **sputum culture:** if bacterial infection suspected; **serum electrolytes:** if dehydration and/or electrolyte disturbance suspected; **theophylline level:** for prior, chronic administration and acute dosing scheme; **CBC:** pharmacologic treatment will affect differential white blood cell count.

Initial evaluation

Spirometry: include response to bronchodilator; asthma is not excluded if β-2-agonist does not reverse obstruction at a single examination.

Serial peak-flow monitoring: establish trends for best result; diurnal variation (> 15%) suggests asthma; useful for documentation of response to medication adjustment or adverse environment and to signal onset of exacerbation.

Body plethysmography: may be necessary to rule out other disorders (restrictive), provide assessment of air trapping, and measures of airway conductance.

Chest radiograph.

Allergen skin testing: >50% patients have significant atopic disorder and environmental triggers require assessment.

Bronchoprovocation testing: increased sensitivity to bronchoconstrictors, such as methacholine or histamine, may help establish diagnosis; exercise challenge can be useful; provocation with allergens can be dangerous.

Clinical response to oral course of corticosteroids: 7–10 days of prednisone usually will elicit a measurable response both clinically and via spirometry.

Differential diagnosis

• Consider causes of cough and wheeze: bronchiolitis, bronchopulmonary dysplasia, immunodeficiency, immotile cilia syndrome, congestive heart failure, bronchiectasis, cystic fibrosis, gastroesophageal reflux, foreign body aspiration, and neuromuscular disorders.

Congenital anatomic defects: Tracheoesophageal fistula, tracheoand/or bronchomalacia, lobar emphysema, bronchogenic cyst, pulmonary sequestration, anomalous blood vessels, and tracheal or bronchial stenosis.

Airway encroachment

Mediastinal tumor or adenopathy, pulmonary tumor, hemangioma, papilloma, recurrent sinusitis, chronic infection, hypersensitivity pneumonitis, allergic bronchopulmonary aspergillosis, α-$_1$-antitrypsin deficiency, visceral larval migrans, carcinoid tumors, pulmonary vasculitis, idiopathic pulmonary hemosiderosis, sarcoidosis, habit cough, upper airway obstruction, pulmonary embolus, pertussis, environmental irritant exposure, and hyperventilation syndrome.

Etiology

• Asthma is a chronic inflammatory disorder; all grades of severity or phenotypes show evidence of airway inflammation: epithelial disruption, increased mucus production and mucus gland hypertrophy, mucosal edema, altered basement membrane matrix, inflammation.

• Airway hyperreactivity, presumably driven by inflammation mechanisms.

• A genetic basis is suspected and multiple phenotypes are likely to exist based on multiple genetic loci.

• Atopy (genetic predisposition to develop IgE-mediated inflammatory responses) is the strongest identifiable predisposing factor for developing asthma.

Complications

Respiratory arrest and death, barotrauma, right middle lobe syndrome, irreversible air flow limitation.

Treatment

Lifestyle management
• Excellent conditioning and a normal lifestyle is encouraged. The patient should not alter goals or activities based on asthma.

• Diet should be altered only if food, food additive (*eg*, sulfite), or drug (*eg*, ASA, nonsteroidal anti-inflammatory drugs) has been identified as a trigger.

Pharmacologic treatment
Long-term control medications
Corticosteroids
Inhaled corticosteroids: anti-inflammatory; dosage dependent on severity and formulation; can be used for daily maintenance routine and at increased dosage for short-term management of exacerbations; use of spacer and mouth rinsing wi

Systemic corticosteroids: anti-inflammatory; for short-term "burst" to control exacerbation and for longer term in severe, persistent cases; main side effects include increased activity, appetite; Cushingoid appearance; growth suppression; osteoporosis.

Cromolyn and nedocromil: anti-inflammatory; safety is primary advantage of these agents; nebulizer delivery of cromolyn (20 mg/ampule) may be more effective than MDI (1 mg/puff).

Methylxanthines: predominantly bronchodilator mechanisms; standard dosage adjusted to yield blood concentration of 1015 mg/L; has a narrow therapeutic margin, multiple drug interactions; oral dosing may aid compliance; additive benefit with inhaled steroids.

Long-acting β-2-agonists
Salmeterol (inhaled): bronchodilator; not to be used for acute symptoms or exacerbations because of slow onset of action; does not replace anti-inflammatory medication; tolerance can occur, but clinical significance is unknown.

Oral agents: inhaled route is preferred.

Leukotriene modifiers: new classes of anti-inflammatory drugs with great potential advantages; clinical experience in children is just beginning; leukotriene-receptor antagonists (multiple entities) and a 5-lipoxygenase inhibitor (Zileuton); *special note*: age indications vary.

Quick-relief medications
Short-acting inhaled β-2-agonists
Albuterol, bitolterol, pirbuterol, terbutaline: bronchodilator mechanism; drugs of choice for intermittent symptom control and management of acute bronchospasm; regularly scheduled daily use not recommended; oral route not recommended.

Anticholinergics
Ipratropium bromide: bronchodilator mechanism (reduces vagal tone); may provide some additive effect to β-2-agonist as supplement but not indicated as a primary drug.

Corticosteroids
Systemic (methylprednisolone, prednisolone, prednisone): anti-inflammatory mechanism; for moderate to severe exacerbations (usually 3–5 day courses; up to 10 may be indicated); tapering the dose following improvement not indicated.

• Severe attacks should be treated in hospital with careful monitoring, oxygen, hydration, aerosol β-2-agonist (intermittent or continuous), systemic corticosteroid (oral or parenteral, but initiated early); theophylline for those on maintenance.

Treatment aims
To find minimum treatment necessary to suppress symptoms and limit side effects.

To maintain (near) "normal" pulmonary function.

To avoid loss of time from school and other activities; avoid parental loss of work time (quality of life measures).

To enable patient and/or family to take responsibility for day to day management of asthma.

To reduce the frequency of exacerbations and to avoid hospital admissions.

To exercise optimal environmental control measures.

Prognosis
• Most patients with asthma cope well, have normal lifestyles, and achieve normal life expectancies.

• The natural history of childhood asthma is varied with many patients showing remissions during the first and second decades of life.

• Patients in remission from childhood asthma may see symptoms reappear in the fourth and fifth decades.

• Severely ill or unstable asthmatics can do well with appropriate monitoring, environmental control, adequate anti-inflammatory medication, and appropriately enacted action plans for exacerbations.

Follow-up and management
• Measurements of the following are recommended:

Signs and symptoms of asthma.

Pulmonary function.

Quality of life/functional status.

Pharmacotherapy, including adverse effects.

Provider–patient communication and patient satisfaction.

General references
National Asthma Education Program: Expert Panel Report 2: *Guidelines for the diagnosis and management of asthma.* US Department of Health and Human Services, Public Health Service, National Institutes of Health: Washington, DC; 1997 [NIH Publication

O'Byrne PM, Thomson NC (eds): *Manual of Asthma Management.* WB Saunders Co., Ltd: London; 1995.

Ataxia, acute

Diagnosis

Symptoms

Disturbed coordination: affecting amplitude and velocity of intended movements, and sparing strength; tremor may be present.

Hypotonia: in some cases but usually mild.

Truncal ataxia: unsteadiness in sitting, standing, or walking; titubation.

Limb ataxia: often accompanied by tremor.

Other symptoms depending on etiology: *eg*, headache, neurologic deficits.

Recent infection or immunization: *eg*, resolving varicella.

History of medication use: *eg*, antiepileptic drugs.

The pace of onset and the most common etiologies

Onset	Most common etiologies
Sudden (minutes to hours)	Intoxication, some metabolic diseases, vascular disease (stroke or hemorrhage)
Days to weeks	Tumor, inflammatory (postinfectious or demyelinating)
Months or years, with slow progression	Neurodegenerative disease
Intermittent	Metabolic disorders

Signs

Sensory ataxia

Areflexia: with diminished proprioception and vibratory sense.

Romberg's sign: exacerbation of truncal instability with eye closure.

Cerebellar ataxia

Truncal: hyporeflexia, unsteady stance or gait; Romberg's sign is absent; when severe, sitting and/or speech may be affected.

Appendicular (limb): dysmetria and dysdiadochokinesia (impaired rapid alternating movements) ipsilateral to the affected cerebellar hemisphere.

Signs of raised intracranial pressure.

Other neurologic signs according to etiology: altered mental status, cranial nerve palsies, hemiparesis, sensory deficits.

Skin lesions: *eg*, evidence of resolving varicella.

Investigations

• Investigation may occasionally be deferred (*eg*, classic, acute cerebellar ataxia clearly following a bout of varicella); additional studies are often required:

Neuroimaging (cranial CT, MRI, or MRA): for tumor, vascular malformation, hydrocephalus, vasculitis (and generally performed prior to lumbar puncture).

Toxin screen of urine and/or blood: for drug intoxication.

Blood chemistries, including ammonia, pyruvate, lactate; and urine amino and organic acids: for inborn errors of metabolism.

CSF analysis: for infection and postinfectious syndromes (*eg*, Guillain–Barré).

Antibody titers against specific infectious agents: *Mycoplasma*, Epstein–Barr virus.

Nerve conduction studies: for Guillain–Barré syndrome; early, absent F-waves may support diagnosis; in 1 wk most patients show slowed or blocked nerve conduction.

Complications

Herniation of the cerebellum (upwards or downwards) in cases of posterior fossa mass lesion.

Respiratory failure: in Guillain-Barré syndrome.

Complications of drug ingestion and inborn errors of metabolism: *eg*, cardiac dysrhythmia with severe carbamazepine intoxication.

Treatment

Diet and lifestyle

Specific inborn errors of metabolism require appropriate dietary restriction and/or avoidance of certain medications (*eg*, low-protein diet in hyperammonemia syndromes).

Pharmacologic treatment

- Intoxications should be managed according to the offending agent.
- Bacterial infections require appropriate antibiotic therapy and/or surgical drainage.
- In ADEM, steroid therapy should be considered; controlled trials are lacking and not all patients respond, but anecdotal reports strongly support the notion of a steroid-responsive subgroup.
- In genetic disorders causing episodic ataxia, specific therapies, such as acetazolamide, may be effective.

Nonpharmacologic treatment

Surgical intervention in posterior fossa tumor, expanding hematoma, abscess, empyema, Dandy-Walker cyst.

Radiotherapy (and/or chemotherapy) in selected patients with malignant posterior fossa tumors.

Treatment aims

To promptly and specifically manage disease according to etiology.
To prevent recurrence in intermittent ataxia.

Prognosis

- In postvaricella ataxia, complete resolution occurs in nearly all cases within 3 to 5 weeks; recovery is less predictable in ADEM.
- Cerebellar astrocytoma can often be managed definitively by surgery alone with excellent outcome; prognosis is variable with other posterior fossa tumors, which may require irradiation, chemotherapy, or both.

Follow-up and management

- Acute ataxia is usually a monophasic illness, and follow-up is based on the etiology.
- If deficits persist, physical occupational therapy is indicated.
- If no cause is evident, careful follow-up for recurrence (which would suggest metabolic disease) is required.

General references

Connolly AM, Dodson WE, Prensky AL, Rust RS: Course and outcome of acute cerebellar ataxia. *Ann Neurol* 1994, **35**:673–679.

Gieron-Korthals MA, Westberry KR, Emmanuel PJ: Acute childhood ataxia: 10-year experience. *J Child Neurol* 1994, **9**:381–384.

Atrioventricular block

Diagnosis

Definition

• Complete atrioventricular (AV) block is defined as the inability of an atrial impulse to be conducted to the ventricle.

• Second-degree AV block occurs with progressive slowing of AV conduction (progressive PR prolongation) and eventual loss of conduction (P wave with no QRS complex). Second-degree AV block may be labeled Mobitz type I or Wenckebach block; block occurs in the AV node proximally after progressive slowing of AV conduction evidenced by PR prolongation until conduction is completely blocked.

• Mobitz type II AV block occurs in the His bundle with either relatively normal conduction or AV block; more commonly progresses to complete AV block.

• First-degree AV block results in delayed conduction from the atrium to ventricle with a prolonged PR interval, but no loss of conduction (*see* figure).

Symptoms

First-degree AV block: patients are usually asymptomatic.

Second-degree AV block: patients are only symptomatic if block results in a long pause (>2–3 seconds); this is seen only in high-grade AV block.

Third-degree or complete AV block: dizziness, presyncope, syncope:(secondary to low cardiac output and hypotension); fatigue, exercise intolerance (secondary to blunted cardiac output response to exercise, limited by inability to increase heart rate normally).

Sudden death: prolonged pauses or asystole lead to ventricular fibrillation or cardiac standstill.

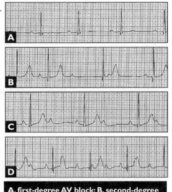

A, first-degree AV block; B, second-degree AV block (Mobitz I); C, second-degree AV block (Mobitz II); D, third-degree AV block.

Signs

First degree: none.

Second degree: in Mobitz type I, irregular pulse with pauses; in Mobitz type II, irregular pulse with occasional dropped complexes; bradycardia, signs of congestive heart failure (tachypnea, retractions, rales, hepatomegaly, jugular venous distension, edema).

Third degree: bradycardia; signs of congestive heart failure (tachypnea, retractions, rales, hepatomegaly, jugular venous distension, cannon waves, edema), hydrops in the fetus.

Investigations

• Complete AV block is associated with congenital heart disease, most commonly L-transposition of the great arteries, ventricular inversion or corrected transposition, or heterotaxy syndromes; these defects can be identified by cardiac ultrasound.

ECG: to evaluate degree of block and location of escape rhythm; block in the AV node usually results in a narrow QRS escape complex; block in the His–Purkinje system may result in a wide QRS escape complex.

24-Hour ambulatory monitoring (Holter): to evaluate extent of AV block. Second-degree AV block is common in adolescents during sleep and is usually benign unless pauses are excessively long (>3–4 seconds) or block is high grade (>3:1). With complete AV block, the low rate should be noted as well as pauses (>3 seconds), ventricular ectopy and prolongation of the QT interval, all of which are associated with increased incidence of syncope and sudden death.

Differential diagnosis

Diagnosis is made by ECG. Care should be taken to distinguish AV dissociation with accelerated junctional rhythm or sinus slowing from AV block. Differential is in determining etiology.

Etiology

Digoxin toxicity, inflammatory cardiovascular diseases (viral myocarditis, rheumatic fever, collagen vascular diseases, Kawasaki disease), long QT syndrome, neuromuscular (muscular dystrophy, myotonic dystrophy, Kearns-Sayre syndrome, metabolic, hematologic (hemosiderosis), and infectious disorders (diphtheria, Rocky Mountain spotted fever, bacterial endocarditis), tumors, congenital heart defects, L-transposition of the great arteries, heterotaxy syndrome, Ebstein's anomaly, atrial septal defects, AV canal defects, postoperative repair of ventricular septal defect (VSD), tetralogy of Fallot, or AV canal defects.

• Congenital heart block is associated with collagen vascular disease in the mother who has positive serology for anti-Ro or anti-La antibodies [1,2].

Epidemiology

• Congenital complete heart block (CCHB) [3] and postoperative heart block [4] are the most common causes. Congenital heart block occurs with an incidence of 1:15,000 live births. In two thirds of cases, CCHB is associated with maternal collagen vascular disease (positive anti-Ro or anti-La antibodies) and in patients with complex congenital heart disease, especially heterotaxy syndrome.

• Postsurgical complete AV block occurs in ~1% of cases in which a VSD is repaired. Some form of AV block occurs in 30%–60% of patients with L-transposition of the great arteries.

Complications

Syncope: may be associated with injury as there is little warning of impending syncope in this condition.
Cardiac arrest.
Sudden death.

Treatment

Diet and lifestyle

• No dietary restrictions. For first- and second-degree AV block that is asymptomatic, restrictions depend on underlying cause. Those patients with myocarditis or inflammatory heart disease should restrain from vigorous activity. Patients with complete heart block may be allowed to set their own level of activity. Excessive fatigue or exercise limitation may be an indication for pacemaker implantation. Pacemaker implantation may result in restriction from contact sports, including wrestling and football. Location of the pacemaker, chest, or abdomen may result in additional limitation.

Pharmacologic treatment

Acute treatment

Standard dosage	Atropine, i.v. bolus, 0.02–0.04 mg/kg (maximum, 1–2 mg).
Contraindications	Hypersensitivity to anticholinergic drugs; narrow-angle glaucoma; tachycardia; myocardial ischemia; obstructive gastrointestinal disease; obstructive uropathy; myasthenia gravis.
Special points:	Lessens AV block when increased vagal tone is a major contributor. Can be given every 1–2 h.
Main drug interactions:	Amantadine increases anticholinergic side effects; atenolol increases β-blockade effects; phenothiazines decrease antipsychotic effects; tricyclic antidepressants increase anticholinergic effects.
Main side effects	Gastrointestinal: altered taste, nausea, vomiting, constipation, dry mouth; genitourinary: urinary retention ocular: blurred vision, dilated pupils, increased intraocular pressure; cardiovascular: palpitations, tachycardia; central nervous system: headaches, flushing, nervousness, restlessness; other: decreased sweating.

Standard treatment

Standard dosage	Isoproterenol, 0.1–2.0 µg/kg/min i.v.
Contraindications	Relative: preexisting ventricular arrhythmias. Elevation of heart rate may suppress ventricular ectopy.
Special points	Should be used as a temporary bridge until temporary or permanent pacing can be achieved.
Main drug interactions:	Use with other sympathomimetic bronchodilators or epinephrine may result in exaggerated sympathetic response Effects of isoproterenol in patients on monoamine oxidase inhibitors or tricyclic antidepressants may be potentiated.

β-Blocking agents and isoproterenol inhibit the effects of each other.

Main side effects	Central nervous system: nervousness, headache, dizziness, weakness; gastrointestinal: nausea, vomiting; cardiovascular: tachycardia, palpitations, chest pain; other: flushing, tremor, sweating.

• There are no effective drugs for chronic AV.

Other treatment options

• Temporary pacemaker used in emergent situations until more permanent pacing can be achieved or in situations deemed to be temporary (myocarditis, drug toxicity).

Treatment aims

To return patient to normal activity and normal life.
To prevent syncope and sudden death.

Prognosis

Incidence of sudden death in postoperative complete heart block that is not paced is as high as 50%. In congenital heart block, incidence of sudden death is 5%–10%. Prognosis is excellent in both groups once pacer is implanted. A small number of congenital heart block patients develop a dilated cardiomyopathy. The prognosis in postoperative heart block is related to the underlying congenital heart defect and any residual lesions.

Follow-up and management

Patients with first- and second-degree AV block should be followed at least yearly to observe for the development of higher grade or complete AV block.
Patients with a pacemaker need monthly to bimonthly transtelephonic checks and twice yearly office checks with complete analysis of the pacemaker function.
Permanent pacemaker generators require replacement every 5–15 y. Wires may fracture or require replacement secondary to growth when placed in a small child.

Key references

1. Chameides L, Truex RC, Vetter VL, et al.: Association of maternal systemic lupus erythematosus with congenital complete heart block. N Engl J Med 1977, **297:**1204–1207.

2. Bunyon JP, Winchester RJ, Slade SG, et al.: Identification of mothers at risk for congenital heart block and other neonatal lupus syndromes in their children. Arthritis Rheum 1993, **9:**1263–1273.

3. Pinsky WW, Gillette PC, Garson A Jr., McNamara DG: Diagnosis, management and long-term results of patients with congenital atrioventricular block. Pediatrics 1982, **69:**728–733.

4. Driscoll DJ, Gillette PC, Hallma GL: Management of surgical complete atrioventricular block in children. Am J Cardiol 1979, **43:**1175–1180.

Diagnosis

Symptoms and signs [1]

History: high risk of completed suicide

Presence or previous history of major mental illness: especially endogenous depression, mania, chronic disease, previous attempts, and schizophrenia.

Evidence of planning: time spent in preparation of the means of death, *eg*, buying and hoarding tablets, precautions taken against discovery or intervention by others, acts in anticipation of death, *eg*, making or updating will, writing suicide note.

Continuing wish to die: no help sought after attempt, continued wish to die after resuscitation, hopelessness.

Violent method chosen: *eg*, hanging, jumping from height, firearms.

History: low risk of completed suicide

No history or presence of major mental illnesses or chronic disease.

Little or no preparation or precautions: decision to attempt suicide taken within 1 h of the act or after conflict; act performed in front of another.

No continuing wish to die: help sought after act, no wish to die after resuscitation, optimism about future.

Nonviolent means: method perceived by patient as having a low risk of real harm; patients may not understand the toxic effects of drugs taken and may mistakenly consider acetaminophen and aspirin harmless because they are available over the counter and benzodiazepines dangerous because they are prescription-only drugs.

Mental state

• Orientation and memory must be checked first because the toxic effects of drugs or alcohol must be allowed to wear off before further assessment is attempted.

• An acute organic brain syndrome, including visual hallucinations can be caused by overdose of drugs.

Features of major mental illness, especially endogenous depression or psychosis: patient should be asked about persistent low mood, worse in mornings, sleep disturbance with early morning wakening, appetite and weight loss, lack of energy, pessimism, low self-esteem, guilt, excessive worrying, delusions, and hallucinations.

Investigations

• Available databases should be checked for evidence of previous or present psychiatric care.

• Further history should be obtained from available family informants. Look for signs of withdrawal.

• Physical investigations appropriate for the type of self-harm should be made.

• Assess family competence to protect child.

Complications

• No overall physical complications are seen; complications depend on the nature of the self-harm.

Differential diagnosis

Self-cutting or self-damage to relieve tension: often multiple superficial cuts on forearms.

Self-mutilation in context of psychotic illness: especially schizophrenia.

Accidental ingestion of toxic substances: eg, tablets that look like sweets to children, weedkiller stored in a lemonade bottle.

Etiology

• Causes include the following:

Major depression, schizophrenia, mania.

Drug or alcohol abuse.

Chronic physical ill health.

Recent bereavement.

Identity crisis.

Poorly developed coping skills.

Relationship problems.

Social stressors, peer pressure.

Epidemiology [1]

• The rate of adolescent suicide has increased in the US 44% since 1970.

• An estimated 1:50–100 attempts succeed.

• Suicide is the third leading cause of death among children aged 15–24.

• Many motor vehicle crashes may be unrecognized suicide attempts.

• Trends vary widely over time and across different cultures.

• Risk factors for completed suicide are male sex, poor physical health, being isolated, positive family history.

Factors associated with repetition

• Factors that indicate a greater risk of repetition include previous psychiatric treatment, substance problems, previous deliberate self-harm, sociopathic traits, family history, and unchanged problems and circumstances.

• Chronic repeaters invariably have severe personality difficulties, chaotic lifestyles, deprived backgrounds, and great difficulty in engaging in any form of therapy.

Treatment

Diet and lifestyle

• Family stress, social isolation, positive family history, and depression are all high risk factors for repetition of suicide attempts, so efforts should be made to change the lifestyle of the patients and families through therapeutic intervention.

Pharmacological treatment

• The physical consequences of self-harm must be treated first.

• Except in emergencies, psychotropic drugs should be given only for treatment of specific mental illness under close psychiatric supervision, usually as an inpatient.

• Tranquillizing drugs must be avoided unless absolutely necessary for the safety of patients or others.

• For the emergency management of violently mentally disturbed patients, a short-acting antipsychotic, eg, droperidol or haloperidol in 5 mg increments i.m. every 15 min, should be used until symptoms are controlled, unless seizures are a risk. An antiparkinsonian drug, eg, procyclidine, 5–10 mg i.m., can be added to avoid dystonic reactions. Drugs should not be given i.v. when the cause of the mental disturbance is not known.

• When seizures are a risk, a benzodiazepine, eg, diazepam in 5 mg increments i.v. or lorazepam, 2–5 mg i.m., can be used. Benzodiazepines must be avoided in patients with severe respiratory impairment. Antipsychotic agents and benzodiazepines combined have an additive tranquillizing effect.

Nonpharmacological treatment [2]

Psychiatric referral [3]

• High-risk patients need psychiatric referral.

• Patients with major mental illness need urgent psychiatric treatment, usually on an inpatient basis.

Detention and emergency treatment [2]

• Patients or parents threatening discharge who have not been assessed or who have been assessed and are considered to be at immediate risk may have to be detained for further assessment or treatment.

• If a patient refuses to talk, information to make an assessment must be obtained from other informants before the patient can be discharged.

• Compulsory detention in hospital must be considered in cases of psychiatric illness or serious suicide risk.

• Emergency action in the patient's best interest is legally sanctioned in virtually every state; failure to act may be construed as negligence.

• Family must be assessed for their ability to protect the child and to stabilize the situation.

Counseling

• Most patients are cooperative, and many are not suffering from mental illness. Low-risk patients should be offered brief problem-orientated counseling, where available.

• Patients with alcohol or substance abuse problems should be referred to the relevant specialist services.

• Open access or a telephone help-line may be offered, if available.

Treatment aims

To treat any underlying mental disorder.
To help patient to solve problems and to provide support through current crisis.
To strengthen patient's future coping skills.
To help family provide support.

Prognosis

• Repetition occurs most often within the first 3 months of an episode.
• Repetition with increased suicidal intent may herald completed suicide.
• Long-term risk of completed suicide overall is ~1% at 1 y, ~2.8% at 8 y.
• ~7% of patients make 2 or more attempts, 2.5% 3 or more, and 1% 5 or more.

Follow-up and management

Low-risk patients: no special care.
High-risk patients and those with mental illness: need close monitoring.

Dealing with violent mentally disturbed patients

• Aggressive patients are often frightened.
• Keep calm and gentle in voice and actions.
• Do not corner, crowd, or threaten the patient.
• Give clear explanations of what is happening.
• Do not see or leave the patient alone.
• Call for adequate extra staff, porters, security staff, or police as necessary backup.

Key references

1. Hodas GR, Sargent J: Psychiatric emergencies. In *Textbook of Pediatric Emergency Medicine*. Edited by Fleisher G, Ludwig S. Williams and Wilkins: Baltimore; 1993.

2. Brent DA: Depression and suicide in adolescents and children. *Pediatr Rev* 1993, **14:** 380–388.

3. Henden H: Psychocynamics of suicide with particular reference to the young. *Am J Psychiatry* 1991, **148:** 1150–1158.

Diagnosis

Symptoms

Developmentally inappropriate symptoms of either inattention, or of impulsivity or hyperactivity or both for 6 months or more.

Onset before 7 years of age.

Symptoms present in two or more settings (eg, at home and at school).

Symptoms cause significant impairment in social or academic function.

Symptoms not exclusively associated with certain other disorders, including pervasive developmental disorder; mood, anxiety, or personality disorder; or psychosis.

• Mental retardation is not an exclusionary criterion for attention deficit–hyperactivity disorder (ADHD).

• ADHD is classified as predominantly inattentive, predominantly hyperactive or impulsive, or both (see table).

• Comorbidity (eg, learning disability, tics, or Tourette syndrome, mental retardation) is common and may dominate the clinical picture.

Criteria for diagnosis

Inattentiveness (at least 6)

Frequent mistakes in or failure to attend to details of schoolwork, or home or play activities

Difficulty sustaining attention in tasks or play activities

Appearance of not listening when spoken to directly

Poor follow-through with school assignments, chores, and so on

Difficulty organizing tasks and activities

Excessive avoidance of tasks requiring sustained mental efforts

Frequent losing of items necessary for school (or play) activities

Distractibility by extraneous stimuli

Forgetfulness in daily activities

Impulsivity/hyperactivity (at least 6)

Frequent fidgeting and squirming

Frequent leaving of seat where inappropriate

Frequent, inappropriate running, climbing, and so on

Difficulty engaging in quiet play

Physical activity appears driven

Excessive talking

Blurting answers before question completed

Difficulty awaiting turn

Frequent interrupting

Signs

• The diagnosis of ADHD is primarily one of history, and signs are often absent.

• Behavior in the office setting may not be representative.

• "Soft" neurologic signs may be present, including poor fine or gross motor skills, mild choreiform movements, and so on.

• Other signs relating to comorbidity may be present.

Differential diagnosis

Developmentally appropriate behavior.
Childhood absence epilepsy.
Depression.
Conduct or anxiety disorder.

Etiology

• Genetic predisposition appears to play a major role in ADHD.

• Environmental factors, including child-rearing techniques, may ameliorate or exacerbate symptoms.

• The concept of ADHD as a medical disorder is significantly influenced by culturally determined expectations for sustained attention and quiet behavior in children.

Epidemiology

• Precise prevalence is difficult to gauge because of the subjective nature of diagnosis and different methods of ascertainment.

• Several studies suggest a prevalence of 3%–5% of school-age children, with boys affected more frequently than girls.

Investigations

• Behavioral questionnaires for teachers and parents (eg, Connors or McCarney scales) may be helpful.

• IQ and achievement testing is often indicated, especially if there is academic underachievement, because ADHD may be associated with or exacerbated by learning disorders.

• Electroencephalography should be considered if the pattern of inattentiveness suggests absence epilepsy.

• Additional psychometric tests may aid diagnosis (eg, the Connors Continuous Performance Test, which evaluates attention and impulsivity by assessing ability to respond or inhibit response to letters presented serially on a computer screen).

Complications

Depression, aggressive behavior, poor self-esteem, chronic underachievement.

Treatment

Diet and lifestyle

• Claims that specific foods, dyes, additives, etc. exacerbate ADHD symptoms have generally not been substantiated by careful controlled trials.

• Caffeine-containing foods and beverages should be consumed in moderation.

Pharmacologic treatment

• Medications are not a substitute for behavioral measures and are not always required (*see* below).

• A stimulant (methylphenidate, dextroamphetamine, or pemoline) is generally used first; clonidine may be used when tics are present or exacerbated by stimulant therapy, but is less effective.

• Antidepressants should be considered if depression aggravates or results from ADHD symptoms.

• The following dosages of stimulants refer to children ≥6 y of age.

Methylphenidate (Ritalin)

Standard dosage	Methylphenidate, 0.3 mg/kg/dose or 2.5–5.0 mg/dose given before breakfast and lunch; occasionally, a third dose in the mid to late afternoon is helpful, but evening doses tend to produce insomnia.
	Increase dosage by 0.1–0.3 mg/kg/dose or by 5–10 mg/d at weekly intervals to obtain optimum response
	Maintain dosage at 0.3–2.0 mg/kg/d (typically 10–40 mg/d); should not exceed 60 mg/d.
Special points	Convert to sustained-release formulation if appropriate.

Dextroamphetamine sulfate (Dexedrine)

Standard dosage	Dextroamphetamine sulfate, 2.5 mg/dose once or twice daily (slightly longer acting than methylphenidate).
	Increase by 2.5–5 md/d at weekly intervals to obtain optimum response.
	Maintain at 0.1–1.0 mg/kg/d (typically 5–30 mg/d); should not exceed 40 mg/d.
Special points	Convert to sustained release formulation if appropriate.

Pemoline (Cylert)

Standard dosage	Pemoline, 18.75 mg/d as a single morning dose.
	Increase by 18.75 mg/d every 2–3 weeks to obtain optimum response.
	Maintain at 1.0–2.5 mg/kg/d (typically 18.75–75.0 mg/d); should not exceed 112.5 mg/d.

Clonidine (Catapres)

Standard dosage	Clonidine, 0.05 mg/d (*ie*, half of a 0.1-mg tablet) as a single evening dose.
	Increase by 0.05 mg/d in one or two doses every 1–2 weeks to obtain optimum response.
	Maintain at 8.0 µg/kg/d (0.10–0.40 mg/d); should not exceed 0.5 mg/d.
Special points	Transdermal formulation (Catapres TTS) available.
Main side effects	*Stimulants:* insomnia, anorexia, end-of-day "rebound," dysphoria.
	Clonidine: sedation, orthostatic hypotension.

Treatment aims

To control symptoms and/or mimimize resulting functional impairment.

To maintain self-esteem and healthy family dynamics.

To identify and correctly manage comorbidity.

Prognosis

Stimulant therapy response rate is 70%.

Long-term follow-up studies limited, but 10%–60% persistence into adulthood is reported.

Follow-up and management

Periodic follow-up (semiannual or more often) is indicated to optimize behavioral management and pharmacotherapy.

Uncertainty of therapeutic response should prompt trial off medication.

Referral for psychiatric evaluation and/or family counseling is helpful in some instances.

Nonpharmacologic treatment

Provide additional, individualized supervision in school.

Break down assignments, chores, into smaller tasks with reinforcement at each stage.

Token economies.

Minimize environmental distractions (especially during homework).

Provide ample opportunity for physical activity.

Set reasonable limits on television, video games, and so on, and ensure appropriateness of content.

Provide child with an opportunity to engage and excel in one or more extracurricular activities of interest.

Family counseling.

General references

Wilens TE, Biederman J: The stimulants. *Psychiatr Clin North Am* 1992, **15:**1.

Cantwell DP: Attention deficit disorder: a review of the past 10 years. *J Am Acad Child Adolesc Psychiatr* 1996, **35:**978–987.

Reiff MI, Banez GA, Culbert TP: Children who have attentional disorders: diagnosis and evaluation. *Pediatr Rev* 1993, **14:**455–465.

Autistic spectrum disorders (pervasive developmental disorders)

Diagnosis

Definition

• Autistic spectrum disorders, or pervasive developmental disorders, are characterized by qualitative impairment in several areas of development, most typically social interaction and, in most cases, verbal and nonverbal communication; a restricted repertoire of interests and activities; peculiar habits, unusual response to specific sensory stimuli, and/or self-stimulating behavior; frequent coexistence of mental retardation but with the above deficits disproportionate to the degree of cognitive impairment.

Symptoms

Autistic disorder

Includes symptoms from each of the following three categories with onset of at least some symptoms prior to 3 years of age (see *Diagnostic and Statistical Manual of Mental Disorders*, for details).

Qualitative impairment in social interaction: poor eye contact, poor peer relationships, no emotional reciprocity.

Qualitative impairment in communication: delay in spoken language or inability to sustain conversation; idiosyncratic use of language; lack of make-believe or social imitative play.

Restricted repertoire of interests and activities: marked preoccupation with a small number of specific activities; rigid adherence to routine (ritualism); stereotyped motor activity (rocking, spinning, head-banging).

Pervasive developmental disorder not otherwise specified

Severe impairments in one or more of the above areas, but not meeting criteria for autism or other specific pervasive developmental disorder, childhood schizophrenia, avoidant personality disorder.

Asperger's syndrome

• Language and cognitive skills are normal, but there is severe impairment in social interaction, with restricted interests activities.

Rett's syndrome

Regression of communication/cognitive skills by 6–18 months.

Loss of purposeful hand use.

Appearance of hand automatisms despite loss of purposeful hand use.

Affects females exclusively.

Prominent postnatal deceleration of head growth.

Jerky, unstable gait: half of patients never walk.

Common: seizures, hyperventilation/apnea, scoliosis, small hands and feet.

Signs

• Signs may be absent or relate to underlying etiology.

• Emphasize head circumference; eyes, including funduscopy (*eg*, congenital infection); muscle tone, coordination; dysmorphic features.

Investigations

• Investigations occasionally help define the cause, aid prognosis, or generate useful information for genetic counseling, but the overall yield is low.

Neuroimaging (cranial CT, MRI, or MRA): cerebral dysgenesis is occasionally identified, and nonspecific findings (*eg*, mild ventriculomegaly) are common.

Electroencephalography: for seizures and Landau–Kleffner syndrome.

Cytogenetic studies and DNA analysis: autistic features are sometimes prominent in fragile X syndrome and some chromosomal disorders.

Metabolic studies: serum chemistries, plasma and urine amino/organic acids, blood lactate and pyruvate may reveal an inborn error of metabolism.

Differential diagnosis

Deafness.

Developmental language disorder.

Avoidant personality disorder.

Reactive attachment disorder (associated with history of severe neglect or abuse).

Landau-Kleffner syndrome of acquired epileptic aphasia.

Childhood schizophrenia.

Selective mutism (*i.e.*, situational inhibition of language).

Otherwise uncomplicated mental retardation.

Etiology

• Autism is usually idiopathic, but may be associated with a variety of underlying cerebral insults or abnormalities, including chromosomal and genetic disorders, inborn errors of metabolism, congenital infections, and so on.

There is an increased risk of autism and related disorders in siblings of patients, suggesting a significant genetic component, even in idiopathic cases.

Epidemiology

Two to five cases per 10,000 individuals for autism; higher for pervasive developmental disorder, depending on precise criteria and vigor of ascertainment.

One to two cases per 20,000 females for Rett's syndrome.

Complications

• Comorbid conditions, such as epilepsy or mental retardation, are common.

Treatment

Diet and lifestyle
• Dietary factors are not clearly relevant.

Pharmacologic treatment
• No pharmacologic treatment has been shown to be effective in improving overall development. However, in individual patients, symptoms such as disabling repetitive activities, severe hyperactivity or distractibility, or anxiety, should prompt consideration of drug therapy.

For hyperactivity or severely impaired attention
• Consider stimulants or clonidine (*see* Attention Deficit–Hyperactivity Disorder).

For severe, aggressive, or self-injurious behavior.
• Consider neuroleptics, which are best used in conjunction with intensive behavior therapy, or selective serotonin reuptake inhibitors (*eg*, fluoxetine [Prozac]).

For anxiety
• Consider benzodiazepines (best used intermittently) or neuroleptics.

For disabling ritualistic behavior or repetitive activities
• Consider fluoxetine or other drugs that augment central serotonergic activity.

Nonpharmacologic treatment
Special education.

Behavioral modification program for management of unacceptable or disabling behaviors (*eg*, aggression, self-injury, disruptive activities).

• Based on unproven theories about the fundamental neurodevelopmental defect in autism, a variety of complex therapies have been proposed, including various regimens of desensitization, vestibular stimulation, and "facilitated communication" (in which communication, *eg*, via a letter board, is promoted by stabilization of the child's hand by a therapist or parent). Controlled trials of these therapies have generally not demonstrated efficacy.

Treatment aims
To minimize disruptive behavior.
To maximize function and social integration given the limitations of the illness.
To recognize and treat comorbidity, including epilepsy.

Prognosis
• A small percentage of children with autism live completely independently as adults; a much larger number achieve varying degrees of partial independence. The most useful predictor of long-term prognosis is language development.

Follow-up and management
• After initial diagnostic evaluation, periodic medical follow-up is not always necessary, especially if appropriate social supports have been established.
• Selected patients may require intensive inpatient management for development of appropriate pharmacologic and behavioral treatment regimens.

General references

American Psychiatric Association: Diagnostic and Statistical Manual of Mental Disorders, edn 4. Washington, D.C.: American Psychiatric Association; 1994. **34:**1124–1132.

Bauer S: Autism and the pervasive developmental disorders: (part 2). *Pediatr Rev* 1995, **16:**168–176.

Campbell M, Cueva JE: Psychopharmacology in child and adolescent psychiatry: a review of the past seven years: (part I). *J Am Acad Child Adolesc Psychiatr* 1995.

Diagnosis

Symptoms
• Symptoms generally include the following, alone or in combination:

Headache, papilledema, visual failure, vomiting: alone or in combination indicate raised intracranial pressure due to either intracranial mass or hydrocephalus secondary to obstruction.

Diplopia, facial droop, or drooling: cranial nerve abnormalities.

Irritability, drop in school performance, personality changes.

Seizures: focal seizures suggest localization of tumor.

Hemiparesis.

Signs
Papilledema, impaired visual acuity, visual field defects.

Diplopia: with or without clear III or VI nerve palsy.

Facial weakness.

Dysphasia.

Hemiparesis, hyperreflexia, extensor plantar response, hemisensory loss.

Investigations
Neuroradiography: primarily CT and MRI of brain; more invasive procedures (*eg*, angiography or positron emission tomography) sometimes needed for further aspects of management.

Resection or biopsy: in all cases except diffuse brain stem tumors and optic nerve tumors, biopsy with attempt at gross total resection should be performed both to establish the histologic diagnosis and to debulk the tumor.

Blood tests: possibly needed to clarify differential diagnosis, *eg*, blood cultures when metastatic brain abscess suspected.

Lumbar puncture: to identify meningeal spread of malignancy.

Complications
Blindness: papilledema due to progressive raised intracranial pressure leads to blindness if unrelieved.

Herniation: brain shift due to increasing mass of cerebral tumor can lead to central or transtentorial brain herniation, with irreversible ischemic brain damage and fatal apnea due to failure of brain stem function.

Cognitive impairment from radiation therapy (particularly whole brain irradiation): most severe in the youngest patients. Careful consideration of the risks and benefits is essential.

Differential diagnosis
Cerebrovascular disease.
Other organic brain disease (*eg*, encephalitis or demyelination).

Etiology
• The cause of most cerebral tumors remains unknown, although the incidence is increased after exposure to radiation, in patients with neurofibromatosis, and in some rare inherited immunodeficiency diseases.

Epidemiology
• The most common solid tumor in children accounting for over 20% of all pediatric malignancy.
Highest risk in infants.
Slight male predominance.

Treatment

Diet and lifestyle

- No special diet is necessary for patients with primary brain tumors.
- Impaired cognitive function and fatigue may affect schooling.

Pharmacologic treatment

For raised intracranial pressure and stabilization of brain function

Standard dosage	Dexamethasone, 0.5 mg/kg divided every 6 hours.
Contraindications	None.
Special points	Steroids should be weaned as quickly as possible, either shortly after surgical debulking, or shortly after initiation of adjuvant therapy.
	All patients should be placed on an H_2 antagonist such as ranitidine.
Main drug interactions	None.
Main side effects	Gastritis, weight gain, psychosis, hyperglycemia.

For acutely raised intracranial pressure

- In patients who are unconscious as a result of raised intracranial pressure from cerebral tumor or in those who have herniated, with respiratory arrest: artificial ventilation, mannitol as an osmotic diuretic, and i.v. dexamethasone may be needed in an emergency department or intensive care unit setting.

Chemotherapy

- For children less than 3 years of age, chemotherapy is the primary modality of treatment, usually using a combination of cyclophasphamide or ifosfamide, carboplatin or cisplatin, and etoposide. MOPP (mechlorethamine, Oncovin [vincristine], procarbasine, and prednisone) has also proven effective.
- For older children, histology dictates treatment, which usually follows irradiation.
- Medulloblastoma and primitive neuroectodermal tumor (PNET): cisplatin and/or cyclophosphamide, often combined with lomustine, etoposide, or vincristine.
- Glioma: lomustine and vincristine, with or without procarbazine.
- Ependymoma: no defined role for chemotherapy.

Other treatments

- Surgery is curative for low-grade astrocytoma that can be completely excised (defined as the absence of tumor on postoperative MRI).
- Radiotherapy is used in all but the youngest patients. Whereas glioma and ependymoma are treated with irradiation to the tumor volume, medulloblastoma and PNET require prophylactic irradiation to the entire brain and spine.

Treatment aims

- Cure is possible in over half of children with brain tumors. Children with low grade astrocytoma, ependymoma, and medulloblastoma, which can be completely excised, have a better prognosis. Outlook is less good for high-grade gliomas and disseminated tumors.

Prognosis

- Prognosis is related to tumor type, extent of resection, and presence or absence of metastases. Infants with malignant tumors fare poorly.
- For medulloblastoma that is completely excised without metastases, 70%–80% of patients can be cured. For other medulloblastoma patients, and patients with supratentorial PNET, cures are possible in 30%–50% of cases.
- For ependymoma patients with complete surgical excision, 70% of patients are cured; for those with metastases or incomplete excision, cures are rare.
- For malignant glioma, cure is possible for 20%, primarily those with completely excised anaplastic astrocytoma. Patients with glioblastoma multiforma and brain stem glioma are rarely cured.

Follow-up and management

- Clinical assessment of neurological and performance is used to monitor progress with follow-up brain scanning at intervals of 3–6 months.
- If disease progresses, further surgery is considered in 10%–15% of patients, as well as experimental treatments, eg, focused radiation, immunotherapy, or high-dose chemotherapy with stem cell support.
- The terminal phase can vary in duration. Most patients can be managed in the home, with the support of a home hospice program.

General references

Cohen ME, Duffner PK: *Brain tumors in children*, ed 2. New York: Raven Press; 1994.

Heideman RL, Packer RJ, Albright LA, et al.: Tumors of the central nervous system. In *Principles and Practice of Pediatric Oncology.* Edited by Pizzo PA, Poplack DG. Philadelphia: JB Lippincott; 1997.

Bronchiolitis and respiratory syncytial virus

Diagnosis

Symptoms

Prodrome: 1–2 days of fever, rhinorrhea, milder cough.

Apnea: may occur early before full intensity of chest symptoms.

Persistent, increased cough: may later be productive.

Rapid respirations.

Skin color changes: rashes (rare).

Poor feeding, lethargy.

Signs

Findings of rhinitis: occasionally otitis, conjunctivitis.

Pharyngitis, hoarseness.

Tachypnea with usually shallow respirations.

Tachycardia: especially when hypoxemia present.

Fever: usually milder later in course.

Nasal flaring, retractions, and hyperinflation.

Wheeze, increased expiratory phase, and rales and/or rhonchi.

Palpable liver and/or spleen: secondary to hyperinflation.

Cyanosis: *Note*: poor correlation with hypoxemia.

Vomiting (posttussive).

Evidence for dehydration may be present: secondary to poor oral intake.

Investigations

Complete blood count: with differential (no specific findings).

Pulse oximetry.

Arterial blood gas if respiratory failure appears imminent: severe hypoxia, raised or rising partial pressure of carbon dioxide.

Rapid viral identification: usually a "respiratory panel" is available to include common seasonal respiratory pathogens by antigen detection.

Viral culture: results delayed but may be useful to identify causative organism.

Serologic diagnosis: paired samples needed; rarely indicated as clinical diagnosis is usually evident.

Chest radiograph

Interstitial pneumonitis: the most typical finding; usually diffuse but may be segmental.

Hyperaeration: also typical and may be the only finding.

Peribronchial thickening: common but may not be related to the primary infection.

Consolidation: occasional in hospitalized patients; usually is subsegmental.

Complications

Otitis media: is most common (secondary; bacterial).

Pneumonia: secondary, bacterial; occurs in < 1% of hospitalized cases.

Apnea.

Respiratory failure.

Cardiac failure: secondary to pulmonary disease or rarely myocarditis.

Bronchiolitis obliterans: rare; usually associated with adenovirus-induced bronchiolitis/pneumonia.

Differential diagnosis

Pneumonia (viral, bacterial), *Chlamydia pneumonitis*, asthma, foreign body, cystic fibrosis, and pertussis.

Gastroesophageal reflux.

• The diagnosis is evident when, during an epidemic period, an infant presents with tachypnea, diffuse wheeze, and hyperinflation (radiograph) after a febrile upper respiratory illness.

Etiology

• Bronchiolitis is an acute inflammatory process causing obstruction of the small conducting airways and a manifestation of lower respiratory tract obstruction. RSV is the most common cause (70% of bronchiolitis cases and 40% of pneumonia in younger children). Other infectious etiologies include parainfluenza virus (second most common cause of bronchiolitis; more often associated with croup, tracheobronchitis, and laryngitis), influenza virus, adenovirus, rhinovirus, *Mycoplasma pneumoniae*, *Chlamydia*, and ureaplasma. *Pneumocystis carinii* is rarely associated with wheezing in infancy.

• RSV causes epithelial damage and elicits a mononuclear cell infiltrate and peribronchiolar edema. Those predisposed to the development of reactive airways (asthma) may develop RSV-specific immunoglobulin-E (IgE) responses, presumably because of a high IgE-responder phenotype. Notably, 30%–40% of patients who develop severe wheezing with RSV (ie, hospitalized) later show a tendency to wheeze repeatedly.

Epidemiology

• RSV epidemics peak from late fall to early spring. Up to 40% of primary infections result in febrile pneumonitis, but only 1% require hospitalization. Family studies indicate that nearly 70% of children are infected in the first year of life; by 24 months, nearly all children have been infected at least once. Beyond the first year, the clinical severity diminishes, changing from bronchiolitis and pneumonia to predominantly tracheobronchitis and reactive airway events.

• Transmission is by droplets or fomites. The virus can remain infectious for hours on surfaces. Hospital-acquired infections are common.

Treatment

Lifestyle management

• During the acute illness, routine health maintenance and respiratory care is provided at home or in hospital.

• Home management for mildly symptomatic patients is recommended.

• Adequate hydration should be assured.

• For significant wheeze or work of breathing, bronchodilator treatment (*eg*, albuterol) may be tried.

• Reassess infant with increased respiratory distress and tachycardia (oxygen saturation).

Hospital care

Pharmacologic treatment

Corticosteroids: although controversial, a trial is reasonable for hospitalized patients in whom bronchodilator responsiveness is documented.

Theophylline: not useful as a bronchodilator but may be helpful for management of apnea.

Antibiotics: not indicated unless secondary bacterial infection detected.

Ribavirin (antiviral) treatment: this is controversial because of concerns regarding cost, benefit, safety and quite variable clinical efficacy (conflicting chemical trials); may be considered for patients who are at risk for severe or fatal infections (*see* Other information), but no definitive indications have been established [1].

Immunoprophylaxis: RSV–intravenous immunoglobulin (RSV-IVIg) is approved for prevention of RSV disease in 1) children less than 2 years of age with bronchopulmonary dysplasia (BPD) who have been oxygen dependent at least 6 months prior to oncoming RSV season, and 2) selected infants with prematurity (gestational age < 32 weeks at birth) without BPD.

Intravenous hydration: monitor intake and output; avoid excessive hydration and aspiration.

• Consider use in severely immunodeficient patients (primary disorder such as severe combined immunodeficiency or severe HIV)

• RSV-IVIg is given at a dose of 750 mg/kg once per month beginning just before and monthly during the RSV season.

Nonpharmacologic treatment

Infant showing inability to feed, severe respiratory distress, and/or hypoxemia should be hospitalized (*see* Other information).

Supplemental oxygen for saturation < 92%; titrate inspired oxygen to achieve >95% saturation. *Note:* nasal cannula may not effectively deliver oxygen if nasal passage not patent or patient mouth breaths.

Bronchodilator trial: all hospitalized patients should receive a trial of an aerosolized β-2-agonist for potential relief of obstruction. Monitor oxygen saturation concurrently as hypoxemia may worsen in some patients. Improvement suggests continuation may be beneficial, and that airway hyperreactivity associated with asthma may be present.

• Careful monitoring of vital signs and clinical status as patient may worsen during inpatient stay; use both electronic instruments and direct visual contact; include oximetry, and confirm progression to respiratory failure with arterial blood gas.

• Hospitalized patients should be isolated and may be cohorted in the same room. Use gown, gloves, and careful hand washing.

• Additional control measures may be advisable beyond patient isolation measures. Consider laboratory screening for RSV infection in patients, cohorting medical staff, exclusion of infected staff from contact with high-risk patents, and limitations on visitation.

Treatment aims

To adequately monitor until resolution.
To maintain oxygenation.
To assess reversibility of airway obstruction (bronchodilator response).
To avoid complications of treatment.
To identify high-risk patients.

Prognosis

• Acute severe obstructive symptoms usually resolve in 3–5 days, but cough and fatigue may last up to 14 days. Complete recovery expected for most patients.

• Patients with recurrent episodes of wheeze (obstruction) often found to have reactive airway disease. • Chronic lung disease or other complications are rare in otherwise normal hosts.

Follow-up and management

• Most cases are uncomplicated and require no follow-up unless reactive airway disorder is uncovered, complications arise, or the patient has another disorder that causes increased risk for severe or fatal RSV infection.

Key reference

1. American Academy of Pediatrics: Respiratory syncytial virus. In *1977 Red Book: Report of the Committee on Infectious Diseases*, ed 24. Edited by Peter G. American Academy of Pediatrics: Elk Grove Village, IL; 1997:443–447.

General reference

Hall CB: Respiratory syncytial virus. In *Textbook of Pediatric Infectious Diseases*, ed 3. Edited by Feigin RD, Cherry JD. W.B. Saunders, Co.: Philadelphia; 1992:1633–1656.

Holberg CJ, Wright AL, Martinez FD, *et al.*: Risk factors for respiratory syncytial virus-associated lower respiratory illness in the first year of life. *Am J Epidemiol* 1991, **133:**1135–1151.

Shaw KN, Bell LM, Sherman NH: Outpatient assessment of infants with bronchiolitis. *Am J Dis Child* 1991, **145:**151–155.

Welliver JR, Welliver RC. Bronchiolitis. *Pediatr Rev* 1993, **14:**134–139.

Diagnosis

Symptoms
• Pain is the primary symptom of burn injury.

Signs
First-degree burns: present with redness, mild tenderness, and, occasionally, slight swelling of the involved skin.

Superficial second-degree (partial-thickness) burns: may have intact, thin-roofed bullae; red, moist, denuded areas that are tender; or both.

Deep partial-thickness burns: appear paler, drier, and more mottled than superficial second-degree burns; they are not always tender and may be difficult to distinguish from third-degree burns.

Third-degree burns: usually appear white or charred, dry or leathery, and are anesthetic.

• Surrounding areas of second-degree burn may be tender.

• Percentage of total body surface area (BSA) of burns (second- and third-degree only) are estimated using a chart. Proportions change with age, with younger children having a relatively larger head with smaller torso and legs [1]. The area of the palm (without digits) is approximately 1% BSA.

• Electrical burns may appear as small areas of first- or second-degree burn or, in severe injuries, a deep, depressed entry wound and blown-out exit wound.

Investigations
Minor burns (<10% BSA)
• Minor burns require no laboratory studies.

Larger and major burns (>10% BSA)
Complete blood count with differential: to insure that over time oxygen carrying capacity is maintained and infections are identified early.

Blood urea nitrogen and serum creatinine: measurements can be helpful in fluid management and to identify renal impairment.

Type and hold for possible blood transfusion.

Urinalysis: for myoglobinuria in third-degree and electrical burns.

Arterial blood gases: to monitor pulmonary function and acid base status.

Cooximetry: to identify and quantitate carbon monoxide poisoning.

Chest radiograph: if inhalation injury is suspected.

Measurement of central venous pressure: can guide fluid management in major burns.

Bladder catheterization with measurement of urine output: for fluid management.

Culture of burn: to identify potential pathogens and guide antimicrobial treatment should an infection develop.

Electrocardiogam: for serious electrical burns.

Complications
Burn shock (>20% BSA).

Inhalation injury: airway burn/obstruction; pulmonary injury; carbon monoxide poisoning, cyanide poisoning, or both.

Infection.

Scarring/contractures.

Etiology
• Thermal, electrical, or chemical energy damages the skin and underlying tissues.

• Temperature, duration of exposure, and thickness of skin determine the depth of a thermal injury.

• Large surface-area burns result in failure of the skin to preserve fluid, regulate temperature, and provide a barrier to infection.

• Mediators released from large burns cause systemic effects, including diffuse capillary leak, myocardial depression, and hypotension.

• Hair follicles and sweat glands in the deep dermis provide cells for reepithelialization and healing of burn wounds.

• Full-thickness and some deep partial-thickness burns require grafting.

Epidemiology
• Burns and smoke inhalation are the third leading cause of death in childhood.

• Scalds account for 80% of injuries. Reducing maximum tap water temperature to under 125°F reduces the risk of deep scald burns [2].

• House fires cause 75% of deaths. Cigarettes, children playing with matches, heaters, and faulty electrical systems in homes without smoke detectors are the most common causes of fatal house fires.

• Electrical burns in infants and toddlers most often result from extension cords in the mouth.

• Child abuse is the cause of 10%–20% of burns, particularly scalds.

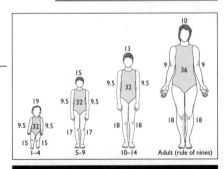

Burn assessment chart depicting changes in bodily proportions with age.

Treatment

Diet and lifestyle
• Not applicable.

Pharmacologic treatment

Major burns

• Estimated total fluid for first 24 hours (BSA >15%): 4 ml/kg/%BSA (add maintenance if < 5 years [3]) and 5000 ml/m^2/%BSA (add 2000 ml/m^2/day maintenance [4]).

• Give half of fluid in first 8 hours, half in next 16 hours in addition to constant maintenance rate.

• Use crystalloid (Ringer's lactate) in first 24 hours. Do not add potassium because potassium may be released from damaged tissues, and renal failure may develop.

• Follow urine output and peripheral perfusion. Revise fluid rate as needed.

• Administer analgesia:

Standard dosage   Morphine sulfate 0.1–0.2 mg/kg intravenously as needed for pain.

• Cardiovascular status should be stable before administering.

• Nothing by mouth if >15% BSA because ileus is common. Consider NG tube for larger burns.

Nonpharmacologic treatment

Major burns

• Stop burning by removing burned clothing and irrigating caustic exposures.

• Cover burns with clean or sterile sheet.

• Intubate early for stridor, signs of inhalation injury, or burn shock.

• Administer 100% oxygen if burned in a house fire or closed space, or if the child is in shock.

• Gain vascular access. For burns > 10% BSA, use peripheral intravenous catheter; > 40%, central venous catheter; > 65%, two central venous catheters. If possible, place catheters through intact skin.

Minor burns

• Wash with soap and water.

• Debride broken bullae by wiping with gauze. Intact bullae should be left unless they are in areas that will rapidly rupture (hands, flexion creases).

• Dress minor partial-thickness burns with antibiotic cream/ointment (silver sulfadiazine, bacitracin) and dress with layer of absorbant gauze.

Minor burns

Analgesia.

Tetanus prophylaxis.

Treatment aims

To keep child warm.
To maintain intravascular volume.
To minimize risk of infection.
To keep child as comfortable as possible.

Prognosis

• Burns of >30% BSA are life threatening; >50% are frequently fatal.
• Superficial second-degree burns heal with minimal scarring. Deep second-degree and third-degree burns usually result in scarring. Skin grafting usually improves the cosmetic result.

Follow-up

• Minor second-degree burns require once- or twice-daily dressing changes.
• Larger burns should be assessed for proper healing by a physician during the first week after injury.

Key references

1. Lund CC, Browder NC: The estimate of areas of burns. *Surg Gynecol Obstet* 1944, **79**:352.

2. Feldman KW, Schaller RT, Feldman J, et al>: Tap water scald burns in children. *Pediatrics* 1978, **62**:1–7.

3. O'Neill JA: Fluid resuscitation in the burned child: a reappraisal. *J Pediatr Surg* 1982, **17**:604–607.

4. Carvajal HF: Fluid resuscitation in pediatric burn victims: a critical appraisal. *Pediatr Nephrol* 1994, **8**:357–366.

5. Herndon DN, Thompson PB, Desai MH, Van Osten TJ: Treatment of burns in children. *Pediatr Clin North Am* 1985, **32**:1311–1332.

Cardiomyopathies

Diagnosis

Symptoms

Hypertrophic (a.k.a., HOCM, IHSS, ASH, familial CM)

• Patients may be asymptomatic, with or without history; may occur during childhood, but especially in teenagers, young adults.

Palpitations: premature ventricular contractions (PVCs), ventricular tachycardia (VT); **exercise-induced chest pain; dizziness, syncope:** especially with stress or activity; **dyspnea on exertion:** approximately 50% of patients.

Dilated

Congestive heart failure: exercise intolerance, dyspnea on exertion, altered growth, sweating; palpitations, chest pain.

• May occur in all age groups from infancy on. May get a history of preceding febrile illnesses, viruses, rashes.

Signs

Hypertrophic

Harsh systolic ejection murmur along the left sternal border: diminished with squatting, accentuated by Valsalva maneuver); **systolic murmur of mitral regurgitation (MR) at LV apex; gallop rhythm, ectopic beats on examination (PVCs); rales:** if significant pulmonary edema is present.

Dilated

Tachycardia: with or without Gallop rhythm; **tachypnea for age:** with or withour rales; **systolic murmur of mitral regurgitation (MR) at LV apex; hepatomegaly:** with late dependent edema.

Investigations

Electrocardiogram: *hypertrophic and dilated*: PVCs with normal QT interval, LV hypertrophy by voltage criteria, T-wave flattening or inversions diffusely.

Chest radiography: *hypertrophic*: normal in approx 50% of patients; *dilated*: cardiomegaly with left atrial and LV enlargement, pulmonary edema.

Echocardiography: *hypertrophic:* left atrial enlargement (LAE); MR; systolic anterior motion (SAM) of the mitral valve; asymmetrical, thick ventricular septum or other ventricular wall; abnormal LV diastolic performance. A resting LV outflow tract gradient may or may not be demonstrated by Doppler echocardiography; *dilated:* globular dilated left ventricle with poor systolic contractility, normal LV wall thickness, mitral annular dilation with MR and LAE. Look for valve disease or regional wall motion abnormalities.

Holter monitoring: *hypertrophic and dilated*: check for PVCs, VT, SVT or atrial fibrillation in dilated cardiomyopathy (embolic risk).

Nuclear imaging: may identify myocardial perfusion defects in HOCM.

Cardiac catheterization: *hypertrophic:* 1) to check degree of LV outflow obstruction at rest and provocative testing (*ie*, dobutamine); 2) to perform myocardial biopsy to confirm diagnosis; and 3) to assess LV outflow gradient with verapamil, beta-blockade and ventricular pacing; *dilated:* 1) to check ventricular end-diastolic pressure (worst prognosis >25 mmHg) and cardiac index, 2) to perform myocardial biopsy, and 3) to perform coronary arteriography to rule out congenital or acquired coronary disease (*ie*, anomalous coronary origin or aneurysms).

Complications

• Endocarditis may occur on the mitral valve in either hypertrophic or dilated cardiomyopathies.

Low cardiac output state, pulmonary venous hypertension.

Atrial and ventricular tachydysrhythmias, sudden cardiac death.

Thrombus formation causing stroke or systemic embolization in DCM.

Differential diagnosis

Hypertrophic

Murmur: fibrous subaortic stenosis or valvar aortic stenosis; LVH: secondary effects of systemic hypertension; PVCs or syncope: rule out prolonged QT syndrome.

Storage diseases with cardiac involvement: *ie*, infants of diabetic mothers.

Syndromes associated with HOCM: *ie*, Friederich's ataxia, Noonan's syndrome.

Dilated

Acquired inflammatory carditis (Kawasaki disease, rheumatic fever), anomalous origin of the left coronary artery from the pulmonary artery (ALCAPA).

Acquired LV dysfunction: toxin-mediated post-anthracycline therapy, hemochromatosis, or related to untreated tachyarrhythmias.

Etiology

Hypertrophic

• Inheritance is autosomal dominant. Genetically heterogeneous, at least 4 gene loci (chromosomes 1, 14, 15) cause mutations of the beta-myosin heavy chain contractile protein.

Pathology: asymmetric hypertrophy of the ventricular myocardium, without chamber dilation; microscopic hypertrophy of cardiac myocytes with abnormal intercellular connections; intramural coronary arteries thickened with narrowed lumens; the anterior mitral valve leaflet may abut the septum causing LV outflow obstruction in systole.

Pathophysiology: impaired filling, relaxation; hyperdynamic systolic function. LV outflow tract gradient +/- present.

Dilated

"Idiopathic" postviral (coxsackie B and A, echovirus) myocarditis, mitochondrial disorders, carnitine deficiency; HIV is becoming a more frequent cause of acquired cardiac dysfunction in children.

Epidemiology

Hypertrophic

• Male to female ratio is equal.

• Myocardial hypertrophy occurs during growth spurts. Follow-up negative study prior to completion of growth.

• Annual mortality (sudden death) is ~2.5% in adults, 6% in children and young adults.

Dilated

• In familial cases, there may be an X-linked recessive inheritance. In acquired cases, no clear cut genetic tendency.

Treatment

Diet and lifestyle

Hypertrophic

• Patients should avoid high-level competitive activities, which might stimulate ventricular dysrhythmias.

Dilated

• Avoid excessive salt and fluid intake, avoid high level activities. Infants may benefit from nasogastric feeding to avoid excessive cardiac work.

Pharmacologic treatment

For hypertrophic cardiomyopathy

• Administer beta -blockers to slow heart rate, enhance diastolic filling, decrease ventricular outflow gradients, and suppress PVCs.

Standard dosage	Propranolol, 1–6 mg/kg/d divided every 6 h.
	Nadolol, 20–80 mg/d divided every 12 h.
	Atenolol, 25–50 mg/d given every 12–24 h.
Contraindications	Atrioventricular conduction delay, significant reactive airway disease.

• Calcium channel blockers may enhance ventricular relaxation.

For dilated cardiomyopathy

• Administer digoxin to enhance cardiac contractility.

Standard dosage	Digoxin, load with 30–40 mu g/kg; total digitalizing dose (TDD), p.o. over 24 h divided every 6–8 h (maximum dose, 1 mg); Maintenance *digoxin* dose, 5 mu g/kg/dose given every 12 h.

• Diuretics are given to improve fluid homeostasis.

Standard dosage	Lasix, 1–4 mg/kg/d p.o or i.v. every 12 h.
Special points	Follow for hypokalemia.

• Afterload reducing agents can be used to lower systemic vascular resistance and enhance cardiac output.

Standard dosage	Captopril, 1–6 mg/kg/d divided every 6–8 h.
Side effects	Cough, renal impairment.
Special points	Follow for hyperkalemia, especially with potassium sparing diuretics.

• Antiarrhythmic agents: to suppress ventricular or atrial dysrhythmias.

• Anticoagulants (aspirin, dipyridamole, warfarin): due to the predisposition for spontaneous thrombus formation.

Nonpharmacologic treatment

Hypertrophic

Transvenous pacing: RV pacing may decreas outflow gradient by changing septal depolarization and LV outflow tract configuration.

Automatic implantable cardioverter-defibrillator pacemakers: for intractable VT with syncope.

Open heart surgery: ventricular myotomy–myectomy (Morrow procedure) to relieve LV outflow obstruction; mitral valve replacement may be required.

Dilated

Cardiac transplantation: an option if patient fails optimal medical management.

Treatment aims

Hypertrophic and dilated

To maintain adequate cardiac output and avoid sudden death.

To control potentially lethal ventricular dysrhythmia.

Hypertrophic

To maintain diastolic filling (preload) and avoid lowering systemic vascular resistance (afterload), which can exacerbate LV outflow gradient.

Dilated

To lower circulating volume (preload) and enhance output by lowering afterload.

To avoid intracardiac thrombus formation.

Prognosis

Hypertrophic: variable survival; highest risk of sudden death with positive family history, VT on Holter monitoring, and exercise in young adult years; risk not related to LV outflow gradient.

Dilated: after the age of 2 y, higher incidence of progressive heart failure leading to death; best prognosis for conditions with a treatable cause (ie, carnitine deficiency or inflammatory carditis); prognosis better if echocardiographic ventricular shortening fraction is ≥20% (normal ≥28%).

General references

Benson L: Dilated cardiomyopathies of childhood. *Prog Pediatr Cardiol* 1992, 1:13–36.

Maron B, Bonow R, Cannon R, et al.: Hypertrophic cardiomyopathy: interrelation of clinical manifestations, pathophysiology and therapy. *N Engl J Med* 1987, 316:780–789, 884–852.

Seiler C, et al.: Long term followup of medical versus surgical therapy for hypertrophic cardiomyopathy. *J Am Coll Cardiol* 1991, 17:634–642.

Tripp M: Metabolic cardiomyopathies. *Prog Pediatr Cardiol* 1992, 1:1–12.

Diagnosis

Symptoms

• Prior to cardiopulmonary arrest (CPA), symptoms related to underlying etiology predominate.

• Rarely is CPA a sudden event in children. There is usually progressive deterioration in cardiopulmonary function.

Signs

• Prior to CPA, signs due to underlying etiology will predominate and may include the following:

Tachypnea, dyspnea, bradypnea.

Tachycardia, bradycardia.

Grey, mottled coloring.

Stupor.

• Without intervention, patients may progress to:

Apnea.

Pulselessness/asystole.

Unresponsiveness.

Cyanosis.

Dilated, fixed pupils.

Later findings: dependent lividity, rigor mortis.

Initial investigation

• Laboratory investigations are rarely useful during a resuscitation because even rapidly run tests usually do not alter therapy.

• Whole blood glucose test is mandatory.

• Consider the following:

Arterial blood gases: assess hypoxemia, acidosis

Electrolytes, creatinine, BUN.

Hematocrit, whole blood count.

Blood and urine cultures.

Toxicology screen: if ingestion is suspected.

Liver enzymes: assess end organ damage.

Coagulation studies.

Chest radiograph.

Electrocardiogram: if primary cardiac event is suspected

Cervical spine films: in cases of suspected traumatic injury.

Complications

Failure to reanimate patient.

Pneumothorax: may be related to primary event, chest compressions, vascular access attempts, or high airway-pressure ventilation.

Cardiac arrhythmias: related to primary event, resuscitation medications, hypoxemia, direct cardiac injury.

Completion of cervical spine injury: lack of spine immobilization.

Nosocomial infections: nonsterile techniques

Aspiration pneumonitis.

End organ failure: brain, liver, kidney, intestine due to prolonged hypoxemia.

Rib fracture, chest-wall and pulmonary contusions: related to primary event or chest compressions.

Differential diagnosis

Cardiac lead disconnection.

• Ventricular fibrillation may be mistaken for asystole.

Etiology

Sudden infant death syndrome in 30%–50% of patients.

Drowning in 15%–20% of patients.

Trauma: most common cause after one year of age.

Airway obstruction: foreign body, croup, epiglottitis (rare).

Respiratory disease: asthma, pneumonia.

Smoke inhalation.

Ingestion.

Sepsis/meningitis.

Increased intracranial pressure.

Cardiac disease, arrhythmia.

Treatment

ABCs: airway, breathing, and circulation
• Every patient undergoes a rapid and sequential assessment of the ABCs.

Airway patency
• Insure airway patency, by using positioning, suction, adjunctive airways, removal of foreign body.

Breathing
• Use bag-valve mask ventilation (BVM), with cricoid pressure. Most children can be adequately ventilated with BVM.

Endotracheal intubation: suction, oxygen, equipment, medications, monitors.

Cricothyroidotomy: for a complete upper airway obstruction only, when unable to orotracheally intubate.

Circulation
• Chest compressions for patients in CPA or without a palpable pulse; should be one third to one half the depth of thoracic cage.

• Gain intravascular access. Use quickest, largest, most accessible site. Intraosseous access for ≤6 years: asystolic or severely compromised.

• Treat arrhythmias.

• Expand intravascular volume with 20 mL/kg normal saline.

Pharmacologic treatment
• All intravascular drugs can be given via intraosseous.

• Endotracheal drugs include: epinephrine, lidocaine, atropine, naloxone.

Oxygen; all patients should get 100% oxygen.

Common resuscitation medications

Epinephrine
• Use for asystole, profound bradycardia, pulseless ventricular tachycardia (VT), ventricular fibrillation (VF), hypotension due to myocardial dysfunction.

Standard dosage	Epinephrine, first dose ETT: 0.10 mg/kg of 1:1000.
	First dose i.v.: 0.01 mg/kg of 1:10,000 concentration.
	All subsequent doses: 0.1–0.2 mg/kg of 1:1000, 3–5 min apart.
Contraindication	Hypertension.
Main side effects	Tachycardia, arrhythmias.

Dextrose
• Use for documented or suspected hypoglycemia.

Standard dosage	Dextrose, 0.5–1 g/kg intravascular of D_{25} or D_{10}.
Contraindiations	Intraspinal or intracranial hemorrhage (use D_{10}).
Main side effects	Hyperglycemia, osmotic diuresis, vein sclerosis

Other important resuscitation drugs
Sodium bicarbonate: does not correct respiratory acidosis; use for prolonged CPA or severe metabolic acidosis.

Atropine: symptomatic or vagally mediated bradycardia.

Lidocaine: VT, VF, frequent PVCs.

Naloxone: suspected opiate overdose.

Adenosine: supraventricular tachycardia (SVT).

Antiobiotics: suspected infection.

Electricity

Synchronized cardioversion: hemodynamically unstable SVT, VT, atrial fibrillation/flutter; 1st dose: 0.5 J/kg; subsequent dose: 1 J/kg.

Defibrillation: pulseless VT/VF; 1st dose: 2 J/kg; subsequent doses: 4 J/kg.

Treatment aims
To identify and correct immediate life-threatening physiologic derangements.
To timely terminate adequate resuscitation efforts when unable to reanimate the patient.

Important information
Size of ETT = (age in years ÷ 4) + 4.
Premature newborn 2.5, 3.0.
Term newborn 3.0, 3.5.
• If child is ≥8 y, use cuffed tube.
Normal respiratory rates

Newborn	40–60 breaths/min.
Infant (<1 y)	20–30 breaths/min.
Child (1–8 y)	20 breaths/min.

Rates of chest compression

Newborn	120/min.
Infant (<1 y)	at least 100/min.
Child (1–8 y)	100/min.

Prognosis
• Prognosis for survival is dismal.
• The vast majority or patients who survive have severe neurologic disabilities.
• Patients that have a CPA in a hospital have a better chance of survival (17%–65%) than those who arrest outside the hospital (0%–23%).
• Children with isolated respiratory arrest have better chance of survival (40%–86%).

Follow-up and management
• Post-stabilization care must continue in a pediatric intensive care unit.

General references
Textbook of Pediatric Advanced Life Support. New York: AHA; 1994.

Goetting ME: Mastering pediatric cardiopulmonary resuscitation. *Pediatr Clin North Am* 1994, **41**:1147–1181.

Schlinder MB: Outcome of out-of-hospital cardiac or respiratory arrest in children. *New Engl J Med* 1996, **339**:1473–1479.

Zaritsky A: Pediatric resuscitation pharmacology. *Ann Emerg Med* 1993, **22**:179–189.

Celiac disease

Diagnosis

Symptoms

Classic presentation (1–3 years of age): diarrhea, anorexia, poor growth, abdominal distention, abdominal pain, muscle wasting, irritability [1].

Older children: abdominal pain, bloating short stature, delayed puberty, anemia, joint complaints, constipation, and lassitude.

Other associations: IgA deficiency, diabetes mellitus, chronic active hepatitis, cystic fibrosis, epilepsy, Down syndrome, dermatitis herpetiformis.

Failure to thrive, vomiting, or diarrhea: common in infants.

Other symptoms: behavioral problems, iron-deficiency anemia, edema, arthritis common in infants.

Signs

Failure to thrive: common even in asymptomatic infants and children.

Short stature, fine skin, clubbing, evidence of weight loss.

Pallor: anemia due to iron or folic acid deficiency.

Abdominal distention, muscle wasting.

Dental enamel hypoplasia: 10% to 20% untreated children.

Investigations

Initial

Plot growth curve: (*see* next page) normal growth in first few months of life; deviation from growth curve after introduction of gluten.

Full blood count, serum iron, ferritin, or folate, and erythrocyte folate measurement: to identify microcytic (iron deficiency) or macrocytic (folic acid deficiency) anemia or a dimorphic pattern of anemia due to both.

Serum calcium, albumen, and magnesium measurement: concentration possibly depressed.

Specific

Circulating antibody (antigliadin, antireticulin, antiendomysial) measurement: antiendomysial most specific [2].

Fecal fat estimation: 3-day fecal fat excretion: greater than 15% malabsorption in infants or greater than 8% in older children considered abnormal.

D-xylose test: serum test to evaluate proximal small bowel ability to absorb a simple monosaccharide.

Upper gastrointestinal endoscopy with biopsy of duodenum or proximal jejunum: reveals short (or absent) villi, intraepithelial lymphocytes, and crpyt hyperplasia.

Contrast radiography: small bowel follow-through to assess small intestine; poor sensitivity, luminal dilation, and altered mucosal folds often observed.

Complications

Anemia: due to iron or folic acid deficiency.

Osteomalacia, osteoporosis: due to hypocalcemia (tetany and seizures due to exacerbation by magnesium deficiency).

Short stature: secondary to inadequate nutrition.

Small-intestinal lymphoma: T-cell lymphoma complicating 5%–10% of cases; may be manifest as unexplained small-intestinal perforation [3].

Celiac crisis: severe diarrhea, dehydration, shock in rare patients.

Differential diagnosis

Diarrhea
Irritable bowel disease.
Infections (bacterial, parasites).
Inflammatory bowel disease.
Laxative abuse.
Lactose intolerance.
Drug-induced (antibiotics).
Pancreatic disorders.
Encopresis.
Nonspecific diarrhea of infancy.

Failure to thrive
Cow's milk allergy.
Cystic fibrosis.
Enteritis (postviral inflammatory bowel disease).
Schwachman syndrome (inherited pancreatic insufficiency).
Genetic disorders.
Inadequate dietary intake.
Heart disease.
Renal disease (renal tubular acidosis).
Child neglect syndrome.

Etiology

• In northern Europeans, 98% of cases of celiac disease are associated with the extended haplotype HLA B8, DR3, DQ2, although, in southern Europeans, HLA, DR5/7, DQ2 accounts for one third of cases.
• 10%–20% of first-degree relatives of probands are similarly affected.
• Family history often reveals a Celtic ancestry.

Epidemiology

• Accurate data relating to the incidence and prevalence of celiac sprue in the US are lacking (~1:5000 people).
• The prevalence of celiac disease in the UK is particularly high (1:1200 people, rising to 1:300 around Galway Bay in Ireland).
• Slightly more women than men suffer from celiac disease.
• The incidence of presentation has three peaks: infancy (9–36 mo), on introduction of foods containing gluten; third decade, frequently manifest with minor symptoms of fatigue; fifth decade, normally manifest with a specific nutritional deficiency (eg, iron, folic acid, or calcium).

Treatment

Diet and lifestyle

• A gluten-free diet is the mainstay of treatment and involves avoiding products containing wheat, rye, barley, or oats. Care should be taken to avoid any food contaminated by these cereals or their partial hydrolysates, including beer. Women of childbearing age who experience amenorrhea due to nutritional deficiencies will probably have a return of regular menstruation and may become pregnant. Men who have had long-standing disease may complain of impotence and infertility. These problems normally resolve within 2 years of starting a gluten-free diet.

• Specific nutritional deficiencies should be treated by replacement: iron, calcium, vitamin B_{12}, folic acid, or magnesium.

Pharmacologic treatment

• For most patients, a gluten-free diet is sufficient; extremely ill patients with celiac crisis can be given systemic steroids or parenteral hyperalimentation.

Standard dosage — Prednisone, 1–2 mg/kg daily (maximum 60 mg)

Contraindications — Caution in diabetes mellitus or during pregnancy.

Special Points — Care should be taken to avoid high-dose (prednisone >10 mg/d), long-term steroid treatment because of side effects).

Main drug interactions — Mild antagonism to thiazide diuretics.

Main side effects — Weight gain, fluid retention, osteoporosis, cushingoid facies, diabetes mellitus, changes in behavior.

Follow-up and management

• Outpatients must be reassessed 6–8 weeks and 3–4 months after starting a gluten-free diet, when repeat biopsy should be done.

• A second biopsy should be done 6 months to 1 year after starting treatment, when continued improvement in the structure of the small-intestinal mucosa should be expected.

• Annual hematological screening is rcommended to exclude development of specific nutritional deficiencies.

• When the diagnosis is doubtful, a gluten challenge, with 40 g gluten or 4 slices of normal bread daily for 2 weeks (adults) or 6 weeks (children), may be followed by a repeat jejunal biopsy [4].

• Antiendomysial antibody testing is useful for follow-up screening as the antibody approaches normal values when maintaining a gluten-free diet.

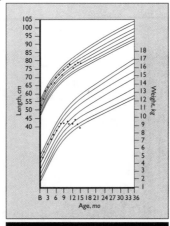

Growth curve of child with celiac disease

Treatment aims

To improve general well-being, small-intestinal mucosal structure, and assocated mutritional deficiencies. To reduce the risk of development of small intestinal lymphoma.

Prognosis

• With a gluten-free diet, general health is improved within a few weeks.
• Untreated patients are at a 5%–10% risk of developing a small intestinal T-cell lymphoma, the incidence of which probably falls if they maintain a strict diet
• Failure to improve suggests incorrect initial diagnosis, failure to adhere strictly to a gluten-free diet, or concurrent disorder (ie, malignancy).

Support groups

• Sprue Association, USA Inc., P.O. Box 31700, Omaha, NE 60131-0700.
• Gluten Intolerance Group of North America, P.O. Box 23053, Seattle, WA 98102-0353.

Key references

1. Walker-Smith JA: Celiac disease. In *Pediatric Gastrointestinal Disease.* Edited by Walker WA, Durie PR, Hamilton JR, Walker-Smith JA, Watkins JB. Philadelphia: BC Decker; 1996:840–861.

2. Chen KN, Endomysial antibody screening in children. *J Pediatr Gastroenterol Nutr* 1994, **14:**316–320.

3. Harris OD, Cooke WT, Thompson H, *et al.*: Malignancy in adult disease and idiopathic diarrhea. *Am J Med* 1967, **42:**889–912.

4. Catassi C, *et al.*: Dose dependent effects if protreated ingestion of small amounts of gliadin in coeliac disease in children: a clinical and jejunal morphometric study. *Gut* 1993, **34:**1515–1519.

Diagnosis

Definition and classification

• Cerebral palsy (CP) is a heterogeneous group of chronic, nonprogressive motor disorders of cerebral origin caused by early brain insult or abnormality.

• CP is classified according to 1) quality of motor abnormality (pyramidal [spastic], extrapyramidal [dystonic, choreoathetotic, hypotonic, ataxic], or mixed) and 2) distribution of symptoms (quadriparesis, hemiparesis, diparesis, monoparesis).

• The underlying cerebral abnormality is by definition nonprogressive, but symptoms typically develop during the first postnatal year.

Motor symptoms

Delay in acquisition of one or more motor skills.

Unusual postures and abnormalities of muscle tone.

Early strong hand preference: especially when CP is asymmetrical.

Comorbid symptoms: variable; include mental retardation, behavioral problems, epilepsy, visual impairment, hearing impairment, strabismus, feeding disorders.

Signs

General: lag in development of relevant postural reflexes.

Spastic CP: hypertonia, hyperreflexia, and evolution of characteristic postures (*eg*, exaggerated asymmetric tonic neck reflex or leg scissoring due to excessive adductor tone).

Upper extremity in spastic CP: shoulder adduction/internal rotation, elbow flexion, forearm pronation, wrist/finger flexion, thumb adduction.

Lower extremity in spastic CP: hip extension/external rotation, knee extension, foot plantar flexion, Babinski sign.

Dystonic CP: cocontraction of agonist and antagonist muscle groups with resultant rigidity and unusual postures.

Athetotic or choreoathetotic CP: intrusive movements (twisting, writhing, or fragmentary jerks); dysarthria.

Hypotonic CP: *See* Hypotonia.

Ataxic CP: dysmetria, dysdiadochokinesia, and truncal instability.

Investigations

• Investigation, including the following, is aimed at defining the underlying cause, excluding alternative diagnoses, and detecting comorbidity.

Neuroimaging (cranial CT, MRI): for tumor, hydrocephalus, developmental brain defect.

Titers of specific antibodies: for TORCH infections.

Electroencephalography: for seizures.

Ophthalmologic evaluation: to detect visual impairment and to diagnose congenital infection or anomalous development of eye structures.

Audiologic evaluation: to detect hearing impairment.

Metabolic studies (serum chemistries, blood lactate and pyruvate, urine and plasma amino and organic acids, lysosomal enzymes, and so on): for inborn errors of metabolism.

Karyotype: to detect underlying chromosomal abnormality.

CPK, electromyography, muscle biopsy: *see* Hypotonia.

Differential diagnosis

• Active underlying neurological disease must be excluded when the cause of the motor disability is inapparent. In some instances, this requires that the diagnosis of CP be tentative until sufficient time has elapsed to establish the nonprogressive nature of the disorder.

• Neurodegenerative and neurometabolic disease cause progressive symptoms.

• *See* Hypotonia for neuromuscular diseases such as congenital myopathies.

Spinal cord syndromes: relatively uncommon.

Tumor and hydrocephalus in infancy: typically cause progressive macrocephaly with sutural diastasis.

Orthopedic disease: congenital arthrogryposis or joint deformity, congenital hip dislocation.

Etiology

Hypoxic-ischemic encephalopathy.

Periventricular/intraventricular hemorrhage: frequent cause of CP, especially in premature infants.

Chromosomal disorders.

Cerebral dysgenesis (anomalous brain development evident on neuroimaging).

Stroke: usually idiopathic, but sometimes resulting from underlying heart disease, hemoglobinopathy, etc.

Acute, transient metabolic disturbance: severe hypoglycemia or hyperbilirubinemia.

Infection: either congenital or acquired.

• Many cases remain unexplained.

Epidemiology

• The prevalence of CP has increased over the past 15 y in most countries due to improved survival of premature infants.

Complications

Fixed contracture: in spastic or dystonic CP.

Pain: due to hip or other joint dislocation, pressure-induced ulceration, etc.

Scoliosis: in nonambulatory patients.

Depression and other psychological problems: adolescents are particularly susceptible to these symptoms, engendered by frustration and poor self-image.

Constipation: due to relative immobility, poor abdominal muscle tone, and impaired toileting skills.

Treatment

Pharmacologic treatment

• In general, pharmacologic treatment is reserved for palliation of severe spasticity or rigidity. A variety of drugs have been advocated, including baclofen, benzodiazepines, dantrolene, and other muscle relaxants. In most cases, however, long-lasting muscle relaxation can only be achieved at the expense of sedation or other side effects, and function is not improved. Intrathecal administration of baclofen is available in special centers and is claimed to improve function in some cases. In carefully selected cases, injection of botulinum toxin into specific muscle groups may improve function.

Nonpharmacologic treatment

Physical measures

• Physical and occupational therapy are the mainstay of CP management. However, complex, expensive regimens that impose a significant family burden should be avoided, as controlled trials documenting efficacy are lacking.

• Therapy involves range of motion and muscle-stretching exercises to prevent contracture and reduce resting muscle tone; encouragement of postural reflexes; positioning and seating to improve feeding, optimize function, and prevent complications such as pressure ulcers, scoliosis, and respiratory and gastrointestinal problems; bracing in certain situations (eg, ankle–foot orthoses in spastic CP involving the lower extremities) to help prevent contractures and improve function.

Orthopedic and neurosurgical treatment

• Tendon lengthening, tendon transfer, or tenotomy can improve function and may play an important palliative role where function is severely limited; for example, diapering and perineal care of children with severe spastic CP may be facilitated by adductor tenotomy, and fixation may prevent or eliminate hip pain due to dislocation.

• Selective posterior rhizotomy is claimed to improve function in highly motivated patients with significant gait impairment due to diplegia, but results are inconsistent.

Treatment of comorbidity

• Recognition and management of comorbid conditions may greatly improve function, and may be more important than the treatment of CP proper.

• Treatment should be considered for a number of conditions (listed below).

Epilepsy: antiepileptic drugs, ketogenic diet, surgery (focal resection, corpus callosotomy).

Feeding disorders: gradual introduction of more challenging foods; in some cases, permanent gastrostomy is indicated.

Gastroesophageal reflux: positioning, thickened feedings, antacids, agents to increase motility, fundoplication.

Constipation: dietary measures, fluids, laxatives.

Behavioral disorders: program of behavior management, appropriate psychopharmacologic agents (eg, stimulant therapy for attention deficit/hyperactivity disorder).

Visual impairment: special education or training.

Strabismus: patching or surgery.

Hearing impairment: amplification, specialized education.

Depression: support, antidepressant medication.

Treatment aims

To preserve and maximize function and independence.
To minimize the impact of comorbidity.
To minimize discomfort.
To discourage ineffective and unnecessarily burdensome treatments and minimize parental guilt.

Prognosis

• Although the motor abnormalities of CP are permanent, the functional consequences are determined by subtype, cause, nature and extent of comorbidity, and management.

• In general, patients with hemiparetic CP are ambulatory and have average or near-average intelligence. Individuals with spastic quadriparesis usually are more significantly disabled motorically and have more extensive comorbidity, but the range is broad.

Follow-up and management

• Periodic follow-up is indicated to verify diagnosis, prevent complications, monitor management, and assess and minimize comorbidity.

• When the diagnosis is firm, comorbidity minimal, and family support good, frequent specialty evaluation is unnecessary.

General references

Pellegrino L: Cerebral palsy: a paradigm for developmental disabilities. Dev Med Child Neurol 1995, 37:834–839.

Taft LT: Cerebral palsy. Pediatr Rev 1995, 16:411–418.

Diagnosis

Symptoms

Localized symptoms

Tender swelling of single or regional group of cervical lymph nodes: often associated with symptoms of earache, sore throat, rhinorrhea, or toothache.

Systemic symptoms

Fever, malaise, anorexia, lethargy: in cases of adenitis associated with cellulitis, suppuration, bacteremia, or viremia.

Signs

Unilateral or bilateral swelling of one or more of the cervical lymph glands.

Overlying erythema and warmth: may indicate accompanying cellulitis.

Fluctuance with suppurative adenitis or abscess formation.

Impetigo of the face/scalp or acute otitis media.

Granulomas or ulcer of the conjunctivae: cat scratch disease.

Torticollis: associated with tender or very large glands.

Drainage: occasionally accompanies mycobacterium infections.

Investigations

• Physical examination with special concentration on upper respiratory tract, overlying skin, scalp, and dentition.

• History of travel, animal/insect exposure, trauma, tuberculosis risk factors and constitutional symptoms.

Acute localized adenopathy

Throat culture.

• If initial presentation includes moderate fever, fluctuant node, or if initial empiric antibiotic treatment has not reduced symptoms within 48–72 hours:

CBC, ESR, blood culture, needle aspiration for gram stain and culture.

• Any infant less than 1 month of age should have a full work-up for sepsis.

Subacute/chronic localized adenopathy

• Investigations to distinguishing infectious from noninfectious/ oncologic etiologies.

CBC, ESR, PPD placement, IFA or PCR assay for *Bartonella henselae*, HIV test, toxoplasmosis titers, chest radiography; ultrasound or CT scan, and excisional or partial biopsy.

Acute/subacute generalized adenopathy

• Evaluation of possible systemic infections with CBC, ESR, liver function test, chest radiography, PPD placement, HIV test, RPR, serologic tests for EBV and CMV.

Complications

Cellulitis, bacteremia, or metastatic foci of infection.

Very rarely: mediastinal abscess, purulent pericarditis, thrombosis of the internal jugular, poststreptococcal acute glomerulonephritis

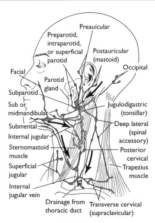

Preauicular
Preparotid, intraparotid, or superficial parotid
Postauricular (mastoid)
Facial
Occipital
Parotid gland
Subparotid
Sub or midmandibular
Jugulodigastric (tonsillar)
Submental
Deep lateral (spinal accessory)
Internal jugular
Sternomastoid muscle
Posterior cervical
Superficial jugular
Trapezius muscle
Internal jugular vein
Drainage from thoracic duct
Transverse cervical (supraclavicular)

Lymphatic flow of the head and neck.

Differential diagnosis

Neoplasms: painless, firm, noninflamed posterior cervical or supraclavicular masses.
Congenital: cystic hygroma, thyroglossal duct cyst, branchial cleft cysts, lymphangiomas, hemangiomas.
Sternocleidomastoid hematomas or fibromas.
Parotitis.
Kawasaki syndrome.
Sarcoidosis.
Chronic granulomatous disease.
Histiocytic necrotizing lymphadenitis.
Phenytoin-induced adenopathy.

Etiology

Acute localized adenitis

Viral: adenovirus, herpes simplex virus, enteroviruses, human herpesvirus 6, rubella, mumps.
Bacterial: *Staphylococcus aureus*, *Streptococcus pyogenes*, group B *Streptococcus* sp, anaerobes, *Mycoplasma pneumoniae*, *Francisella tularensis*, *Yersinia pestis*.
Protozoal: toxoplasmosis.

Subacute/chronic localized adenitis

Mycobacteria (atypical and tuberculosis), *Bartonella henselae* (causes cat scratch disease), toxoplasmosis

Generalized adenitis

Viral: Epstein–Barr virus, HIV, measles, varicella, adenovirus, cytomegalovirus.
Bacterial: syphilis, tuberculosis, brucellosis.
Fungal/protozoal: histoplasmosis, toxoplasmosis.

Epidemiology

• Adenitis is a very common diagnosis in children. The etiologic agents of adenitis vary with age:
Neonates and young infants: Group B *Streptococcus* sp. or *Staphylococcus aureus*.
Infants and young children: *Staphylococcus aureus*.
Preschoolers (1–4 y): adenitis due to *Streptococcus pyogenes*, *Staphylococcus aureus*, atypical mycobacterium, or *Bartonella henselae*.
Older children (5–15 y): anaerobic bacterial infections, *Mycobacterium tuberculosis*, as well as the agents responsible for infections in preschool aged children.

Treatment

Diet and lifestyle

• Promoting good dental hygiene and limiting kitten exposure could prevent some cases of adenitis.

Pharmacologic treatment

• Treatment is directed toward the etiologic agent. Acute viral adenopathy and isolated adenopathy due to *Bartonella henselae* are managed conservatively with spontaneous resolution expected. Pharmacologic treatment of acute bacterial adenitis is outlined below. Incision and drainage is indicated if abscess formation is identified at initial examination or develops after antibiotic therapy has begun. Fluctuant collections suspected to be from mycobacterium or cat scratch disease should be treated with aspiration (rather than incision) to avoid fistula formation. Analgesics and antipyretics may be used in any form of adenitis for comfort.

For acute bacterial adenitis

• Parenteral antibiotic therapy should be instituted in any child under 1 month of age or any age child with moderate to severe systemic symptoms of infection.

Staphylococcal or streptococcal infections

Standard dosage	Oxacillin 150 mg/kg/d i.v. in divided doses every 6 h.

Anaerobic infections

Standard dosage	Penicillin G 100,000–250,000 U/kg/d i.v. divided every 4 h, or
	Clindamycin 25–40 mg/kg/d i.v. in 4 divided doses.

• Oral antibiotic therapy may be instituted for children without systemic signs or symptoms of illness.

Staphylococcal or streptococcal infections

Standard dosage	Cephalexin 50–100 mg/kg/d p.o. in 4 divided doses.

Group A β-hemolytic *Streptococcus* sp infections

Standard dosage	Penicillin VK 15–40 mg/kg/d p.o. in 4 divided doses, or
	Erythromycin 30–50 mg/kg/d p.o. in divided doses.

Anaerobic infections associated with dental or periodontal source

Standard dosage	Penicillin VK 15–40 mg/kg/d p.o. in 4 divided doses, or
	Clindamycin 15–25 mg/kg/d p.o in 4 divided doses.

Contraindications

Penicillins and cephalosporins: should be avoided in any patient with a history of hypersensitivity reaction.

Clindamycin: contraindicated in any patient with a history of pseudomembranous colitis or clindamycin hypersensitivity.

Other treatment options

• The treatment of chronic, localized, or generalized adenopathy is dependent on the causative agent and may include antibiotics, antivirals, antifungals, surgical excision (especially for atypical mycobacterial infections), and/or chemotherapeutic agents.

Treatment aims

To treat and prevent further spread of underlying infectious agents.

Prognosis

• Prognosis is dependent on the etiologic cause of the lymphadenitis. However, most cases of acute bacterial adenitis have resolution of fever, erythema, and systemic symptoms within the first 72 h of appropriate therapy.

• Complete resolution of lymph node swelling may take up to 4–6 wk.

• Suppuration and drainage of the lymph node may occur despite appropriate therapy.

• Lymphadenopathy associated with cat scratch disease usually resolves spontaneously within 2–6 mo.

Follow-up and management

• Follow-up is individualized by etiologic agent. Acute infections should be assessed after 48–72 h of therapy for initial response and then again in 2–4 wk for resolution of lymphadenopathy.

Key references

1. Burton, DM: Practical aspects of managing non-malignant lump of the neck. *J Otolaryngol* 1992, **21**:398–403.

2. Chesney, PJ: Cervical lymphadenitis and neck infections. In *Principles and Practice of Pediatric Infectious Diseases*. Edited by Long SL, Pickering LK, Prober CG. New York: Churchill Livingstone; 1997:186–197.

3. Marcy, SM: Infections of lymph nodes of the head and neck. *Ped Inf Dis J* 1983, **2**:397–405.

4. Midani S: Cat-scratch disease. *Adv Pediatr* 1996, **43**:397–422.

Diagnosis

• Child abuse is pervasive in society and may present with many different signs and symptoms depending on the specific injury to the child or adolescent. A unifying definition is that abuse is a symptom of family dysfunction in which there is a physical, sexual, emotional, or developmental injury to the child caused by acts of commission or omission on the part of the parents.

Signs and symptoms

• The most common injuries occur to the soft tissues in the form of bruises, abrasions, lacerations, and burns.

• The most severe injury with the most long-lasting effects is the psychological injury and the tendency for abuse to cycle into the next generation.

• Even if old enough and developmentally capable, the child may not reveal the cause of the injuries.

Any infant who is bruised should be evaluated for abuse.

Any child <2 years of age who is burned should be carefully evaluated.

Multiple bruises in varying stages of healing and bruises in unusual places: *eg*, trunk, buttocks, inner thighs.

Patterns of injury: *eg*, slap marks, strangulation marks, ligatures around wrists and ankles.

Other common injuries include fractures, head injury, abdominal injury, and injury to the sensory organs, mouth, eyes, and ears.

Starvation, poisoning, underwater submersion, homicide: less common.

Investigations

• It is important to collect data in four areas: history of injury, physical findings, laboratory/radiographic findings, and observation of the parents;

add these data bits together to determine if there is a suspicion of abuse.

• Check to see if the injury matches the history and the developmental capabilities of the child.

• Look for parental interaction that shows lack of concern for the child, lack of knowledge about the injury, or a changing history of injury.

• Any child who has a suspicious fracture should have a complete skeletal survey for trauma to rule out other fractures.

• Other laboratory tests are guided by the injury, *eg*, multiple bruises may require coagulation studies to rule out a bleeding problem; a CT of the head for suspected intracranial injury.

• Observe the parents' interaction with the child and their interaction with you.

• If possible check old records to note pattern of injuries.

• Social work or child protective services consultation should be requested for further family assessment.

Complications

• Failure to diagnose and report abuse may lead to more serious injury to the child or even to death.

• If injuries are misdiagnosed, they may go unrecognized and untreated.

Differential diagnosis [2]

Accidental or noninflicted injury.

Rare medical conditions, eg, hemophilia, osteogenesis imperfecta, or Ehlers-Danlos syndrome.

• There is a differential diagnosis list associated with each form of injury.

• The differential diagnosis list must be considered carefully because the diagnosis of suspected abuse may have social and legal ramifications. State laws require the reporting of only the suspicion of abuse, not a proven case; however, the condition continues to be under-reported by most physicians.

Etiology [1]

• Causes of abuse are many: family stress, isolation, societal violence, inadequate preparation for parenting, widespread use of corporal punishment, and substance abuse by the parents.

• Abuse is common enough that it effects all strata of society, all economic groups, and all subsets of the population.

Epidemiology

• There are about 3 million cases of abuse reported each year in the U.S.

• There are over 1000 deaths per year in the U.S.

• The incidence of physical abuse is about 23:1000 population.

• Almost every type of medical specialist has the potential to encounter abuse.

• Of all the reported cases of suspected abuse, only 50% are verified.

• There are indistinct lines separating corporal punishment from child abuse.

Other information

• Most locales have regional child abuse referral centers. If you encounter difficulties in case identification or management, consult you local center.

Treatment [4]

General information

• The cornerstone of treating abuse is suspecting it and reporting it to the local child protective service agency. In some jurisdictions, the initial report may also go to the police department.

• Each physician should be aware of the prevailing local law and reporting procedures.

• The other roles of the physician are to treat the injuries to aid in making a scientific diagnosis if possible.

• Once the child has been diagnosed and reported and the specific injures attended to, then the physician must determine if the child will be adequately protected from further injury. If the home is deemed unsafe and the child welfare system is unable to provide emergency placement, then the child should be protected by an acute care hospitalization even if the injuries do not normally warrant hospitalization.

The physician should approach the parents in a nonaccusatory way and should stress their concern for the child and the need to determine the extent of injury and the possibility of recurrence.

• Confrontation with the parents will be counterproductive and will place the child at further risk.

• The use of a multidisciplinary team is most helpful. This may be a well-organized regularly functioning team within the hospital or an ad hoc group of physicians, nurses, and social workers gathered around a single case.

• In any setting, whether the hospital emergency department or in a primary physician's office, it is good to have a prepared protocol to follow when suspected abuse is encountered. This will guide the physician in taking the appropriate steps during a period of high interpersonal stress while working with the abusive family.

• Remember that most parents do not wish to or intend to abuse their child. Abuse often happens at a moment of frustration and stress. There is a small but dangerous subgroup of parents who repeatedly inflict trauma on their child and have the potential to cause severe injure or death. Initially, it may be impossible to tell these two types of parents apart, thus the first goal of treatment is to always protect the child.

• One subset of abused children are those suffering the Munchausen syndrome by proxy (MSBP) [5]. These are children whose parents exaggerate illness or actually produce signs and symptoms of illness in order to gain admission to the hospital. This form of abuse is difficult to diagnose as it takes many different forms and is usually performed by an intelligent and medically sophisticated parent. MSBP has its own special keys to diagnosis and therapy.

• Long-term therapy for the child and family may involve psychotherapy, developmental stimulation programs, therapeutic nursery school, or other forms of individual, group, or family therapy.

Treatment aims

To recognize abuse and report it.
To reat injuries.
To protect the child.
To preserve families when possible.
To effectively prosecute when family cannot be rehabilitated.

Prognosis

• Overall prognosis is good if family services are available.

• Where services do not exist, there are higher rates of foster care placement and higher rates of reinjury.

Follow-up and management

• Children who have been abused need to be closely followed for repeat injury and for psychological and developmental manifestations of their abuse.

• Siblings of abused children also need to be followed closely.

Key references

1. Ludwig S, Kornberg AM, eds.: *Child Abuse: A Medical Reference*, edn 2. New York: Churchill Livingstone; 1992.
2. Giardino AP, Christian CW, Giardino ER: *A Practical Guide to the Evaluation of Child Physical Abuse and Neglect.* Thousand Oaks: Sage Publications; 1997.
3. Wissow LS: Child abuse and neglect. *N Engl J Med* 1995, **21:**1425–1431.
4. Reece RM, ed. *Child Abuse: Medical Diagnosis and Management.* Philadephia: Lea & Febinger; 1994.
5. Levin A, Sheridan M: *Munchausen Syndrome by Proxy.* New York: Lexington Press; 1995.

Diagnosis [1]

Definition

• Child sexual abuse is a complex and potentially damaging problem for children of all ages. The term *sexual misuse* may better apply because abuse has a connotation of direct physical injury and force that are not the dynamics of the misuse of a child for the sexual gratification of an adult. In child sexual abuse, the offender uses his relationship to control the child and gain what he wants. Perpetrators can be very clever in their manipulative techniques and very determined to meet their sexual gratification needs.

Symptoms

• The symptoms of child sexual abuse may be very varied and dependent on what the perpetrator did to the child. Often there are no physical complaints or, at most, transient complaints until injured tissue heals. Children often tell about their sexual abuse at a time distant from when it occurred.

• Symptoms may be acute or chronic. They may relate to specific physical findings or be psychological representations of what occurred, *eg*, vaginal pain in the absence of an abnormal examination. Sexual abuse should be considered as one element in the differential diagnosis list of common complaints such as enuresis, encopresis, and constipation. Symptoms may relate to sexually transmitted diseases acquired during the abusive encounter.

• Most often the diagnosis is based on the child giving a history of contact with an adult or a person significantly older than they are and in a position of control. The more detailed and specific the history, the more credible the story. The history must be evaluated in light of the child's age, their developmental abilities, and the method they use to disclose their history.

Signs

Vaginal or anal bruising or bleeding: occurs in the minority of cases [2].

Careful vaginal examination using a colposcope may show signs of old, healed injury that has left a pattern of scarring.

Vaginal discharge, erythema, rash, ulcerative lesions, or other findings specific to sexually transmitted diseases (STDs).

Pregnancy: may be the result of sexual abuse.

• The child may also show signs of psychological distress and exhibit new fears, phobias, sleep disorders, distrust or desire to avoid certain people or situations.

• Adolescents may express their sexual abuse encounters with a variety of symptoms and signs, including substance abuse, running away, promiscuous behavior, suicide attempts, or depression.

• When physical abuse is present in the genital area, one must consider attempted sexual abuse.

Investigations

• If the child has been abused within 72 hours or if there is any evidence of bleeding, the child must be referred to a local emergency department so that investigations and forensic specimens are obtained. Otherwise, careful history taking and physical examination are the central forms of investigation.

Complications

• These will vary with the nature and extent of the abuse; they include acute hemorrhage and destruction of normal anatomical structures due to the effects of any of the STDs.

• The greatest concern is that of long-term psychological impairment.

• Some have called sexual abuse a "psychological time bomb" that can produce anything from acute findings of posttraumatic stress syndrome to chronic complaints and somatization that becomes manifest in adult life.

Differential diagnosis

• Many of the complaints that a sexually abused child may have are consistent with long differential diagnosis lists.

• There may be instances in which children fabricate their stories of abuse, but these are very rare.

• Some parents (often those who have been abuse victims themselves) may over-interpret their child's signs and symptoms.

• Caution must be taken when evaluating a child whose parents are in the midst of a custody suit wherein one parent alleges that the other sexually abused the child; this is a very difficult and entangled situation.

Etiology

• The cause of child sexual abuse rests with the pathology of the perpetrator. Pedophiles are generally of two types: those who fail to advance to adult sexuality and remained fixed in being attracted to youth, and those who do achieve adult status but then undergo regression.

• The widespread availability of explicit sexual portrayals in the mass media and the abundance of child pornography may add to the problem.

Epidemiology

• The rates of child sexual abuse have increased dramatically over the past 15 y.

• Our children are the first generation of youth who have been able to describe their abuse and have someone believe them.

• Currently the rates of child sexual abuse match those of physical abuse reports in some states.

• On a national scale, sexual abuse accounts for 12%–13% of all abuse but its rate of rise has been the steepest over the three national incidence studies.

• Both boys and girls are abused, although girls report abuse more often. Estimates are that 1:4 girls has had some type of abusive encounter and 1:10 boys.

Other information

• Many regions have child sexual abuse evaluation centers that accept referrals if you are considering this diagnosis and lack the expertise to manage all the details.

Treatment [3,4]

General treatment

• As with physical abuse, the first step in the treatment process is the identification of the possibility of child sexual abuse and reporting it to the proper authorities.

• In most states, child sexual abuse is reported to law enforcement officials. If the abuse occurred at the hands of a parent or a person acting in the role of a parent it is also reported to the child protective service agency.

• The physician must have the time, skill, and motivation to getting a detailed history from the child and recording it in a factual, nonjudgmental way

• It is important to do a complete physical examination with careful attention to the areas of the body involved in the abusive act.

• If there are signs or symptoms referable to an STD(s), obtain cultures and other relevant specimens. Treat STDs according to existing guidelines for pharmacologic therapy.

• The physician must all take steps to reassure the child and the parents that the sexual encounter does not necessarily result in any ongoing problems, determination of sexual preference, or tendency toward repeated behaviors provided a healthy secure environment can be provided for the child in the context of an accepting, supportive family.

• Some children will evidence immediate psychological dysfunction and may require psychiatric referral for depression or posttraumatic stress disorder.

Treatment aims

To recognize and report the abuse.

To carefully document findings, as your evaluation will possibly be used in court.

To treat the child for injury and/or infection.

To reassure the family.

To refer the child to mental health services if needed.

Prognosis

• Prognosis will depend on the nature and extent of the abuse, whether it is intra- or extrafamilial, and the strength and supportiveness of the surrounding family.

• Most children do well in the short term, but some have reemergence of symptoms later in life.

Follow-up and management

• Follow the children and families closely. They will require a great deal of support.

• Your efforts in court may also be required in order to convict a child sexual abuse offender. Often the offenders are involved with many children before they are apprehended and convicted.

Key references

1. Ludwig S: Child abuse. In *Textbook of Pediatric Emergency Medicine*, ed 3. Edited by Fleisher G, Ludwig S. Baltimore: Williams & Wilkins; 1993: 1429–1463.

2. Heger AH, Emans SJ: *Evaluation of the Sexually Abused Child: a Medical Textbook and Photographic Atlas*. New York: Oxford University Press; 1992.

3. Green AH: Child sexual abuse: immediate and long term effects and intervention. *J Am Acad Child Adolesc Psychiatry* 1993, **32**:890–902.

4. Sgroi SM: *Handbook of Clinical Intervention in Child Sexual Abuse*. Lexington, MA: Lexington Books; 1982.

Colic and crying

Diagnosis

Definition
Colic is defined as a period of sustained crying on the part of an infant. This condition is exasperating to parents and often stressful to the physician trying to guide the young parent.

Symptoms
• The primary symptom of colic is crying for no apparent reason. The normal 1-month-old infant may cry for a mean of 2 hours a day. Crying that exceeds this amount is defined as colic.

• Characteristically the crying occurs at a regular time each day, often at the dinner hour. The child cannot seem to be soothed or comforted over a sustained period. Some maneuvers of rocking and walking with the baby will calm him temporarily.

• The age range for colic is 4–8 weeks; this time period is altered by prematurity and occurs at 4–8 weeks from the estimated day of full-term delivery.

Signs
• The baby is often noted to turn red in the face, to draw up his legs, and to pass excessive amounts of flatus. These symptoms initiate the logical concern that there is something wrong with the child's gastrointestinal system. All of these signs may in fact be epiphenomenon that result from the excessive crying rather than the cause of it.

• On the physical examination, no abnormal finding are demonstrable. The child has usually gained weight appropriately (ie, 0.5–1 oz per day after an initial period of weight loss after birth). Often the baby has had excessive weight gain as parents very naturally respond to the crying by giving more feedings and, in fact, over-feeding.

• It is important to go through the list of possible differential diagnoses as colic is a diagnosis of exclusion once the child's examination is deemed normal and the other causes ruled out.

Investigations
• No investigations need to be performed other than a complete history, physical examination, and assessment of the child's growth since delivery.

• Colic should not be diagnosed over the telephone as there are several important mimics of colic that need to be ruled out.

Complications
• The only complications of colic are iatrogenic and come from unnecessary changes in the formula and stigmatization of a normal baby as being in some way abnormal or defective. These early impressions of the baby may take on a life of their own and be felt for years to come.

Differential diagnosis
The following conditions should be considered in making the diagnosis of colic:
Central nervous system infection.
Otitis media or otitis externa.
Corneal abrasion.
Acute glaucoma.
Thrush.
Hyperthyroidism.
Fractures.
Torsion testis.
Incarcerated hernia.
Bowel obstruction.
Urinary tract infection.
Hair tourniquet.
Diaper rash.
Rectal fissure.
Medications or immunization.
Maternal diet if child is breast-fed.
Virtually all of these diagnoses can be ruled out on the physical examination.

Etiology
• The cause of colic remains illusive. Many theories have been considered, including gastrointestinal illness, allergy, milk intolerance, and others.
• Colic may be a reflection of the changing neurodevelopmental status of the child. It is a state of overarrousal that renders the baby unable to get the sleep it needs.

Epidemiology
• Almost all babies have at least a few periods of colic in their early weeks of life. For some infants (15%–30%), the symptoms are more severe and thus will be brought for medical attention. The severity may relate to their underlying temperament and to the ability of the parents to cope with their state of arousal.

Other information
• If parents can be forewarned about colic through anticipatory guidance, they often can stave off the severe form of the condition.

Treatment

General Treatment

• The main forms of treatment are behavioral suggestions aimed at the parents.

• First, the parents need to be reassured by the pattern of normal growth and the normal physical examination. A review of the differential diagnoses that have been ruled out is also reassuring.

• For breast-feeding mothers, eliminate sources of caffeine and cow's milk from the mother's diet, particularly if you find excessive amounts of intake of coffee, cola, or chocolate. Some mothers will note that certain spices seem to cross into breast milk and make their baby more uncomfortable. These too should be eliminated.

• Next, encourage the parents to avoid over-feeding and over-stimulation. When the baby cries for no apparent reason, it is likely due to a need for sleep. After checking to be sure all their physical needs are met, it is important to place the baby in a safe environment and allow them to cry until they fall asleep. Baby will often wake up refreshed and happy. Keep the baby on an approximately every 2- to 3-hour feeding schedule. Crying 1 hour after feeding is not the cry of hunger.

• Parents may need to be refocused on supporting one another through this process, as fatigue and uncertainty may have them working at cross purposes.

• There is no place for pharmacological therapy in the treatment of colic. There is also no place for frequent formula changes, although these often have a temporary placebo effect.

• In very rare circumstances, a child may need to be hospitalized for colic if the parents have become overstressed and dysfunctional. Often relatives can assume the same role in giving parents some respite.

Treatment aims

To gain parental understanding.
To decrease overfeeding.
To decrease over stimulating.
To break the cycle of crying.

Prognosis

The prognosis is excellent in all cases.

Follow-up and management

During the period of most active colic, the family needs to have close and regular contact with their physician. Telephone contact is often sufficient. Families will often need support in allowing the baby to cry until he or she falls asleep.

Key references

Adams LM, Davidson M: Present concepts of infant colic. Pediatr Ann 1987, 16:817–820.

Carey WB: Colic. In Developmental and Behavioral Pediatrics, ed 2. Edited by Levine MD, Carey WB, Crocker AC. Philadelphia: W.B. Saunders; 1992: 350–353.

Henretig F: Crying and colic. In Textbook of Pediatric Emergency Medicine, ed 3. Edited by Fleisher GR, Ludwig S. Baltimore: Williams & Wilkins; 1993: 1527–1534.

Taubman B: Parental counseling compared with elimination of cow's milk or soy milk protein for treatment of infant colic syndrome. Pediatrics 1988, 81:756–761.

Diagnosis

Definition

• Congestive heart failure (CHF) is defined as the inability of the heart to meet the metabolic needs of the body.

Symptoms

Infants: poor feeding, irritability, listlessness.

Children and adolescents: dyspnea, shortness of breath, exercise intolerance or easy fatigability, loss of appetite.

Signs

Infants

Tachypnea, retractions, rales, tachycardia, hypotension with pallor, diaphoresis, poor perfusion with cool extremities, hepatomegaly, fever in severe congestive heart failure; cyanosis in association with alveolar edema; cough; vomiting.

Children and adolescents

Tachypnea, use of accessory muscles for breathing, orthopnea, rales, cough, tachycardia, jugular venous distention, hepatomegaly, edema (uncommon in children), hypotension, poor perfusion with cool extremities and weak peripheral pulses, pallor, diaphoresis.

• Cardiac examination may show right ventricular or LV heave, displaced point of maximal impulse, and cardiac murmurs dependent on the underlying lesion; a gallop rhythm (S3 or S4) is often audible.

Investigations

ECG: sinus tachycardia, atrial or ventricular hypertrophy depending on underlying cause of CHF, ST-T wave elevation, depression or inversion.

Echocardiography: findings depend on underlying cause for structural abnormalities. Functionally, the atria and/or ventricles are enlarged with increased LV end-diastolic dimensions and decreased shortening fraction.

Chest radiography: generally, cardiac enlargement is noted along with pulmonary venous congestion. Specifics depend on underlying lesion (*see* Figure).

Cardiac catheterization: in specific cases of suspected congenital heart disease, to define the specific structural details of the congenital heart lesion and determine the hemodynamic impairment. In cases of dilated cardiomyopathy, to rule out coronary artery anomalies, to obtain hemodynamic information, specifically regarding pulmonary vascular resistance if cardiac transplantation is being considered and to obtain endomyocardial biopsy, especially if myocarditis is suspected, to clarify cause and help determine prognosis.

24-Hour ambulatory monitoring: to determine possible arrhythmia as cause of cardiac dysfunction, as in chronic automatic atrial tachycardia or to identify associated ventricular arrhythmias.

Laboratory blood tests

Arterial blood gases: to determine acid–base status and potential need for oxygen.

To identify associated dysfunction of other organs such as hepatic or renal and to identify electrolyte abnormalities, which is important when diuretics or digoxin are being considered as therapy.

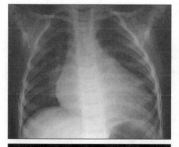

Chest radiography revealing cardiac enlargement.

Differential diagnosis

Infants: sepsis, respiratory infection or insufficiency, severe anemia, pericardial effusion; large thymus may be interpreted as cardiomegaly on chest radiography.

Children and adolescents: overwhelming sepsis, toxic shock syndrome, anemia, leukemia or lymphoma, pericardial effusion.

Etiology

Congenital heart defects

• These lesions more commonly cause congestive heart failure in infancy [1].

Left to right shunting lesions or increased pulmonary blood flow: ventricular septal defect, atrioventricular (AV) canal defects, patent ductus arteriosus, complete or d-transposition of the great arteries, total anomalous pulmonary venous connection, systemic AV fistulae or vein of Galen malformations.

Left heart obstructive lesions: hypoplastic left heart syndrome, aortic stenosis, coarctation of the aorta.

Right heart obstructive lesions: severe or critical pulmonic stenosis.

Atrioventricular valve insufficiency: severe mitral or tricuspid regurgitation.

Semilunar valve insufficiency: severe pulmonary or aortic insufficiency.

Other structural heart defects: Ebstein's anomaly of the tricuspid valve, end-stage congenital heart disease with pulmonary vascular disease.

Left ventricular inflow/right ventricular inflow obstruction: mitral stenosis, cor triatriatum, tricuspid stenosis.

Functional heart abnormalities

Ardiomyopathy: hypertrophic or dilated.

Inflammatory heart disease: myocarditis, rheumatic carditis, endocarditis.

Myocardial infarction, cardiac arrhythmias, muscular dystrophy, severe anemia, upper airway obstruction.

Complications

Arrhythmias; poor growth and development; pulmonary infections and reactive airway disease/bronchial constriction; exercise intolerance; pulmonary artery hypertension; renal failure; hepatic dysfunction.

Epidemiology

As many as 80% of infants who present with congenital heart defects have congestive heart failure as a major component of their clinical presentation [2].

Treatment

Diet and lifestyle

For moderate-to-severe congestive heart failure, a low-salt diet should be followed. Breast milk or a low-salt formula is advised for infants.

Daily activities may be allowed as tolerated, but for more marked CHF, little recreational activity is tolerated. During intercurrent illnesses, patients should rest. Excessive heat or cold should be avoided.

Pharmacologic treatment

Digoxin

Standard dosage	Digoxin, load: 30 µg/kg i.v. total digitalizing dose (TDD); maximum dose, 1 mg. Initial dose, one-half TDD; second dose, one-quarter TDD; third dose, one-quarter TDD. Maintenance, 8–12 mug/kg i.v. in two divided doses.
Contraindications	Relative: hypokalemia, hypocalcemia, renal failure.
Special points	Second and third doses may be given every 2 h if supraventricular tachycardia (SVT) still present; usually given every 6–8 h; a fourth additional dose may be given if patient still in SVT; i.v. dose should be 75%–80% of oral dose; digitalize infants i.v.
Main side effects	Cardiovascular: bradycardia, AV block, ventricular arrhythmias; central nervous system: lethargy, drowsiness, vertigo, disorientation; gastrointestinal: vomiting, nausea, feeding intolerance, abdominal pain, diarrhea; ocular: blurred vision, photophobia, yellow or green vision, flashing lights.

Diuretics

Standard dosage	Furosemide, 1–2 mg/kg every 6–12 h to 6 mg/kg/d or 600 mg/d.
	Aldactone, *infants and children*: 1.5–3.5 mg/kg/d in 2 divided doses; *older children and adolescents*: 25–200 mg/d in 2 divided doses.
	Metolazone, *infants and children*: 0.1–0.2 mg/kg/d in 1–2 divided doses; *older children and adolescents*: 2.5–20 mg daily.
Special points	*Aldactone*: may result in hyperkalemia; should not be used in presence of hyperkalemia.
	Metolazone: potent diuretic; may cause profound diuresis, hypotension, hyponatremia and hypokalemia, especially when used with other diuretics.

ACE inhibitors and afterload-reducing agents

Standard dosage	Enalapril, *infants and children*: 0.1–0.5 mg/kg/d in 2 divided doses; *adolescents*: 2–5 mg/d increased to 10–40 mg/d as tolerated in 1–2 divided doses.
	Captopril, *infants and older children*: 0.05–0.5 mg/kg/dose every 6–8 h initially titrated to maximum of 6 mg/kg/d; *older children and adolescents*: 6.25–12.5 mg/dose to maximum of 450 mg/d.
Contraindications	Worsening renal failure, hypersensitivity.
Special points:	Lower dosage in patients with renal impairment, severe CHF. Administration in volume-depleted patients may cause severe hypotension.
Main side effects	Cough, renal failure, hypotension, dizziness.

Treatment aims

To alleviate symptoms, correct underlying cause when possible, return the patient to as normal a lifestyle as possible, promote normal growth and development and allow for normal childhood activities.

Other treatments

Antiarrhythmics: used to treat specific arrhythmias including SVT and VT (see specific sections).

Oxygen or ventilator support: O$_2$ may be used when alveolar edema is present to improve oxygenation. Use with care in left to right shunting lesions and ductal dependent lesions or those in whom increased pulmonary blood flow could be detrimental.

Surgical correction of underlying congenital heart defect.

Extracorporeal membrane oxygenation: used as bridge to correction, improved function, or cardiac transplantation.

Left ventricular assist device: used as bridge to transplantation.

Intra-aortic balloon pump.

Cardiac transplantation.

Prognosis

Excellent when underlying lesion can be corrected. Symptomatic improvement usually gained when correction not possible. With cardiac transplant, 2-y survival for infants is 69%. For older children and adolescents, 5-y survival is 81%.

Follow-up and management

Depends on underlying cause. Close, continued follow-up is necessary.

Key references

1. Artman M, Graham TR: Congestive heart failure in infancy: recognition and management. *Am Heart J* 1982, **203**:1040–1055.

2. Tyler DC, Buckley LP, Hellenbrand WE, *et al.*: Report of the New England Regional Infant Cardiac Program. *Pediatrics* 1980, **65(suppl 2)**:375–461.

3. Chang AC, Atz AM, Wernovsky G, *et al.*: Milrinone: systemic and pulmonary hemodynamic effects in neonates after cardiac surgery. *Crit Care Med* 1995, **33**:1907–1914.

Diagnosis

Symptoms [1]

• The normal stooling pattern varies greatly between individuals, from several bowel movements per day to one movement every 3 days. Constipation occurs when the normal stool pattern is prolonged, when stooling becomes difficult and painful, or when stools become hard or large.

Decreased bowel movements, painful defecation (straining), abdominal pain: most common symptoms.

Fecal soiling: "encopresis;" watery, involuntary stool leakage; "dirty underwear;" can occur at any age.

Withholding behavior: behaviors associated with leg crossing, "hiding" and refusing to use the toilet; occurs mainly in toddlers.

Unacceptable and inappropriate stool odor: secondary to frequently soiled underwear.

Extremely large stools clogging toilet: common in functional constipation.

Rectal bleeding: secondary to hard, painful bowel movements.

Difficulty with toilet training: fear of using toilet; parents forcing children to use toilet; toddlers.

Signs

Abdominal distention or mass: in severely constipated children, stool can be palpated in the hypogastric and left lower quadrant regions.

Anal fissure.

Delayed meconium passage: if meconium is not passed by the newborn within 48 hours strongly consider Hirschprung's disease.

Rectal prolapse: associated with straining.

Investigations

Blood tests: thyroid function tests.

Rectal examination: arguably the most important investigation to be performed. On digital examination, large amounts of stool palpated within 2 to 4 cm of the anal verge associated with a dilated rectum suggests functional constipation. No palpable stool along with a "tight" rectum indicates Hirschprung's disease. Poor anal tone and lack of an anal "wink" suggests a neurologic etiology.

Abdominal radiography (flat plate): identifies the degree and location of colonic stool; large amounts of stool in the rectosigmoid suggests functional constipation.

Unprepped barium enema: the presence of a "transition zone" (small caliber to large caliber bowel) indicates Hirschprung's disease. In infants with Hirschprung's disease, a transition zone may not be observed. Digital manipulation of the rectum prior to performing a barium enema will open the "transition zone" and may give a false-negative result.

Anorectal manometry: assessment of pressure waves in the rectum. Measurements include contraction and relaxation of internal and external anal sphincters.

Rectal suction biopsy: approximately 3 to 5 mm in diameter deep biopsy into submucosa (taken 3 to 5 cm from anal verge). Biopsy specimens are stained for the presence of ganglion cells and for acetylcholinesterase. The absence of ganglion cells along with increased enzyme activity is diagnostic for Hirschprung's disease.

Complications

Hirschprung's enterocolitis: frequent, bloody diarrhea in a toxic appearing, febrile infant secondary to fecal stasis. Affected patients require hospitalization, IV fluids and parenteral antibiotics, and a surgical consultation.

Sigmoid volvulus: typically occurs in neurologically impaired patients with a history of severe constipation. Associated symptoms include fever, abdominal distention, vomiting, abdominal mass and pain. Barium enema is diagnostic and may reduce volvulus; however, surgery is often required.

Differential diagnosis

Functional constipation.

Hirschprung's disease.

Anorectal disorders: imperforate or ectopic anus; anterior anus.

Neuromuscular disease: primary or secondary to nerve compression from pelvic mass, myelomeningocele.

Endocrine: hypothyroidism, hyperparathyroidism.

Metabolic: hypokalemia, hypocalcemia; hypomagnesemia, diabetes mellitus.

Lead toxicity.

Connective tissue disease: scleroderma, systemic lupus erythematosus.

Intestinal pseudoobstruction.

Infant botulism.

Anatomic disorders: gastrointestinal strictures (Crohn's disease), malrotation, adhesions, necrotizingenterocolitis, prune-belly syndrome, gastroschisis.

Medications: calcium supplements, aluminum-containing drugs, barium, opioids.

Definitions

Functional constipation: ineffective colonic peristalsis and defecation with no underlying cause. Self-perpetuating, with retained rectal stool associated; loss of defecation "urge" and associated with "withholding" behavior.

Organic constipation: constipation secondary to underlying disease process.

Epidemiology

• Approximately 10% to 25% of children have an abnormality associated with defecation.

• Encopresis ("soiling") ranges from 1% to 5% of all children; ratio of boys to girls is 6:1.

Hirschprung's disease [2]

• Congenital absence of ganglion cells in both the myenteric and submucosal plexus.

• The affected colon always begins at the internal sphincter but varies in length proximally; 80% sigmoid; 3% entire colon.

• Rarely, the small intestine is affected.

• Male:female ratio, 3:1; incidence, 1:5000.

Treatment

Diet and lifestyle
• Dairy products, diets deficient in fiber, and foods containing caffeine can be constipating. Whenever possible, children should be encouraged to increase their fiber intake (grains, vegetables) and their fruit intake. Some fruits act as laxatives (apricots, prunes, pears). Juices containing these fruits (in small amounts) can be given to infants.

• Inactivity is also associated with constipation; physical activity should be encouraged.

Pharmacologic treatment
• For moderate to severe constipation, the goal is to achieve a rapid lower bowel clean-out (in a matter of days) along with maintenance therapy with oral medication (which can take months to years).

Oral therapy: various lubricants (mineral oil), osmotic agents (lactulose) and laxatives (magnesium and senna containing compounds) are commercially available for the treatment of constipation. These medications are mandatory for the maintenance of constipation. The goal of treatment is to promote one to two soft, painless stools each day in order to achieve resolution of the megacolon and to restore the defecation "urge" to the patient. Large doses (one to three tablespoons one to three times per day) are often required.

Enemas, suppositories, and rectal stimulation: in general, these medications and maneuvers should be avoided unless prescribed or instructed by a physician. When enemas are indicated, hyperphosphate enemas (saline) are the mainstay of treatment. Mineral oil enemas are useful when "rock-hard" rectal stool is present. Pediatric enemas are used in children less than 2 years of age; adult-sized enemas are used in children older than 2 years of age. In cases of extreme rectal impaction, daily enemas should be administered for 3 to 7 successive days.

Polyethylene glycol solutions (GoLytely): in cases of failed management with enemas and vigorous oral medication, the large-volume oral administration of a polyethylene glycol solution can be used to "clean-out" stool from the colon. Approximately 2 to 4 L need to be administered over a 3- to 5-hour period to achieve adequate colonic cleansing. The majority of pediatric patients require nasogastric administration [3].

Prokinetic agents (Cisapride): promotility agents, typically used for gastroparesis and vomiting, have been shown to improve stool consistency and eliminate soiling [4].

Nonpharmacologic treatment
Toilet training: issues of "toilet" training should be addressed. In infants younger than 2 years of age, toilet training should be discouraged until the symptoms of constipation improve and until soft, painless stools frequently occur. In older children with stool "withholding," the use of the toilet may need to be stopped until any impaction is treated and until soft, painless, normal volume stools are produced.

Family counseling: in severe cases, family counseling by a therapist trained in pediatrics is necessary in order to promote both the child's and parent's understanding of the normal stooling process and to alleviate the anxiety surrounding bowel movements.

Rectal training: young children and adolescents should be encouraged to "toilet" sit in an attempt to defecate one to three times each day for short periods (5 to 10 minutes). This is necessary secondary to the loss of rectal "urge" that occurs in cases of rectal impaction and the need to retrain the body to recognize a full rectum. Often, a reward system can be used to aid in this process.

Rectal biofeedback: electromyographic method for eliminating paradoxical contraction of the external sphincter (not readily available for children) [5].

Surgery: indicated for patients with Hirschprung's disease.

Treatment aims
To alleviate the symptoms of constipation and improve behavioral abnormalities associated with constipation.

Prognosis
• For children with functional constipation the prognosis is good. In cases of organic constipation, the prognosis depends on the underlying cause.

Follow-up and management
• For patients with rectal impaction secondary to functional constipation, initial frequent follow-up is important to be sure that an adequate lower bowel clean-out is achieved. Once maintenance therapy is begun in these patients, intermittent visits (3–6 mo) are needed. Follow-up for organic causes depends on the etiology.

Key references
1. Rosenberg AJ: Constipation and encopresis. In Pediatric Gastrointestinal Disease. Edited by Wyllie R, Hyams JS: Philadelphia: W.B. Saunders; 1993:198–208.
2. Kleinhaus S, Boley SJ, Sheran M, et al.: Hirschprung's disease: a survey of the members of the Surgical Section of the American Academy of Pediatrics. J Pediatr Surg 1979,14:588–597.
3. Ingebo KB, Heyman MB: Polyethylene glyco-electrolyte solution for intestinal clearance in children with refractory encopresis. Am J Dis Child 1988,142:340–342.
4. Murray RD, et al.: Cisapride for intractable constipation in children: observations from an open trial. J Pediatr Gastroenterol Nutr 1990,11:503–508.
5. Riboli EB, et al.: Biofeedback conditioning for fecal incontinence. Arch Phys Med Rehabil 1988,69:29–31.

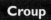

Diagnosis

Symptoms
Drooling.
Hoarseness or muffled voice.
Irritability and/or anxiety.
Fever.

Signs
Pulsus paradoxicus.
Stridor: at rest.
Tachypnea.
Retractions.

Investigations
Lateral neck radiography.
Anteroposterior radiography of neck: should show "steeple sign."
Arterial blood gas: very rarely indicated.

Complications
Respiratory failure.
Hypoxia.
Dehydration.

Differential diagnosis
Infection: epiglottitis, bacterial tracheitis, retropharyngeal abscess, diphtheria.
Immunologic: spasmodic croup, allergic angioedema.
Trauma: foreign body, laryngeal fracture, thermal injury.
Congenital: tracheomalacia, hemangioma, vocal cord paralysis, vascular ring.
Metabolic: hypocalcemia.
Tumor: subglottic hemangioma, lymphoma.

Etiology
• Viral: parainfluenza, RSV, influenza, adenovirus, mycoplasma pneumonia.

Epidemiology
• Peak age: 6 months to 3 years.
• 80% in children less than 5 years.
• Fall and winter predominate.

Treatment

General guidelines

Use humidity.

At home: steam filled bathroom or humidifier.

Hospital: cool mist tent.

Comfort measures: do not agitate child as can cause laryngospasm and deterioration of clinical status.

Fluids: if signs of dehydration.

Pharmacologic treatment

Standard dosage	Racemic epinephrine, 0.05 ml/kg/dose diluted to 3 cm^3 in normal saline via nebulizer with oxygen. Maximun dosage, 0.50 mL given over 15 min. Do not administer more frequently than every hour. Dexamethasone (steroid), 0.60 mg/kg, i.m. in single dose.
Main side effects	Rebound phenomenon can occur with use of racemic epinephrine with worsening of symptoms.
Special points:	If patient has received racemic epinephrine in office or emergency department, he or she will generally be admitted to hospital. If racemic epinephrine is not available, can use L-epinephrine. Patients will have preference for sitting position over lying position.

Other treatment options

• Intubation is required in less than 1% of hospitalized patients. Tube size is smaller than ordinarily used for age due to swelling.

Treatment aims

To improve clinical status as rapidly as possible.

Prognosis

• Patients generally improve over 3–5 days without sequelae.

• Patients with recurrent croup may have underlying anatomical abnormality.

• Some children with spasmodic croup may have a higher likelihood of increased bronchial reactivity. If patient has recurrent stridor, he or she may require otolaryngological evaluation.

General references

Super D: A prospective randomized double-blind study to evaluate the effect of dexamethasone in acute laryngotracheitis. *J Pediatr* 1989, **115**:323–329.

Ledwith SE: Efficacy of nebulized racemic epinephrine in conjunction with oral dexamethasone and mist in outpatient treatment of croup. *Ann Emerg Med* 1995, **25**:331–337.

Winch R: Viral croup and bronchiolitis. *Immunol Allergy Clin North Am* 1993, **13**:133–140.

Diagnosis

Symptoms
• Patients present as newborns with clinical evidence of cyanosis, with or without respiratory symptoms, such as rapid breathing.

Signs
• Central, perioral and peripheral cyanosis is noted, but intensity varies.
• Lungs are clear with normal or elevated respirations.
• A cardiac murmur is generally present in most conditions.
• Peripheral pulses and capillary refill are usually normal.

Investigations

Chest radiography
• Lung fields appear "oligemic" (hypoperfused, dark), without infiltrate or effusion.
• Overall heart size may be normal or slightly increased.
• Right aortic arch presents in approx 25% of patients with tetralogy of Fallot (TOF).
• Classic "boot-shaped" configuration described for TOF may not be seen well in neonates if thymic shadow is present.

Electrocardiography
• If "normal" for a newborn (rightward axis [90°–150°] with right ventricular [RV] dominance), think of TOF, Ebstein's malformation of the tricuspid valve, or single ventricle with PS.
• If axis is 0°–80° with decreased RV force, think of critical pulmonary valve stenosis, pulmonary valve atresia with intact ventricular septum.
• If axis is "leftward" (<0°) with LV dominance, think of tricuspid valve atresia.

Pulse oximetry/arterial blood gas sampling
• Pre- and post-ductal oxygen saturations should be checked in room air. In the absence of a primary lung problem, a pulse oximeter reading, at rest, ≤ 93% is abnormal. Visible cyanosis, however, is not usually obvious until the pulse oximeter reads ≤85–87%. Systemic hypoxemia and respiratory symptoms may start at saturations <65–70%.
• A hyperoxia test should be performed. The patient is placed in 100% oxygen for 10 min, followed by pre- and postductal arterial blood gases (not oxygen saturations!), to assess 1) acid-base status, 2) ventilatory status, 3) response of pO_2 to oxygen (in a cyanotic cardiac defect, the pO_2 will not change; if a pulmonary process is present, the preductal pO_2 will increase >150–200 torr), and 4) compe pre- and postductal pO_2 to delineate a right-to-left ductal shunt to the body.

Echocardiography
• Echocardiography is able to accurately define the anatomy and physiology of most cyanotic heart disease, thus guiding treatment. Gradients across the pulmonary outflow tract, pulmonary valve annulus, and right ventricular size and pressure can be measured.

Cardiac catheterization
Used to assess size and continuity of hypoplastic pulmonary arteries, distribution of aortopulmonary collateral vessels, and the coronary arteries in pulmonary atresia with intact ventricular septum (which may be RV dependent).

Complications
Hypercyanosis ("spells"), metabolic acidosis, death.

Endocarditis.

Arrhythmias or sudden death.

Intracardiac right-to-left shunt: stroke, embolus, brain abscess.

Polycythemia according to degree of cyanosis.

Differential diagnosis
Limited pulmonary blood flow with CHD: TOF with or without pulmonary valve atresia, critical PS, tricuspid valve atresia, pulmonary valve atresia with intact ventricular septum, Ebstein's malformation of the tricuspid valve with pulmonary valve stenosis or atresia, or single ventricle with PS or atresia.

Limited pulmonary blood flow without CHD: persistent fetal circulation.

Cyanosis due to noncardiac causes: infiltrates, effusions, pneumothorax, congenital diaphragmatic hernia, cystic adenomatoid lung malformations, and airway anomalies.

Etiology
• The etiology is felt to be multifactorial, with a strong genetic influence (ie, some familial cases of TOF, the high percentage of patients with TOF in VATER syndrome, gastrointestinal anomalies (eg, omphalocele), and significant environmental influence (ie, the high incidence of Ebstein's malformation in fetuses with maternal Lithium ingestion).

• Recent molecular biology investigations have localized the Di George region to chromosome 22, which has a high linkage with TOF and other forms of CHD. Also, TOF occurs in patients with trisomy 21.

Epidemiology
TOF: accounts for approximately 10% of congenital heart lesions; slight male predominance; high incidence of other extra-cardiac malformations.

Tricuspid valve atresia: accounts for approximately 2% of congenital lesions; slight male predominance.

Pulmonary valve atresia: accounts for 1%–3% of congenital heart lesions.

Critical PS: overall, valvar PS accounts for approximately 10% of CHD, but "critical" PS associated with cyanosis is only a small percentage of that group.

Ebstein's malformation: rare; accounts for 0.5% of CHD; incidence equal in males and females.

Treatment

Diet and lifestyle

- No specific dietary interventions are necessary.
- After surgery, patient's activity level is dictated by the presence or absence of arrhythmias, ventricular dysfunction, or residual shunting.
- Teenagers with palliated single ventricles or repaired complex heart disease may have limited exercise capacity.

Pharmacologic treatment

For neonates

- If oxygen saturation is low (< 70%) and does not improve with supplemental oxygen, then the ductus arteriosus must be reopened.

Standard dosage	Prostaglandin E1 (PGE), as a continuous infusion 0.05 to 0.1 μ/kg/minute.
Side effects	*PGE*: apnea, jitteriness, vasodilation, tachycardia, seizures, fever, thrombocytopenia; for transport, the airway must be secure.

For postoperative patients

- Digoxin and diuretics are common in patients with single ventricle after aortopulmonary shunt, and similarly after complete repair of TOF.

Standard dosage	Digoxin (maintenance dose) 5 μ/kg p.o. every 12 h (i.v. dose is 75% of oral dose).
	Furosemide, range is 1–4 mg/kg/d every 12 h (i.v. or p.o.)
Special points	*Furosemide*: check electrolytes; hypokalemia is associated with cardiac arrhythmias.

Nonpharmacologic treatment

Interventional cardiac catheterization

Indicated for patients with critical pulmonary valve stenosis with adequate sized right ventricular cavity; balloon dilation of the stenotic valve is highly successful.

Surgical treatment

Palliative shunts: in patients dependent on PGE to maintain pulmonary blood flow, a modified Blalock-Taussig (aortopulmonary) shunt precedes later surgical intervention; a 3.5–4.0 mm Impra-Graft or Gore-Tex shunt is anastomosed between the innominate artery and its corresponding branch pulmonary artery (right-sided in a left arch; left-sided in a right arch) or onto the central confluence of the branch pulmonary arteries ("central shunt"); this is usually performed without cardiopulmonary bypass through either a lateral thoracotomy or central sternotomy incision.

Tetralogy of Fallot: complete surgical repair (VSD closure, relief of right ventricular outflow obstruction) is generally accomplished within the first 6–12 months of life. A transannular patch may be needed.

Tricuspid atresia: the right ventricle is hypoplastic, so after an initial shunt procedure, the patient later undergoes a Fontan operation by 2–4 years of age; some institutions advocate further staging with a "hemi-Fontan" at 6–12 months of age.

Pulmonary atresia with intact ventricular septum: early surgery includes a neonatal aortopulmonary shunt; occasionally, if the coronaries are independent of th RV, the pulmonary outflow tract is opened with a biventricular repair (ASD closure, takedown of shunt) performed later; otherwise, the patient is staged toward a Fontan palliation.

Treatment aims

To optimize pulmonary blood flow with "acceptable" oxygen saturation of 75% to 85% (palliated).

To protect the pulmonary vascular bed from high pressure and flow.

- The ultimate goal is to separate systemic venous ("blue") and pulmonary venous ("red") circulations, optimize oxygenation, and decrease cardiac workload.

Prognosis

Follow-up of surgically repaired TOF over the past 20 y: overall good prognosis for late survival, although dysrhythmias, ventricular dysfunction, and limitation of exercise capacity has been noted in older patients with late reparative surgery; with repair of TOF in the first year of life, the long-term risks of cyanosis and RV hypertension are lessened, but pulmonary insufficiency and RV volume overload may be a limiting factor later on.

- Adult survivors of Fontan's operation for single ventricle (since the 1970's) have significant exercise limitations, but may lead functional lives and even reproduce. Atrial arrhythmias (SVT, atrial flutter, sick sinus syndrome) are common postoperative complications following Fontan surgery.

General references

Calder A, Barratt-Boyes B, Brandt P, et al.: Postoperative evaluation of patients with tetralogy of Fallot repaired in infancy. *J Thorac Cardiovasc Surg* 1979, **77**:704–720.

Fontan F, Deville C, Quaegebour J, et al.: Repair of tricuspid atresia in 100 patients. *J Thorac Cardiovasc Surg* 1983, **85**:647–660.

Gillette P, Yeoman M, Mullins C, et al.: Sudden death after repair of tetralogy of Fallot. *Circulation* 1977, 56:566–571.

Hanley F, Sade R, Blackstone E, et al.: Outcomes on neonatal pulmonary atresia with intact ventricular septum: a multi-institutional study. *J Thorac Cardiovasc Surg* 1993, 105:406–427.

Kirklin JW, Blackstone E, Jonas R, et al.: Morphologic and surgical determinants of outcome events after repair of tetralogy of Fallot and pulmonary stenosis. *J Thorac Cardiovasc Surg* 1992, 103:706–723.

Cyanotic heart disease (normal or increased pulmonary blood flow)

Diagnosis

Symptoms

• Patients present as newborns with clinical evidence of cyanosis, with or without respiratory symptoms. Limitation of cardiac output may occur in a few cyanotic lesions.

Signs

• Central, perioral, and peripheral cyanosis is noted, but intensity varies.

• Respiratory rate is normal or elevated, according to amount of cyanosis.

• A cardiac murmur is variably present.

Investigations

Chest radiography

• The lung fields appear normally perfused or overcirculated.

• Heart size may be normal or slightly increased. Right arch present in approximately 25%

• 35% of patients with truncus arteriosus. Also, thymus may be absent in Di George syndrome.

• A narrow mediastinum ("egg on a string") may be seen in truncus arteriosus and dextrotransposition of the great arteries (dTGA).

Electrocardiography

"Normal" for a newborn with rightward axis (90°–150°) and right ventricular (RV) dominance: think of dTGA, truncus arteriosus, total anomalous pulmonary venous return, and Ebstein's malformation of the tricuspid valve.

"Abnormal" for a newborn and axis is "superior": think of single ventricle without pulmonary stenosis.

Pulse oximetry/arterial blood gas sampling

• In the absence of a primary lung problem, a pulse oximeter reading (at rest) ≤93% is abnormal. Cyanosis is not usually obvious until oximeter reads ≤85%–87%.

• A hyperoxia test should be performed. The patient is placed in 100% oxygen for 10 minutes, followed by pre- and postductal arterial blood gases (if a fixed cyanotic cardiac defect is present, the pO_2 will not change; if a pulmonary process is responsible for hypoxemia, the preductal pO_2 will generally increase to >150–200 torr). Comparison of pre- and postductal pO_2 will show right-to-left ductal shunting.

Echocardiography

• The pulmonary outflow tract can be evaluated for patency. The size and location of atrial and ventricular septal defects, the presence or absence of a patent ductus arteriosus, and sites of cardiac mixing can be determined.

Complications

Hypercyanosis, metabolic acidosis, death: in dTGA with inadequate mixing.

Cyanosis, respiratory insufficiency, acidosis: in obstructed anomalous pulmonary venous return.

Endocarditis.

Stroke, systemic embolus, brain abscess: due to intracardiac right-to-left shunt.

Pulmonary hypertension or congestive heart failure: with pulmonary overcirculation lesions.

Hypocalcemia, seizures, immune deficiency with Di George syndrome (ie, truncus arteriosus).

Differential diagnosis

Cyanotic CHD with normal or increased pulmonary blood flow
dTGA, with or without ventricular septal defect (VSD).
Truncus arteriosus.
Total anomalous pulmonary venous connection (TAPVC).
Ebstein's malformation of the tricuspid valve without pulmonary stenosis.
Hypoplastic left heart syndrome.
Cyanosis due to noncardiac causes
Must rule out pulmonary infiltrate, effusion, pneumothorax, congenital diaphragmatic hernia, cystic adenomatoid lung malformations, airway anomalies.

Etiology

• Congenital heart defects occur randomly (8:1000 live births), with cyanotic heart lesions accounting for a small percentage. The etiology is multifactorial, with influences that are both genetic (ie, familial cases of truncus arteriosus and anomalous pulmonary venous drainage) and environmental (ie, increased incidence of Ebstein's malformation with maternal lithium ingestion or heart defects in infants of diabetic mothers). Recent investigations have localized the Di George region to chromosome 22 (seen often with truncus arteriosus.

Epidemiology

dTGA: approx 5%–7% of congenital heart lesions; strong male predominance; without treatment, 30% mortality in 1 wk; extracardiac anomalies are rare.
Truncus arteriosus: rare; approx 1%–4% of congenital lesions in autopsy specimens; slight male predominance; associated with Di George syndrome.
Total anomalous pulmonary venous connection: rare; accounts for <1% of autopsy specimens with CHD; infradiaphragmatic drainage more common in males.
Ebstein's malformation: rare; accounts for 0.5% of CHD; incidence equal in male and female population.

Treatment

Diet and lifestyle

• Activity level is dictated by the presence or absence of ventricular dysfunction, valve disease, and pulmonary pressure. A "prudent diet" without excessive fat intake is recommended, especially following coronary reimplantation in the arterial switch procedure.

Pharmacologic treatment

Neonates

• If oxygen saturation is low (<70%) despite supplemental oxygen and if pulmonary blood flow is present on chest radiograph, then intracardiac mixing is inadequate. Cautious use of prostaglandin E1 (PGE) will increase pulmonary venous return to the left atrium and enhance atrial and ductal level mixing in some patients with dTGA.

Standard dosage	PGE, 0.05–0.10 μ/kg/min infusion.
Side effects	*PGE*: apnea, jitteriness, vasodilation, tachycardia, seizures, fever, thrombocytopenia.
Contraindications	Obstructed anomalous pulmonary venous drainage.
Special points	For transport, the airway must be secure.

Postoperative patients

• After surgical intervention for cyanotic heart disease, patients may require digoxin and diuretics.

Standard dosage	Digoxin, oral maintenance, 5 μ/kg every 12 h (i.v. dose, 75% of oral dose)
	Furosemide (Lasix), 1–4 mg/kg/d divided every 12 h (i.v. or p.o.).
Special points	Check potassium level because hypokalemia is associated with arrhythmias.

Nonpharmacologic treatment

Rashkind procedure (balloon atrial septostomy): indicated for patients with dTGA and intact ventricular septum and restrictive foramen ovale; this nonsurgical creation of an atrial septal defect (ASD) allows oxygenated blood from the left atrium to cross into the right heart and go to the systemic circulation, improving circulation.

Surgical treatment

dTGA: without fixed LV outflow tract obstruction, the preferred surgical procedure is an arterial switch operation (ASO); the aorta and PA are "switched" back to their appropriate ventricle; the coronary arteries are transferred from the anterior native aortic root to the posterior "neo-aortic" root; associated ASD, VSD, patent ductus arteriosus are also repaired.

• Repair is early in life (first 2 weeks of life) when the LV is "prepared" to pump against a high afterload.

Truncus arteriosus: complete surgical repair (VSD closure, placement of a RV–PA conduit) is accomplished within the first few months of life; later repair is associated with pulmonary hypertension and high mortality.

TAPVC: the confluence of pulmonary veins is anastomosed to the posterior aspect of the left atrium, which may need augmentation, and the obligatory ASD is closed; in patients with partial or complete obstruction, surgery is mandated in the neonatal period; in patients with unobstructed TAPVC, surgical repair occurs within the first few months of life.

Treatment aims

To achieve "acceptable" systemic oxygenation prior to definitive surgical intervention.

To protect the pulmonary vascular bed from high pressure and/or high flow.

The ultimate goal is to "normalize" intracardiac flow patterns when two ventricles are present.

Prognosis

• Earlier "atrial inversion" procedures (Senning and Mustard operations) for dTGA resulted in high incidence of cardiac arrhythmias, RV dysfunction, and tricuspid regurgitation.

• Intermediate term results after ASO show a low risk for arrhythmias or "late" cardiac dysfunction, but neo-aortic valve insufficiency and coronary ostial growth need ongoing assessment.

• Many truncus patients survive to young adulthood. Late problems include neo-aortic valve stenosis and/or insufficiency as well as stenotic RV–PA conduits.

• Obstructed total anomalous pulmonary venous return has a high operative mortality (up to 30%) and problems with recurrent pulmonary venous obstruction and pulmonary hypertension.

General references

Ebert P, Turley K, Stanger P, et al.: Surgical treatment of truncus arteriosus in the first six months of life. *Ann Surg* 1984, **200**:451–456.

Cobanglu A, Menashe V: Total anomalous pulmonary venous connection in neonates and young infants: repair in the current era. *Ann Thorac Surg* 1993, **55**:43–49.

Norwood WI, Dobell AR, Freed MD, et al.: The Congenital Heart Surgeons Society: intermediate results of the arterial switch repair: a 20-institution study. *J Thorac Cardiovasc Surg* 1988, **96**:854–863.

Paul M, Wernovsky G: Transposition of the great arteries. In *Moss and Adams' Heart Disease in Infants, Children and Adolescents*, ed 5. Emmanouilides G, Allen H, Riemenschneider T, Gutgesell H. Williams and Wilkins: Baltimore; 1995:1154–1224.

Diagnosis

Symptoms

Chronic cough, recurrent pneumonia, bronchorrhea, nasal polyps, and chronic pansinusitis.

Pancreatic insufficiency: occurs in 85% of patients. Fat malabsorption may lead to failure to thrive or pancreatitis.

Rectal prolapse: occurs in 2% of the patients.

Meconium ileus: 15%–20% of patients present with this symptom.

Distal obstruction: of the large intestine may be seen in older children.

Hyponatremic dehydration.

Hypochloremic metabolic alkalosis.

Signs

Cough (frequently productive of mucopurulent sputum), **rhonchi, rales, hyperresonance to percussion, barrel-chest deformity of thorax in severe cases, nasal polyps, and cyanosis** (in later stages).

Digital clubbing, hepatosplenomegaly in patients with cirrhosis, growth retardation, hypertrophic osteoarthropathy, and delayed puberty, amenorrhea, irregular menstrual periods (in teenage patients).

Investigations

Sweat test: "gold standard" for the diagnosis of cystic fibrosis (CF).

• Sweat chloride >60 mEq/L is considered abnormal. False positives are seen in severe malnutrition, ectodermal dysplasia, adrenal insufficiency, nephrogenic diabetes insipidus, hypothyroidism, hypoparathyroidism, mucopolysaccharidoses. False negatives are seen in patients with edema and hypoproteinemia.

Genetic testing: over 600 identified CF genotypes, but only 20–70 of the most common are tested; thus, the lack of a positive genotype reduces (but does not eliminate) the possibility that a CF sample can be obtained from blood or buccal cell scraping.

Sputum cultures: frequent pathogens include *Staphylococcus aureus*, *Pseudomonas aeruginosa* (mucoid and nonmucoid), *Burkholderia cepacia*.

Pulmonary function tests: usually reveal obstructive lung disease.

Pancreatic function tests: 72-hour fecal fat measurement, measurement of serum para-aminobenzoic acid (PABA) levels, stool trypsin levels, serum immunoreactive trypsin (IRT).

Chest radiography: typical features include hyperinflation, peribronchial thickening, atelectasis, cystic lesions filled with mucus, and bronchiectasis.

Sinus radiography: typically shows pansinusitis.

Complications

Respiratory: recurrent bronchitis and pneumonia, chronic sinusitis, pneumothorax, hemoptysis

Gastrointestinal: include pancreatic insufficiency; patients usually have steatorrhea; decreased levels of vitamins A, D, E and K; poor growth and failure to thrive; meconium ileus equivalent; rectal prolapse; and clinically significant hepatobiliary disease (cirrhosis of the liver, esophageal varices and splenomegaly).

Reproductive: include sterility in 98% of males and 75% of females.

Endocrine: abnormal glucose tolerance; diabetes mellitus.

Differential diagnosis
Pulmonary
Recurrent pneumonia.
Chronic bronchitis.
Immotile cilia syndrome.
Severe asthma.
Aspiration pneumonia.
Gastrointestinal
Gastroesophageal reflux.
Celiac sprue.
Protein-losing enteropathy.
Other
Failure to thrive (secondary to neglect, poor caloric intake or feeding problems).
Immune deficiency syndromes.
Nasal polyposis.
Male infertility.
Hyponatremic dehydration.

Etiology
• The most common severe inherited disease in the Caucasian population (autosomal recessive in inheritance).
• Cystic fibrosis transmembrane regulator (CFTR): functions as a cyclic AMP-activated chloride channel, which allows for the transport of chloride out of the cell. It is accompanied by the passive passage of water, which keeps secretions well hydrated.
• In cystic fibrosis, an abnormality in CFTR blocks chloride transport and inadequate hydration of the cell surface results in thick secretions and organ damage.
• The CFTR gene is 250,000 base pairs long and located on the long arm of chromosome 7. The most common deletion is three base pairs, which results in the absence of phenylalanine at codon 508 (seen in over 70% of the cystic fibrosis population in North America).

Epidemiology
Incidence of abnormalities in the CFTR gene
1:25 individuals in the Caucasian population
Incidence of cystic fibrosis
1:2500 in Caucasian population
1:17,000 in African-American population (rarely seen in African blacks and Asians)

Treatment

Diet and lifestyle

High calorie diet with nutritional supplements (given orally, via nasogastric tube feedings or through gastrostomy tube feeding).

Vitamin supplements: multivitamins and fat soluble vitamin replacement (usually E and K).

• Pancreatic enzyme-replacement therapy can be used in patients who are pancreatic insufficient. Dosage is adjusted for the frequency and character of the stools and for growth pattern.

• Stool softeners treat constipation or meconium ileus equivalent and include mineral oil, oral N-acetylcysteine, lactulose, enemas.

Pharmacologic treatment

Antibiotic therapy (based on sputum culture results)

Oral antibiotics: cephalexin, cefaclor, trimethoprim-sulfamethoxazole, chloramphenicol, ciprofloxacin

Intravenous antibiotics (given for 2–3-week course)

For *Staphylococcus aureus*: oxacillin, nafcillin

For *Pseudomonas aeruginosa* or *Burkholderia cepacia*: semisynthetic penicillin (ticarcillin, piperacillin) or a cephalosporin (ceftazidime) *plus* an aminoglycoside (gentamicin, tobramycin, or amikacin) to obtain synergistic action.

For aid in clearing pulmonary secretions

Aerosolized bronchodilator therapy (to open airways): albuterol

Mucolytic agents (to help break up viscous pulmonary secretions): N-acetylcysteine, recombinant DNase.

Chest physiotherapy with postural drainage.

Treatment aims

To maintain good nutritional status (good nutrition is associated with a better prognosis).

To slow pulmonary deterioration as much as possible.

To maintain a normal lifestyle.

Prognosis

• Long-term prognosis is poor.

• The course of the illness is variable; it is impossible to predict the course of the disease in a specific person.

• The current mean life span is 29 years.

• Due to new antibiotics, enzyme-replacement therapy, and maintenance of good pulmonary toilet with chest physiotherapy and bronchodilators, the mean age of survival has been increasing for the past three decades.

Follow-up and management

• Routine care should be at a Cystic Fibrosis Center.

• Frequency of visits is dependent on severity of illness: usually every 2–4 m.

• Usually lifelong nutritional support is required.

• Duration of antibiotic therapy is controversial. Chronic use is eventually required as the patient's pulmonary function deteriorates.

• All siblings should have a sweat test.

General references

Boat TF, Welsh MJ, Beaudet AL: *Cystic Fibrosis: The Metabolic Basis of Inherited Disease.* McGraw-Hill: New York; 1989:2649–2680.

Colin AA, Wohl MEB: Cystic fibrosis. *Pediatr Rev* 1994, **15**:192–200.

Fick RB, Stillwell PC: Controversies in the management of pulmonary disease due to cystic fibrosis. *Chest* 1989, **95**:1319–1327.

Mouton JW, Kerrebijn KF: Antibacterial therapy in cystic fibrosis. *Med Clin North Am* 1990, **74**:837–850.

Schidlow DV, Taussig LM, Knowles MR: Cystic Fibrosis Foundation Consensus Conference Report on pulmonary complications of cystic fibrosis. *Pediatr Pulmonol* 1993, **15**:187–198.

Wilmott RW, Fiedler MA: Recent advances in the treatment of cystic fibrosis. *Ped Clin North Am* 1994, **41**:431–451.

Diagnosis

Symptoms
• The most sensitive symptom is a history of decreased urine output.
Thirst in the older child, irritability in babies.
Weight loss.
Poor oral intake.
Symptoms of an illness associated with dehydration (*see* Etiology)

Signs [1,2]
• Clinically important dehydration will have at least three of the signs listed below under moderate dehydration.
• Signs of dehydration may be more pronounced with hyponatremic dehydration or more subtle with hypernatremic dehydration.
• Degree of dehydration is determined by weight or body fluid losses.

Mild dehydration (<5% weight loss or >50 mL/kg body fluid loss)
Vital signs: slight increase in heart rate, normal BP and respiration.
Skin: capillary refill <2 seconds on finger, elasticity normal.
Mucous membranes: moist.
Mental status: normal.
Eyes: tears present.

Moderate dehydration (5%–10% weight loss or 50–100 mL/kg body fluid loss)
Vital signs: increase in heart rate (orthostatic change), normal BP and respiration.
Skin: capillary refill 2 seconds on finger, elasticity normal.
Mucous membranes: dry.
Mental status: altered (ill appearance, headache, lethargy, irritability).
Eyes: tears absent, sunken.

Severe dehydration (>10% weight loss or >100 mL/kg body fluid loss)
Vital signs: markedly increased heart rate, fall in BP and hyperpnea.
Skin: capillary refill >3 seconds on finger, tenting.
Mucous membranes: dry.
Mental status: depressed (toxic or ill appearance, lethargic, irritable).
Eyes: tears absent, sunken.

Investigations

Urine
Output decreased with increasing dehydration to oliguria and anuria.
Specific gravity: >1020; increases with degree of dehydration to >1030.
Osmolarity: >600; increases with degree of dehydration.

Electrolytes
Not drawn with mild dehydration.
Serum sodium characterizes type of dehydration: isotonic (130–150 mEq/L), hypotonic (<130 mEq/L), hypertonic (>150 mEq/L).
Serum bicarbonate decreases with increasing dehydration.
Blood urea nitrogen is elevated with increasing dehydration.

Arterial pH
Not drawn except in cases of severe dehydration.
Decreased with increasing dehydration: >7.1 with severe dehydration.

Differential diagnosis
• Dehydration is not a disease. It is a state of hypovolemic shock. One must determine the cause (see Etiology).

Etiology
Poor intake: anorexia, restriction to fluids, pharyngitis or stomatitis
Increased output: increased insensible losses (fever, sweating, heat, hyperventilation); renal losses (DKA, ATN, diuretic usage, DI, CAH, nephropathies); gastrointestinal losses (diarrhea, vomiting).
Translocation of fluids: burns, ascites, paralytic ileus after abdominal surgery.

Epidemiology
• Dehydration secondary to diarrhea is the leading cause of death world wide in children <4 y of age.
• In the United States, approximately 500 children die from diarrheal illnesses with dehydration, and another 200,000 are hospitalized each year.

Complications
Death: if fail to treat shock and restore circulation to tissues.
Cerebral edema or bleeding with hypertonic dehydration.
Hypocalcemia with hypernatremic dehydration.
Seizures with hyponatremic dehydration.

Treatment

Lifestyle management

- Avoid bundling and leaving children in hot cars.
- Increase fluids in heat and with gastroenteritis.
- Avoid free water in babies <6 months of age.
- Make up baby formula according to directions.

Treating shock

- Administer 10–20 cc/kg aliquots of isotonic solution regardless of serum toxicity or cause of dehydration (normal saline or ringer's lactate) until blood pressure normalizes, heart rate decreases, and end organs are perfusing well (capillary refill < 2 seconds).
- If dextrose is needed for low glucose, it should be given separately as a 0.5 g/kg bolus.

Oral rehydration

In the first 4–6 hours

- Replace entire deficit with high sodium (75–90 mEq/L of sodium) and 2.5% dextrose solution; have caretaker syringe or spoon in small amount every 2–5 minutes.

In the next 16–20 hours

Use maintenance solution of 40–60 mEq/L sodium and 2.5% dextrose or alternate initial replacement fluid with breast milk, water, or low-carbohydrate juices.

Intravenous rehydration

Stock for replacement phase is determined by measured losses

Isotonic dehydration: D51/4NS plus 20/KCl/L.

Hyponatremic dehydration: D51/2NS plus 20/KCl/L.

Hypernatremic dehydration: D51/5NS plus 20/KCl/L.

Rate of replacement

Isotonic or hyponatremic dehydration: half stock replacement over the first 8 hours; half over the next 16 hours.

Hypertonic dehydration: full stock replacement slowly and evenly over 48 hours.

Exceptions: No dextrose initially for DKA; use isotonic solutions for burns; severe electrolyte disturbances require individual calculations.

Maintenance requirements

Maintenance fluids must be given in addition to the deficit

Maintenance requirements per 24 hours:

Weight	Fluids per 24 hours
<10 kg	100 cc/kg.
10–20 kg	1000 cc + 50 cc/kg for each kg >10 kg.
>20 kg	1500 cc + 20 cc/kg for each kg >20 kg.

For example, a 25-kg child needs 1600 cc/day.

Treatment aims

To treat shock (with restoration of normal vital signs for age).

To correct fluid and electrolyte deficits more slowly.

Prognosis

- Prognosis is dependent on the disease process and initial state and type of dehydration.

Follow-up and management

Monitor urine output (>1 cc/kg/hr) .

Monitor vital signs.

Monitor serial weights.

Replace losses (vomiting, diarrhea, insensible).

Other information

Fluid deficit estimates: 1 kg weight loss = 1 L fluid loss.

- Current weight is a percentage of "well" or normal weight (eg, the "well" weight of a 9-kg child who is 10% "dry" = 9 kg/0.9 = 10 kg, meaning that 1 kg of weight has been lost, which corresponds to a 1-L deficit).

Key references

1. Gorelick MH, Shaw KN, Baker MD: Effect of temperature on capillary refill in normal children. *Pediatr* 1993, **92:**699–702.
2. Gorelick MH, Shaw KN, Murphy KO: Validity and reliability of clinical signs in the diagnosis of dehydration in children. *Pediatr* 1997: **99:**e6(www.pediatrics.org).
3. Shaw KN: Dehydration. In *Textbook of Pediatric Emergency Medicine*, ed. 3. Edited by Fleisher GR, Ludwig S. Williams and Wilkins: Baltimore; 1993:147–151.
4. American Academy of Pediatrics Committee on Nutrition: Use of oral fluid therapy and post-treatment feeding following enteritis in children in a developed country. *Pediatr* 1985, **2:**358–361.
5. Finberg L, Kravath RE, Fleischman AR (eds): *Water and Electrolytes in Pediatrics.* Philadelphia: WB Saunders; 1982.

Diagnosis

Symptoms

Fatigue: principally affecting proximal muscles in arms and legs; 15%–30% of these patients have associated arthralgias, Raynaud's phenomenon, or myalgia; painless weakness is common [1]; **dysphagia; unusual, severe manifestations:** interstitial lung disease, pulmonary hypertension, ventilatory failure, heart block or arrhythmias, dysphagia [2]; **skin rashes; draining lesions.**

Signs

Muscle wasting: principally of proximal muscles; **gower's sign:** inability to rise from the floor with use of arms; **loss of muscle reflexes:** in late-stage disease; **heliotrope rash:** lilac discoloration around eyelids (may be faint); **gottron's papules:** small raised reddish plaques over knuckles; **gottron's sign:** an erythematous rash over extensor surfaces of hands and elbows; **cutaneous calcinosis:** may occur in 20% of cases, resulting in tender lesions draining chalk-like material.

Investigations

Key investigations

Creatine kinase, aldolase measurement: concentration 5–30 times upper limit of normal but not disease-specific; concentrations higher in many patients with muscular dystrophy [2].

Electromyography: to check for insertional irritability and small polyphasic potentials.

MRI: to detect inflamed muscles and to guide site of biopsy [3].

Muscle biopsy: needle or open surgical technique; classic changes are inflammation, with mononuclear cell infiltrate composed mainly of lymphocytes (some macrophages and plasma cells), with muscle-fiber necrosis, and, in chronic cases, replacement of muscle fibers by fat and fibrous tissue; changes often patchy, and up to 20% of patients may have relatively normal appearance.

Other investigations

Measurement of other enzymes: *eg,* transaminase concentrations may be raised (also reflecting muscle in inflammation).

Myoglobin measurement: appears to reflect disease activity.

Autoantibody analysis: weak positive antinuclear antibody reaction in 60%–80% of patients with myositis; antibodies to transfer RNA synthetase enzymes, notably the anti-Jo-1 antibody, occur in 30% of patients.

Complications

Interstitial lung fibrosis, arthritis, Raynaud's phenomenon: in patients with Jo-1 antibody.

Aspiration: due to dysphagia.

Cardiac or respiratory failure: rare; caused by rapidly progressive myositis.

Underlying neoplasm: exceedingly rare (unlike in adults).

Differential diagnosis

Muscular dystrophy.
Osteomalacia.
Rhabdomyolysis.
Drug-induced inflammatory disease (including D-penicillamine).
Metabolic myopathies (eg, McArdle's disease).
Inclusion body myositis [1].
Infection (eg, pyomyositis, viral)

Etiology

• Inflammatory muscle diseases are part of the family of autoimmune rheumatic diseases.
• Causes include the following:
Hormonal component.
Immunogenetic predisposition: HLA B8 and DR3 associated with myositis, principally in whites; DR3 linked to Jo-1 antibody.
Environmental factors: increased risk of developing myositis at different times of year found in one study.

Epidemiology

• The annual incidence of dermatomyositis is 4:1,000,000.
• The female : male ratio is 2–3:1 overall.

Polymyositis [1,2]

One case for every 10 cases of dermatomyositis.
No skin rash or microvascular injury.
Perifascicular atrophy uncommon.
Endomysial infiltration common.
Surrounded and invaded fibers frequent.

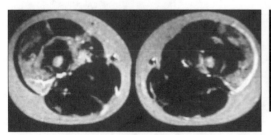

MRI of proximal legs in patient with edema, especially in the vastus lateralis muscles bilaterally.

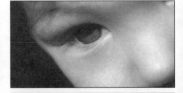

Heliotrope rash in an 18-month-old with erythema and induration around the eyes.

Treatment

Diet and lifestyle
• Exercise and activity are limited during the inflammation.
• Hydration is important in patients with calcinosis to avoid nephrolithiasis.

Pharmacological treatment

Corticosteroids
• After the diagnosis has been established, treatment should be initiated quickly [1,2].

Standard dosage	Methylprednisolone pulse, 30 mg/kg/d (maximum 1 g) for 3 d then Prednisone, 1–2 mg/kg/d initially (up to 60 mg/day); continued until creatine kinase returned to near normal (usually 1–3 mo); then reduced slowly to 5–10 mg daily over following 3 mo.
Contraindications	Severe osteoporosis.
Main drug interactions	None.
Main side effects	Osteoporosis, increased risk of infection, hyperglycemia, hypertension, obesity.

Other immunosuppressants
• These are indicated in patients who have not shown a response to high-dose steroids after 1 month or who cannot tolerate them [1,4,5].

Standard dosage	Azathioprine, 2–3 mg/kg. Methotrexate, up to 15 mg weekly.
Contraindications	*Methotrexate:* abnormal liver function, major renal disease, porphyria.
Main drug interactions	*Methotrexate:* many analgesics and antibacterials.
Main side effects	Bone-marrow suppression, liver damage.

Other options
• Oral or occasionally i.v. cyclophosphamide has been used in severely affected patients, usually combined with steroids.
• Intravenous gammaglobulin may be used [4].
• Colchicine may attenuate calcinosis flares [6].

Nonpharmacological treatment
Physical and occupational therapy.
Orthopedic intervention for flexion contractures.

Treatment aims
To control disease as soon as possible. To maintain reasonable degree of mobility. To reduce treatment to smallest dose needed after 3–4 months of aggressive therapy to avoid side effects (e.g., intercurrent infection or osteoporosis).

Prognosis
• ~80% of patients recover fully.
• <10% die as a direct result of the disease or as a consequence of its treatment.
• Some patients are left with some muscle weakness.
• Patients who respond most slowly to initial treatment have the poorest prognosis.

Follow-up and management
• Patients must be followed for several years.
• Regular clinical examination, creatine kinase measurement, and formal muscle strength testing are needed.
• Physical and occupational therapy help to keep the range of joint movement normal and to maintain muscle power.

Key references
1. Dalakas MC: Polymyositis, dermatomyositis, and inclusion-body myositis. *N Engl J Med* 1992, 325:1487–1498.
2. Pachman LN: Juvenile dermatomyositis. *Ped Clin North Am* 1986, 33:1097–1117.
3. Hernandez RJ, Keim DR, Sullivan DB, et al.: Magnetic resonance imaging appearance of the muscles in childhood dermatomyositis. *J Pediatr* 1990, 117:546–550.
4. Lang BA, Laxer RM, Murphy G, et al.: Treatment of dermatomyositis with intravenous gammaglobulin. *Am J Med* 1991, 91:169–172.
5. Plotz PH, et al.: Current concepts in the idiopathic inflammatory myopathies polymyositis, dermatomyositis and related disorders. *Ann Intern Med* 1989, 111:143–157.
6. Taborn J, Bole GG, Thompson GR: Colchicine suppression of local and systemic inflammation due to calcinosis universalis in chronic dermatomyositis. *Ann Int Med* 1978, 89:648–649.

Diagnosis

Symptoms

Fever, cough, shortness of breath: increased susceptibility to respiratory viral infections (*eg*, adenovirus, parainfluenza, and respiratory syncytial virus) and to opportunistic infections (*eg*, *Pneumocystis carinii*).

Fever, diarrhea, vomiting: increased susceptibility to viral gastroenteritis (*eg*, rotavirus).

Cough, shortness of breath, cyanosis: increased incidence of congenital heart defect (*eg*, tetralogy of Fallot, truncus arteriosis, interrupted aortic arch).

Seizures: hypocalcemic.

Feeding difficulties: increased incidence of palatal abnormalities, congenital heart defect.

Failure to thrive.

Signs

Characteristic facies: hypertelorism, low-set simple ears, micrognathia, short upper-lip philtrum.

Cyanosis, heart murmur: congenital heart defect.

Palatal abnormalities: cleft palate, velopharyngeal insufficiency (hypernasal speech, nasal regurgitation, feeding difficulties).

Nonverbal learning disability.

Investigations

Culture infection site(s): tracheal aspirates, stool cultures.

Complete blood count: with differential and platelet count.

Endocrine evaluation: low calcium, elevated phosphorus, absent-to-low parathyroid hormone.

Cardiology evaluation

Chest radiograph: invisible thymus, cardiomegaly, conotruncal abnormalities.

Electrocardiogram.

Echocardiogram.

Immunologic abnormalities

Cell-mediated immunodeficiency.

Low absolute lymphocyte count.

Diminished total T-cell numbers.

Abnormal T-cell proliferation in vitro: mitogens and/or antigens.

Small proportion have markedly impaired T-cell function.

Humoral immunodeficiency: occasionally.

Hypergammaglobulinemia: rare.

Hypogammaglobulinemia: immunoglobulin-A (IgA) deficiency, delayed development of responsiveness to protein antigens (*eg*, tetanus and diphtheria titers).

Normal immunologic functions.

Complement system.

Phagocytes: neutrophils, monocytes, macrophages, eosinophils.

Complications

Cardiac mortality and morbidity.

Infections.

Seizures.

Increased risk for autoimmune disease.

Differential diagnosis

Cell-mediated immunodeficiency.
Severe combined immunodeficiency (interleukin-2–receptor deficiency, abnormal signal transduction, adenosine deaminase deficiency, purine nucleoside phosphorylase deficiency).
Bare lymphocyte syndrome.
Wiskott–Aldrich syndrome.
Ataxia–telangiectasia.
Cartilage hair hypoplasia.
HIV infection.
Congenital heart defect without immunodeficiency or other possible components of field defect.

Etiology

• Clinical surveys show that up to 90% of patients with Di George syndrome have a deletion of chromosomal region in 22q11. This deletion is described as a field defect that is associated with a range of problems, including immunodeficiency and congenital heart disease.

Epidemiology

• Leading cause is deletion of chromosome 22q11 deletion; occurs in 1:3000–4000 live births (most sporadic mutations, some familial).
• Teratogens (retinoic acid, maternal diabetes).

Treatment

Diet and lifestyle

• Until presence and severity of immunodeficiency are defined, carry out isolation precautions and administer only irradiated, cytomegalovirus-negative blood products.

• Among those with immunodeficiency, most have mild defect (which will normalize by 1 year of age); therefore, a normal lifestyle is recommended for most children.

Pharmacologic treatment

Bactrim: for *Pneumocytis carnii* penumonia prophylaxis in those with severe immunodeficiency.

Varicella zoster immune globulin: consider for chickenpox exposure and acyclovir chickenpox infection.

Other treatment options

Thymic or bone marrow transplant: for severe cases of immunodeficiency
Intravenous gamma globulin.

Treatment aims

To repair cardiac defect.
To aggressively manage infections.
To correct calcium abnormalities.
To correct cleft palate.
To conduct speech and language therapy.
To carefully document immunodeficiency and reassess degree of cell-mediated and humoral abnormalities.

Prognosis

Normalization of immunologic studies by 1 year of age in 90% of patients.

Follow-up and management

• Recommend reevaluation of cellular and humoral immune system at regular intervals until complete function is documented. Once normalization occurs, no further immunologic evaluation or restrictions are warranted. Management of other associated field defects.

Special considerations

No live viral vaccines for at least first year of life.
Decrease exposure to sources of infection.

General references

Bastian J, Law S, Vogler L, et al.: Prediction of persistent immunodeficiency in the Di George anomaly. *J Pediatr* 1989, 115:391–396.

Driscoll DA, Sullivan KE: Di George syndrome: a chromosome 22q11.2 deletion syndrome. *Primary Immunodeficiency Diseases: A Molecular and Genetic Approach.* In press; 1997.

Hong R: Disorders of the T cell system. In *Immunologic Disorders in Infants and Children*, ed 4. Edited by Stiehm ER. WB Saunders: Philadelphia; 1996:339–343.

Diagnosis

Symptoms

• Well-controlled diabetic patients having an operation have no symptoms.

Thirst and polyuria: indicating poor control in patients with any type of diabetes.

Nausea and abdominal pain: indicating very poor control in insulin-dependent patients.

Signs

• Tachycardia, ketosis, dehydration, and hypotension are signs of poor diabetic control in insulin-dependent patients; these will most probably develop after the operation if preoperative control of diabetes was poor.

Investigations [1,2]

For elective surgery

Blood glucose profile: 2 days before patient has major operation; hemoglobin A_{1c}.

• Other investigations are the same as for nondiabetic patients.

For emergency surgery

Blood glucose measurement: to assess hyperglycemia.

Electrolytes, blood urea nitrogen analysis: to assess renal function and electrolyte balance.

Blood gas analysis: to assess acid-base balance.

Complications

Cardiovascular problems: particularly myocardial infarction; the main perioperative causes of death in diabetic patients (rare in childhood).

Infection and poor wound healing: in poorly controlled diabetic patients [3].

Differential diagnosis

Acute surgical abdominal disorders can be confused with severely decompensated diabetes in insulin-dependent patients: a medical opinion is essential.

Etiology

• The stress response to surgery and anesthesia is characterized by hyperglycemia, suppression of insulin release, and insulin resistance.

• This stress response is caused by increases in cortisol, catecholamines, and other counterregulatory hormones.

• The stress response is greater with major surgery.

Epidemiology

• Fifty percent of diabetic patients have operations at some point in their lives.

• Patients with macrovascular disease will probably have several operations.

Treatment

Diet and lifestyle

• Major operations are often followed by a period of relative or absolute starvation: adequate energy intake and insulin must be supplied to diabetic patients because insulin depletion leads to severe catabolic disorders.

• Breakfast and oral agents are omitted if the operation is in the morning.

• If the operation is minor, eating and oral agents can soon be restarted.

Pharmacologic treatment [1,2]

• In most cases children with diabetes will need glucose insulin infusion for 12–24 hours before surgery.

• Regional anesthesia does not produce the same degree of stress response as general anesthesia.

• Infections should be treated aggressively by intravenous antibiotics.

For non–insulin-dependent diabetes (preoperative)

• Metformin (which may cause lactive acidosis) and chlorpropamide (because its long action may lead to hypoglycemia) should be avoided.

Standard dosage	Shorter-acting sulfonylureas (*eg*, glyburide, 2.5–20 mg daily, or glipizide) 2.5–20 mg daily.
Special points	Blood glucose concentration must be monitored.
Main side effects	Hypoglycemia.

For non–insulin-dependent diabetes (perioperative)

• Intravenous solutions containing glucose should be avoided unless hypoglycemia is a risk.

• If the operation is major, treatment should be the same as for insulin-dependent diabetes until the stress response of surgery is finished.

For insulin-dependent diabetes (preoperative)

• Preoperative admission for stabilization may be needed to achieve a blood glucose concentration of 100–180 mg/dL.

• If control is good, the insulin regimen need not be changed until the day of surgery; if control is poor before a meal, short-acting insulin achieves rapid metabolic control.

• Blood glucose concentration must be monitored, *e.g.*, intraoperatively and in recovery room.

• The main side effect is hypoglycemia.

For insulin-dependent diabetes (perioperative)

Standard dosage	Continuous i.v. R insulin by infusion pump at 0.02–0.05 U/kg 1 hour together with D10 at maintenance rates.; monitor blood glucose every 30–60 minutes; adjust insulin infusion to maintain blood glucose 100–180 mg/dL.
Special points	The insulin infusion must be continued until the patient's first full meal, when s.c. insulin should be started 30 minutes prior to cessation of insulin infusion; insulin needs will probably be higher than usual.

Treatment aims

To maintain blood glucose at 100–180 mg/dL during the operation.

Prognosis

Mortality should be similar to that in nondiabetic patients.

Follow-up and management

• Blood glucose should be monitored 3–4 times daily before the operation.

• During and early after an operation, blood glucose should be monitored at least hourly.

• Creatinine and electrolytes should be measured daily, and any deficiencies replaced.

Timing of surgery

• Routine surgery should be postponed in newly diagnosed diabetic patients until good control is attained.

• Acute surgical conditions may lead to ketoacidosis; if possible, surgery should be delayed until metabolic control is achieved.

• Surgery should be done in the morning if possible.

Special situations

Cardiac surgery: Hypothermic bypass surgery with pump priming and inotropic drugs leads to marked insulin resistance and much higher insulin needs.

Pregnancy: control of diabetes during cesaren section is critical for mother and fetus.

• The rapidly changing insulin need makes a separate infusion line for insulin essential.

Key references

1. Clark JDA, Currie J, Hartog M: Management of diabetes in surgery: a survey of current practice by anaesthetists. *Diabetic Med* 1992, **9**:271–274.
2. Gill GV: Surgery and diabetes mellitus. In *Textbook of Diabetes*, vol 2. Edited by Pickup J, Williams G. Oxford: Blackwell Scientific Publications; 1991:820–825.
3. Sawyer RG, Pruett TL: Wound infections. *Surg Clin North Am* 1994, **74**:523–524

Diabetes insipidus

Diagnosis

Symptoms
Polyuria and polydipsia.

Enuresis and nocturnal thirst.

Signs
Urine output: often greater than 2 L/d.

Poor growth and weight gain.

Signs of dehydration: occur quickly in children with diabetes insipidus (DI) if access to water is denied.

Neurologic findings: including decreased visual fields and papilloedema.

Investigations
Biochemical studies: to evaluate glucose, calcium, urea, creatinine as well as sodium and potassium.

Morning urine osmolality twice as great as simultaneously obtained serum osmolality indicates lack of DI.

• Water deprivation over 8 hours, performed in the hospital, demonstrating that urine osmolality is fixed or rises only slightly while serum osmolality continues to increase to levels above 305 mOs indicates DI. A response to vasopressin indicates central DI.

Complications
Hypernatremic dehydration and shock.

Poor growth in inadequately treated children.

Differential diagnosis
Diabetes mellitus.
Renal disease.
Hypercalcemia.
Psychogenic water drinking.
Hypothalamic hypodipsia.
Cerebral salt wasting.

Etiology
Familial vasopressin deficiency (autosomal dominant).
Familial DI associated with diabetes mellitus, optic nerve hypoplasia, and deafness (DIDMOAD).
Histiocytosis.
Brain tumors, especially germinoma, and after brain tumor surgery.
Head trauma.

Epidemiology
• The most common cause of DI in children is due to brain tumor or brain tumor surgery.
• Histiocytosis is also a frequent cause in childhood.

Treatment

Lifestyle

• The child must be allowed access to water and toilet facilities, including permission during school to leave the classroom as needed.

Pharmacologic treatment

Standard dosage	Desmopressin (DDAVP), 0.05 mL (5 µg) nasally at night and increase as needed to twice a day dosing; titrate to a dose sufficient to control polyuria.
Special points	Needs to be titrated to an appropriate dose for control of polyuria.
	DDAVP tablets can be used for children requiring moderate doses (usually < 20 µg/d) and old enough to take tablets. The dose in tablet form is usually 0.1–0.2 mg twice daily but titrate starting with 0.1 mg tablets.

Treatment aims

To prevent hypernatremic dehydration. To permit normal fluid intake and output.

Prognosis

Good as long as medication is taken and water is always available.

Follow-up and management

• Children should be seen at 6-mo intervals to monitor weight gain and linear growth.
• Electrolytes should be monitored during illness.

General references

Robinson AG, Verbalis JG: Diabetes insipidus. *Curr Ther Endocrinol Metab* 1994, **5:**1–6.

Bode HH: Disorders of the posterior pituitary. In *Clinical Pediatric Endocrinology.* Edited by Kaplan SA. Philadelphia: WB Saunders; 1990:63–86.

Diagnosis

Symptoms

• Symptoms usually of short duration (days to weeks), especially at younger ages; may not be mentioned by child or recognized by parents.

Polyuria.

Polydipsia.

Weight loss.

Decreased appetite more common than polyphagia in children.

Lethargy.

Diabetic ketoacidosis or coma: if disease unrecognized, symptoms more severe and progress to coma, vomiting, abdominal pain, air hunger.

Signs

Initially: none present.

Later: mild dehydration, weight loss, fruity odor of ketones on breath, sever dehydration, shock Kussmaul respiration, coma.

Investigations

Urinalysis: shows glucose and (usually) ketones; if positive, immediate follow-up is required.

Blood glucose and serum Na, K, HCO_3, urea: glucose usually >400 mg dL, occasionally >1000 mg/dL; HCO_3 may be <10 mEq/L.

Arterial blood gases: important if severe acidosis suspected; pH may be <7.1.

Complications

Hypoglycemia ("insulin reaction").

Late complications: rare before 10–20 years duration; reduce life expectancy by one third; intensive treatment to achieve improved glycemia control reduces risk, but does not prevent, all late complications.

Retinopathy: may require laser phototherapy.

Nephropathy: microalbuminuria progressing to proteinuria and renal failure; slowed by treatment of hypertension, especially angiotensin-converting inhibitors.

Neuropathy: peripheral sensory, autonomic.

Accelerated atherosclerosis: major cause of death.

Differential diagnosis

Any condition manifest by the following symptoms:

Nausea, vomiting.

Polyuria or frequent urination, relapsed bedwetting.

Polydipsia.

Coma.

Etiology

Genetic susceptibility associated especially with HLA-DR3 and -DR4.

Mechanism involves autoimmune destruction of pancreatic islets.

"Triggering event" (e.g., viral, environmental) not known.

Epidemiology

Prevalence is 1:300 by age 18 y.

Most common in individuals of northern European origin.

Age of onset: 6 mo to 40 y; two thirds before 18 y; peak age, 10–12 y.

Treatment

Diet and lifestyle

• Dietary training is essential: diet should emphasize consistency of carbohydrate intake and timing of meals; usually three meals, bedtime snack, morning and afternoon snacks except in later adolescence.

• Diet composition is similar to standards for nondiabetics.

• There are no restrictions on physical exercise, but precautions needed for possible hypoglycemia.

• Children must always carry glucose tablets in case of hypoglycemia; parents must be taught how to give glucagon for emergency severe hypoglycemia.

Pharmacologic treatment

• Insulin is always needed. Mostly biosynthetic human insulins are available, but pork or beef–pork insulins are still in use.

• The following types of insulin are used:

Ultra-short-acting: lispro (Humalog®)

Short-acting: R (regular).

Intermediate-acting: N (NPH) or L (lente).

Long-acting: U (ultralente).

Premixed: 70/30 (70% N, 30% R).

Standard dosage	Insulin, 3–4 injections per day of mixed short and intermediate-acting insulins with home glucose monitoring 3–5 times per day (*see* types of insulin *above*).
Special points	Selected, highly motivated adolescents may choose continuous subcutaneous insulin infusion by pump.

Treatment aims
To restore normal health and well-being.
To avoid severe hypoglycemia while achieving optimal glycemic control.
To delay onset of late complications.

Prognosis
Morbidity and mortality from diabetic ketoacidosis or severe hypoglycemia are rare.
Excellent and improving in short and middle term.
Late complications associated with one third reduction in life span.
Hypoglycemia is major cause of short-term morbidity.
Major causes of death are coronary artery disease and renal failure.

Follow-up and management
Regular follow-up 3–4 times yearly at diabetes specialty clinic with nurse-educator and dietitian needed.
Monitor glycemic control with hemoglobin A_{1c} 3–4 times yearly.
Patient/family monitoring of blood glucose 3–5 times daily and frequent self-adjustment of insulin doses.
Thorough diabetes training by diabetes-educator and dietitian is essential.

Patient support
Juvenile Diabetes Foundation, 432 Park Avenue South, New York, NY 10016-8103. (800) 533 2873.
American Diabetes Association, 1660 Duke Street, Alexandria, VA 22314; tel: 1-800-ADA-DISC. (800) 232-3472.

General references
DCCT Research Group: The effect of intensive treatment of diabetes on the development and progression of long-term complications in insulin dependent diabetes. *N Engl J Med* 1993, **329:**977–986.

Sperling MA: Diabetes mellitus. In *Pediatric Endocrinology.* Edited by Sperling MA. Philadelphia: WB Saunders; 1996:229–263.

Diabetes mellitus, non–insulin-dependent

Diagnosis

Symptoms

• Fifty percent of patients are symptomatic, 50% found on routine or accidental screening.

• Common symptoms often manifest over many months or years and include the following:

Polyuria, polydipsia.

Pruritus vulvae or balanitis.

Weight loss, tiredness, blurred vision.

Hyperglycemic nonkeratotic coma, with severe dehydration or hyperosmolality: rare manifestation.

Signs

• Generally no signs are manifest.

• Patients may present with the following:

Obesity.

Foot ulceration or infection: rare in children.

Diabetic retinopathy or peripheral neuropathy: rare in childhood.

Signs of secondary causes of diabetes: *eg*, acromegaly, Cushing's disease, thyrotoxicosis.

Investigations

Blood glucose measurement: random capillary/venous blood glucose concentration > mg/dL in symptomatic patient is diagnostic; two random values or any fasting value > mg/dL is also diagnostic.

Glucose tolerance test: needed when diagnosis in doubt. After a 3-day high-carbohydrate (> g/day) diet then overnight fast, patient takes 75 g glucose solution. Plasma glucose is measured before glucose administration then every 30 minutes for 2 hours. Plasma glucose interpretation: ≥ mg/dL at 2 hours and any ; other time diagnostic for diabetes mellitus; ≥ 200 mg/dL before 2 hours but > 140 mg/dL and < 140 mg/dL fasting is defined as impaired glucose tolerance; > 200 mg/dL at 1 hour but < 140 mg/dL at 2 hours is indeterminate and may require retesting.

Measurement of hemoglobin A_{1c}: raised concentration.

Measurement of iron and total iron-binding capacity: to rule out hemochromatosis.

Measurement of thyroxine and thyroid-stimulating hormone: to rule out thyrotoxicosis.

• Glycosuria alone and blood strip readings are never diagnostic.

Complications

• Complications are often present in older adults at the time of diagnosis (after years of hyperglycemia), but not in children.

Diabetic retinopathy: only affects vision if near macula; macular edema frequent with major reduction of visual acuity; proliferative affects fewer but threatens vision by vitreous hemorrhage/fibrosis; both treated by laser.

Diabetic nephropathy: proteinuria is marker for high cardiovascular risk, but not necessarily progressive renal impairment; can be slowed by vigorous antihypertensive treatment especially with angiotensin-converting enzyme inhibitors; end-stage failure can be treated by continuous ambulatory peritoneal dialysis or transplantation.

Large-vessel disease (coronary, cerebrovascular, peripheral: much more common especially when patient has nephropathy; possibly more diffuse than nondiabetic large-vessel disease, but otherwise generally similar; these, especially coronary artery disease, are major causes of premature death.

Differential diagnosis

• Diagnosis is not usually a problem, after diabetes mellitus has been considered; however, possible errors include the following:

Urinary tract infection.

Prostatic hyperplasia.

Vaginal prolapse.

Primary polydipsia.

Diabetes insipidus.

Etiology [1]

• The cause of non–insulin-dependent diabetes mellitus is unknown; the disorder may be part of a constellation with hypertension and hyperlipidemia (Reaven's syndrome, syndrome X).

• Patients may have a mixture of "relative" insulin deficiency and insulin resistance, contributions of the two varying widely among individuals.

• Very rarely, patients have insulin receptor abnormalities, or dormantly inherited defects of insulin secretion (maturity onset diabetes of youth [MODY]).

• A strong familial component is evident, but the disorder is not directly inherited.

• A marked link with obesity is seen.

Epidemiology

• The prevalence varies widely among races, with some populations having a prevalence of > 50% by the age of 50 years.

• The U.S. prevalence of diagnosed diabetes is approx 3%, although an additional 3% may go undiagnosed.

• The disease is six times more common in Asians and about twice as common in Afro-Caribbeans.

• It is probably becoming more common in the developed world, and the frequency in the U.S. is increasing with the increased incidence of obesity.

Treatment

Diet and lifestyle

• The diet should be high in unrefined carbohydrate, low in simple sugars, with high fiber and low fat, spread throughout the day.

• Patients should aim at reducing excess body weight.

• Patients should engage in physical exercise and resume full activities; minimal limitations for those on some drugs include not driving commercial vehicles.

Pharmacologic treatment [2]

Diet modifications alone should be used initially unless the patient is losing too much weight or is seriously symptomatic, in which case diet should be supplemented by pharmacologic treatment.

Sulfonylurea

• These drugs increase insulin response to glucose and tend to cause weight gain.

Standard dosage	Glyburdie, 2.5–20 mg orally daily, given once or twice each day.
	Glipizide, 2.5–20 mg orally daily, given once or twice each day.
Contraindications	Breastfeeding, porphyria, pregnancy; causation in elderly patients and those with renal or hepatic failure.
Special points	Used only in conjunction with a diet.
Main drug interactions	Few of major clinical relevance (*see* manufacturer's current prescribing information).
Main side effects	Hypoglycemia is common; otherwise occasionally rashes, jaundice, headache.

Biguanide

• Metformin reduces hepatic gluconeogenesis and probably decreases carbohydrate absorption.

Standard dosage	Metformin, 1–2.5 g daily in divided doses.
Contraindications	Hepatic or renal impairment (creatinine > 1.4 in men or 1.3 in women), heart failure, pregnancy.
Special points	Does not cause hypoglycemia; may rarely cause lactic acidosis. Should be discontinued 2 days before and 2 days after any radiologic study using i.v. contrast.
Main drug interactions	Alcohol dependence may predispose to lactic acidosis.
Main side effects	Flatulence, anorexia, diarrhea, sometimes transient.

Insulin

Insulin is indicated for symptomatic or uncontrolled diabetes mellitus despite maximal oral agents, in addition to diet. Usually, it is needed only once or twice daily; a longer-acting formulation may be used to control basal hyperglycemia. *See* Diabetes mellitus, insulin-dependent *for details*.

Other options

• Acarbose, 50 mg 3 times daily (alpha-glucosidase inhibitor) decreases rate of glucose absorption, thereby reducing postprandial glycemia; recent introduction.

• Troglitazane increases peripheral insulin sensitivity: recently introduced, little experience in children.

Treatment aims

To restore normal well-being.

To achieve optimal glycemic control without significant hypoglycemia.

To provide patient education and self-care.

To prevent complications.

Prognosis

• Mortality is increased as a result of excess cardiovascular disease, myocardial infarction, stroke, and peripheral vascular disease.

• Morbidity is due to the same causes and also to retinopathy, renal disease, and foot ulceration.

• Oral hypoglycemics have not been proved to reduce mortality or morbidity.

Follow-up and management

• Patients need long-term follow-up for treatment aims and screening for development of complications.

• Glycosylated hemoglobin is an objective marker of glycemic control.

Patient support

American Diabetes Association, 1660 Duke Street, Alexandria, VA 22314; tel: 1-800-ADA-DISC.

Key references

1. Day JF: *The Diabetes Handbook: Non Insulin-Dependent Diabetes.* London: Thorsons; 1992.

2. Tattersall RB, Gale EAM, eds.: *Diabetes: Clinical Management.* **Edinburgh: Churchill Livingstone; 1990.**

3. Glaser NS: Non-insulin-dependent diabetes mellitus in childhood and adolescence. *Pediatr Clin North Am* 1997, **44:**307–338.

Diabetic ketoacidosis

Diagnosis

Symptoms
Polyuria.
Polydipsia.
Abdominal pain or vomiting.
Air hunger.
Lethargy.
Lethargy progressing to coma.

Signs
Hyperpnea (Kussmaul respirations).
Tachycardia.
Dehydration.
Shock.

Investigations
Blood glucose: shows hyperglycemia (may be >1000 mg/dL).

Urinalysis: large glycosuria and large ketonuria.

Electrolyte analysis: low bicarbonate (<10 mEq/L); sodium and potassium may vary, but normal or low potassium may indicate increased risk of hypokalemia.

Arterial blood gas: severe metabolic acidosis with low pH and P_{CO_2}.

Complications
• There is a risk of morbidity or mortality from acidosis or shock.

Cerebral edema: during first 24 hours of therapy; cause unknown, but concerns that it may be related to too-rapid lowering of blood glucose or excessive fluid administration.

Hypokalemia: due to a combination of severe potassium depletion and correction of acidemia; may cause cardiac arrhythmia, arrest.

Differential diagnosis
• Diagnosis is not usually a problem, once possibility of diabetes has been considered.

• Rare variant in childhood is nonketotic, hyperglycemic coma—treatment is similar, but more focus on dehydration and less on acidosis.

• Possible confusion includes stress or epinephrine-induced hyperglycemia and ketonemia.

Etiology
• Primary etiology is insulin deficiency, eg, new-onset diabetes mellitus; onset often associated with a factor that increases insulin requirement, eg, intercurrent infection.

• Rarely caused by purposeful omission of insulin.

Epidemiology
• Illness presents in approximately one third of newly diagnosed diabetes.

• With appropriate management, insulin may be avoided in established diabetes.

• Recurrent episodes of ketoacidosis usually indicate major problems with psychosocial adjustment and/or compliance.

Treatment

Diet and lifestyle

• Patients should remain npo at bedrest until dehydration and acidosis are corrected.

• Intensive care unit admission may be required, depending on severity or risk factors such as hypokalemia or blood glucose >1000 mg/dL.

• Consider cardiac monitor if potassium low.

• Monitor vital signs and state of consciousness (*eg*, Glasgow coma scale) hourly.

Pharmacologic treatment

Intravenous fluid and electrolytes

Standard dosage
For approximate deficits: water, 100–150 mL/kg; potassium, 10 mEq/kg; sodium, 1 mEq/kg.

First hour: 10–30 mL/kg isotonic saline for intravascular volume depletion and shock.

First 8 hours: replace one half of water and sodium deficits plus maintenance; add potassium phosphate or chloride to solutions at 40 mEq/L—higher concentrations may be needed if serum potassium declines; add 5%–10% dextrose when blood glucose <250–300 mg/dL.

Second 16 hours: replace remaining one half of water and sodium deficits plus maintenance; continue potassium and glucose additions as above; replace excessive urinary output over 2 mL/kg/h or over 35 mL/m^2/h.

Bicarbonate therapy

• Bicarbonate therapy is usually not needed, but consider it if arterial pH <7.0–7.1 or respiratory compensation in doubt. If needed, 2 mEq/kg infused over 1 hour will raise serum bicarbonate approximately 4 mEq/L; may epeat if necessary until serum bicarbonate is 10–12 mEq/L.

Insulin

• Begin within first hour of fluid resuscitation a continuous low-dose intravenous infusion of regular aspirin, 0.1 U/kg/h; higher doses are occasionally needed. When recovered enough to begin full meals, administration of subcutaneous regular insulin every 4–6 hours may begin.

Treatment aims

To correct dehydration and shock.
To correct metabolic acidosis.
To identify and treat precipitating cause, eg, infection.
To avoid complications such as cerebral edema, hypokalemia.

Prognosis

• Prognosis for full recovery is excellent.
• Mortality rate is approximately 1%–2%.

Follow-up and management

• Carefully monitor changes in clinical and laboratory status during correction of ketoacidosis as outlined.
• Adjust intravenous therapy as necessary to prevent hypoglycemia or too rapid fall in blood glucose, hypokalemia, excessive urine losses.

General references

Sperling MA: Diabetes mellitus. In *Pediatric Endocrinology*. Edited by Sperling MA. Philadelphia: WB Saunders; 1996:229–263.

Sperling MA: Aspects of the etiology, prediction, and prevention of insulin-dependent diabetes mellitus in childhood. *Pediatr Clin North Am* 1997, **44**:269–284.

Diagnosis

Symptoms
- The neonate may be hypotonic.
- If congenital heart disease is present, symptoms relating to that may occur.

Signs
Congenital heart disease (approximately one third): endocardial cushion defect, ventricular septal defect, patent ductus arteriosus, atrial septal defect.

Dysmorphic features: flat face and occiput, upslanting palpebral fissures, epicanthus, small ears, protruding tongue, single palmar crease (present in 40%), extra nuchal skin, clinodactyly, wide space between first and second toes. It is important to note that no single clinical feature is required or pathognomonic for the diagnosis of Down syndrome.

Hypotonia.

Increased flexibility of joints.

Investigations
- Karyotype is required even if the child has absolutely classic features of Down syndrome in order to determine the type of trisomy 21 in each child (*see* Etiology). A diagnostic index (*see* Rex and Preus in General References) has been developed based on clinical features that may be helpful in assessing infants before the karyotype is completed.

- All individuals with Down syndrome should have a screening echocardiogram because cardiac disease is the major cause of early mortality

- An ophthalmologic examination should be performed to assess for myopia, nystagmus, and strabismus. Cataracts are occasionally congenital but are present in a large number of affected adults.

- Thyroid function tests beginning in childhood and continuing at regular intervals. There is an increased risk for goiter, hyperthyroidism, and hypothyroidism.

Complications
Gastrointestinal anomalies: tracheoesophageal fistula, duodenal atresia, pyloric stenosis, Hirschsprung's disease, imperforate anus. Many of these conditions present in the neonatal period.

Atlantoaxial instability: although asymptomatic atlantoaxial instability is common, it rarely leads to spinal cord compression or other symptoms.

Frequent sinopulmonary infections, otitis media, periodontal disease.

Thyroid dysfunction: hyperthyroidism, goiter, hypothyroidism.

Leukemia: occurs in 1%, most frequently acute lymphoblastic leukemia.

Differential diagnosis
- The phenotype of Down syndrome is distinctive. The clinical features are occasionally subtle, and a karyotype should be performed if the diagnosis is considered. There is some overlap with the clinical presentation of hypothyroidism and Zellweger syndrome.

Etiology
Trisomy for all or a portion of chromosome 21: approximately 97% of cases are due to free trisomy 21 (including mosaics); 3% are due to a translocation in which one of the copies of chromosome 21 is translocated to another acrocentric chromosome (14, 15, 21, 22, or rarely 13); if a translocation is detected in the child, parental chromosomes must be analyzed to assess if one of the parents is a carrier of a balanced translocation.

- Approximately one third of affected children with a translocation will have a carrier parent.

Epidemiology
- The majority of cases of Down syndrome are due to nondisjunction of maternal meiosis I. The risk of having a child with free trisomy 21 increases with maternal age and is 1:909 at age 30 years, 1:394 at age 35, and 1 in 112 at age 40. The recurrence risk for a woman with a child with free trisomy 21 is ~1% plus the age-adjusted risk. The recurrence risk for Down syndrome in a child of a carrier father of a translocation involving chromosome 21 and chromosomes 14 or 22 is 2.5%, and 10% for a carrier mother. If either parent carries a 21/21 translocation, all children will have Down syndrome.

Characteristics of trisomy 13 and trisomy 18

Trisomy 13 occurs at a frequency of 1 in 20,000 births and is characterized by ophthalmologic abnormalities (microphthalmia, colobomas, retinal dysplasia), forebrain abnormalities (including holoprosencephaly), cleft lip/palate, posterior scalp defects, congenital heart disease, polydactyly, and rocker-bottom feet. Most children die in the first month, and those who survive have severe mental retardation.

Trisomy 18 occurs at a frequency of 1 in 8000 births and is characterized by a prominent occiput, short sternum, congenital heart disease, clenched fists with the index finger overlapping the third and the fifth finger overlapping the fourth, and rocker-bottom feet. Many die in the neonatal period, and the majority do not survive beyond 1 year. Survivors have severe mental retardation.

Treatment

General Information

• Treatment is oriented to the specific organ systems involved in each child. The more common problems that become apparent in the neonatal period are described in the Investigations and Complications sections. Beyond the newborn period, children with Down syndrome are at increased risk for several problems, and the pediatrician must monitor for the development of these conditions. There is an increased risk of serous otitis media, and hearing should be checked at least annually. Ophthalmologic abnormalities such as strabismus, cataracts, and nystagmus should also be assessed. Thyroid function tests should be performed regularly.

• The child should be referred to early intervention services so that appropriate physical therapy can be instituted. Families should also be supplied with the names of Down syndrome support groups.

• Although there have been occasional reports of medications that may be of benefit for affected individuals, these results have not been duplicated in well-controlled clinical trials. At the present time, there is no specific pharmacologic therapy that has been reproducibly shown to be beneficial for individuals with Down syndrome.

Prognosis/natural history

Developmental delay/mental retardation: gross motor delay is apparent in infancy, but this improves and the children are able to achieve most early motor milestones. However, cognitive development continues to lag during childhood, and the adult IQ is generally 25–50.

Short stature: generally apparent by age 3.

General references

American Academy of Pediatrics Committee on Genetics: Health supervision for children with Down syndrome. *Pediatrics* 1994, 93:855–860.

American Academy of Pediatrics Committee on Sports Medicine and Fitness: Atlantoaxial instability in Down syndrome: subject review. *Pediatrics* 1995, 96:151–154.

Kallen B, Mastroiaocovo P, Robert E: Major congenital malformations in Down syndrome. *Am J Med Genet* 1996, 65:160–166.

Peuschel SM: Clinical aspects of Down syndrome from infancy to adulthood. *Am J Med Genet* 1990, 7(suppl):52–56.

Rex AP, Preus M: A diagnostic index for Down syndrome. *J Pediatr* 1982, 100:903–906.

Diagnosis

• Earache is one of the most common complaints in childhood; virtually every child has had this problem. Although there is a relatively small set of conditions that cause the complaint, management can become quite difficult.

Symptoms

• The complaint of earache is one that produces an exquisite response on the part of the pediatric patient. A painful ear frequently wakes a child from sleep and produces an abundance of tears. When this presentation occurs it is caused by otitis media and a stretch on the highly sensitive tympanic membrane. The recumbent position may indeed exacerbate the pain.

• Pain that is more gradual in onset may be caused by lesser amounts of middle ear fluid or pus or from one of the other causes of ear pain.

• Fever and nasal rhinorrhea may or may not be present. The child may be lethargic, have altered sleep patterns, and unsteady gait due to an alteration in balance. Parents may also observe an acute decrease in hearing.

Signs

Red, distorted, immobile tympanic membrane: are classic signs of otitis media, but the classic findings are not always seen; the diagnosis should not be based solely on the color of the ear drums.

Pain on motion of the pinna: suggests otitis externa and usually pus will be present in the external auditory canal; finding pus in the canal and a somewhat relieved patient in less pain suggests that the otitis media has perforated and the stretch on the eardrum relieved.

• Other findings include foreign bodies and impacted cerumen that may be causing pain. Parents may attempt to clean the child's ears prior to the visit and unwittingly produce a traumatic abrasion to the external canal. Other causes of ear pain do not relate to the ear and thus a complete examination must be performed.

Investigations

• The vast majority of cases will be diagnosed by the history and physical examination alone, particularly if pneumatic otoscopy is performed. If there are questions about the state of the tympanic membrane, then tympanometry may be used. Hearing screens are not helpful in the acute phase.

Complications

• The most important complication is spread of infection to adjacent structures such as meninges or mastoids. Chronic otitis media can produce hearing loss and chronic speech and language delay.

• Failure to diagnose otitis externa may lead to infection in the adjacent soft tissues.

Differential diagnosis

Beyond otitis media and otitis externa, other causes of ear pain include:
Impacted cerumen.
Trauma to the external canal.
Cholesteatoma.
Foreign bodies.
Tumors.
• There may also be causes outside the ear, where referred pain triggers the sensation of ear pain. These include:
Dental pain from abscess, impacted molars, or gingivostomatitis.
Pharygitis or peritonsillar abscess.
Cervical adenitis.
Sinusitis.
Cervical spine disease.

Etiology

• The most common bacterial causes are *Streptococcus pneumoniae*, non-typeable *Haemophilus influenzae*, and *Moraxella catarrhalis*.
• About one-third of aspirates from the middle ear are viral and are presumed viral in cause.
• Beyond microorganisms, eustachian tube dysfunction and other anatomic considerations also play a role in the cause.

Epidemiology

• Otitis media accounts for more then 20 million office visits per year and 42% of all antimicrobial use. These numbers are increasing over time.
• Some subgroups in the population (Native American, Eskimo) appear to have higher rates as do some individual families.
• The severity and chronicity of otitis is inversely correlated with the age of the first episode.

Other information

• Other factors that may play a role in the etiology include parental smoking, bottle propping, seasonal allergies, and attendance at a daycare center.

Treatment

Lifestyle management
• Smoking cessation in the house and restraint from bottle propping are helpful. If the child has other manifestations of allergic diathesis, then an allergist should be consulted about appropriate and reasonable environmental changes.

Pharmacologic treatment
• Pharmacologic treatment is currently the mainstay of therapy. The antibiotics change depending on resistance patterns that emerge.

Current first-line therapy Amoxicillin, 25–50 mg/kg/d in 3 doses.

Second-line therapies Trimethoprim-sulfamethoxizole, 8 mg/kg/d in 2 doses;

Amoxicillin-clavulanate, 20–40 mg/kg/d in 2 doses;

Azithromycin, 10 mg/kg on day 1 and 5 mg/kg on days 2–5.

Third-line agents Cefaclor, 40 mg/kg/d.

Loracabef, 30 mg/kg/d.

Cefpodoxime, 10 mg/kg/d.

Cefibuten, 9 mg/kg/d.

• Some recent studies have shown spontaneous cure rates of otitis media not much different than cure rates with therapy. With changes prompted by resistance patterns of microorganisms and cost-containment, one strategy that may prevail in the future is to allow simple infections to "run their course."

• If patients respond to the initial therapy and return to normal, no follow-up is needed. If symptoms persist after 2 weeks, they should be reexamined. Some physicians elect to see all their patients younger than 15 months in follow-up because of the implications for developing speech and language.

• For otitis externa, a topical antibacterial otic drop may be prescribed. Other causes of ear pain or referred ear pain will require specific therapy.

• If the recurrent or persistent otitis media is having an impact on speech and language development, then the timetable for referral must be moved forward.

Treatment aims
To diagnose otitis appropriately with care not to over-diagnose.

To use first-line antibiotics when indicated and more broad-spectrum agents with caution.

To follow those children with persistent symptoms.

To refer early when speech and language development is delayed or there is a demonstrable hearing loss.

Prognosis
• The prognosis is very good overall. For those families whose children have frequent and recurrent otitis, the illness can be very frustrating, time consuming, and expensive.

• For a small number of children there is the possibility of life-long hearing impairment and other complications.

• There is still controversy about the long-term impact of myringotomy tubes, so they should not be elected as a quick solution.

Follow-up and management
• Strategy for follow-up should be guided by symptoms, with special care for those children who are in the period of rapid language acquisition.

General references
Klein JO, Bluestone CD, McCracken GH (eds): New perspectives in management of otitis media *Pediatr Infect Dis J* 1994, **13(suppl):**1029–1073.

Swanson JA, Hoecker JL: Otitis media in young children. *Mayo Clin Proc* 1996, **71:**179–183.

Howie VM: Otitis media. *Pediatr Rev* 1993, **14:**320–323.

Potsic WP: The painful ear. In *Textbook of Pediatric Emergency Medicine*, edn 3. Baltimore: Williams & Wilkins; 1993, 369–371.

Eating disorders

Diagnosis

Symptoms

Weight loss more than 15% below normal.

Behavior disguised because of desire to remain undiagnosed.

Preoccupation with diets: in an adolescent of normal weight; self image as overweight.

Vomiting: with atypical symptoms.

Edema: in young women.

Fullness and bloating after meals: especially after binge eating.

Preoccupation with constipation.

Amenorrhea or irregular menstruation.

Low mood, anxiety, drug or alcohol abuse.

Sports injury.

Preoccupation with activity to burn calories.

Signs

Appears too thin.

Tooth enamel loss, caries, prostheses.

Enlarged salivary glands.

Mouth abrasions.

Callus on dorsum of hand: Russell's sign, due to gag reflex causing a bite.

Investigations

History: for psychological, nutritional, and weight-control measures.

Electrolytes: vomiting causes low potassium and high bicarbonate; laxatives cause low sodium, low potassium, and low bicarbonate; blood urea nitrogen increased with dehydration; hypoglycemia.

• Plot height and weight on a standard growth curve. Compare weight over time.

Complications

• Complications rare but may be life threating..

Gastrointestinal bleeding: superior mesenteral artery syndromes.

Cardiac dysrhythmia.

Renal failure.

Adrenal insufficiency.

Leukopenia.

Differential diagnosis

• After the history has been obtained, it is characteristic.

• Rule out physical and other psychiatric illnesses.

Anorexia nervosa.

Depression.

Schizophrenia.

Etiology [1]

• Causes include the following:

Dieting: risk increased 8-fold.

Psychosocial: poor parenting experiences, life events.

Genetic: family history of depression, obesity, and alcoholism.

Epidemiology [2]

• 3% of women between the ages of 15 and 25 y suffer from bulimia nervosa.

• The prevalence is increasing in generations born after 1950.

• The ratio of men to women is 1:10–20.

• Upper socioeconomic classes are disproportionately represented.

Treatment

Diet and lifestyle [3]
• Patients must be helped to eat a regular, well balanced diet; this is achieved by pharmacologic and nonpharmacologic treatment.

Pharmacologic treatment [1–3]
• Drugs are less effective than psychological therapy but can produce a window of remission during which psychological therapy can begin.

Standard dosage	Fluoxetine, 60 mg.
Contraindications	Hypersensitivity, renal failure, lactation, unstable epilepsy; caution in liver failure, renal impairment, cardiac disease, diabetes, pregnancy.
Main drug interactions	Monoamine oxidase inhibitors, tryptophan, tricyclic antidepressants, lithium, flecainide, encainide, vinblastine, carbamazepine.
Main side effects	Asthenia, fever, neurological effects (including headache), pharyngitis, dyspnea, rash, nausea (paradoxically).

Nonpharmacologic treatment [3,5]
• Psychological approaches are the treatment of choice because they are more effective in the short term, probably also in the long term, but hourly sessions of specialist therapy may be needed.

• The effective components include the following:

Educational: nutritional, weight control.

Behavioral: food and purging diary, prescription of regular meals, stimulus control to limit meal size, distraction or relaxation to interrupt symptomatic behaviour.

Cognitive: modification of distorted beliefs about shape and weight, strengthening of coping resources, stress management, problem solving, communication and assertiveness skills.

Treatment aims
To restore normal eating patterns.
To provide psychologic support and treatment.
To reach an early diagnosis, which leads to better outcome.

Prognosis
• 50%–60% of patients are asymptomatic after treatment. 40% have ongoing problems.
• Relapse is common in the first year after treatment.
• After 5 y, one third recover, one third have some symptoms, and one third are still affected.
• Self-harm is common in the 30% of patients with borderline personality disorders (ie, ~30% of these or ~10%–20% of all patients).
• Mortality rate is 5%–18%.

Follow-up and management
• 6-monthly follow-up is needed.

Key references
1. Kreipe RE: Eating disorders among children adn adolescents. *Pediatr Rev* 1995, **16:** 370–379.
2. Ratnasuriya RH, Eisler I, Szwukler GI, *et al.* Anorexia nervosa: outcome and prognostic factors after 20 years. *Br J Psychiatry* 1991, **158:** 495–502.
3. Fisher M, Golden NH, Kutzman DK, *et al.* Eating disorders in adolescents: a review. 1995, **16:** 420–437.

Diagnosis

Symptoms

Headache, altered mental status (delirium, lethargy, confusion), behavioral abnormality: may progress to obtundation, coma.

Speech disturbance, limb weakness, incoordination, involuntary movements: indicating focal cerebral involvement.

Seizures.

Signs

Drowsiness, confusion, irritability, coma.

Nuchal rigidity due to associated meningeal inflammation (may be absent).

Fever (may be absent).

Associated focal neurological findings: *eg*, hemiparesis, dysphasia (especially in herpes simplex encephalitis).

Ataxia, nystagmus, myoclonus, involuntary movements, extensor plantar responses.

Cranial nerve palsies: due to associated meningeal involvement (infrequent).

Evidence of systemic involvement: *eg*, cutaneous lesions in some infants with neonatal herpes simplex encephalitis.

Investigations

Cranial CT or MRI: may help to exclude other causes and may show brain edema; focal inferior temporal and orbital frontal damage with herpes simplex may take several days to become apparent (especially on noncontrast CT).

Lumbar puncture for cerebrospinal fluid (CSF) analysis: CSF is occasionally normal, but may be under increased pressure and usually shows lymphocytic pleocytosis, modestly elevated protein, and normal glucose concentration. Erythrocytes are sometimes present in necrotizing encephalitides (*eg*, due to herpes simplex). Enzyme-linked immunoassays for viral antigens and gene amplification with polymerase chain reaction are increasingly available to aid early specific diagnosis, but are not completely sensitive.

Specific viral antibody titers: showing a significant rise is helpful in retrospect.

Electroencephalography: typically shows widespread slow activity; periodic complexes or focal slowing over temporal region are particularly suggestive of herpes simplex encephalitis. Brain biopsy: is generally not necessary but is occasionally helpful when the diagnosis is in doubt (*eg*, to evaluate for tumor, parasitic or fungal infection, and so on).

Complications

Seizures and status epilepticus: often occur and require vigorous treatment.

Cerebral edema: may cause transtentorial herniation and calls for measures to reduce intracranial pressure.

Chronic neurologic residua: *eg*, mental retardation, motor or behavioral abnormalities, especially in necrotizing forms of encephalitis (*eg*, herpes simplex).

Differential diagnosis

Meningitis: bacterial, tuberculous, fungal, or viral.

Acute disseminated encephalomyelitis (may be triggered by preceding infection or vaccination, but is probably not caused by active infection of the brain).

Encephalopathy with systemic infection (eg, due to hyperpyrexia).

Metabolic encephalopathy: usually no fever, headache, or CSF abnormality.

Cerebral abscess, empyema, subdural hematoma, other mass lesions.

Neoplasm (eg, leukemia) with meningeal involvement.

Etiology

• Viral invasion of brain parenchyma causes an inflammatory reaction of varying intensity, associated with perivascular cuffing with lymphocytes and other mononuclear cells and with destruction of nerve cells and glia; hemorrhagic necrosis may occur.

Epidemiology

• Herpes simplex virus (HSV) is the most common cause of sporadic encephalitis.

• Other herpes viruses, especially herpes zoster, cytomegalovirus, and Epstein-Barr virus, are common causes, particularly when immunity is impaired, as in transplant or AIDS patients.

• Arboviral encephalitides may occur in epidemics in which mosquitoes bite humans.

• Mumps encephalitis and subacute sclerosing panencephalitis have declined in incidence with vaccination; the latter is a progressive late complication of measles infection.

• Progressive multifocal leukoencephalopathy is seen in immunosuppressed patients and is caused by a human polyoma virus.

• HIV infection may cause meningoencephalitis at seroconversion and later, a slowly progressive dementia.

Treatment

Diet and lifestyle
Not relevant.

Pharmacologic treatment
• No effective treatment is available for many of the viruses causing encephalitis; often, the specific causative virus is not identified.

• Seizures require anticonvulsant administration.

• Full supportive measures are necessary during what is often a self-limiting illness with good recovery.

• Ventilation, mannitol, and dexamethasone can be used acutely to manage edema.

• Intravenous acyclovir started early reduces the morbidity and mortality of herpes simplex encephalitis; treatment should not await the outcome of brain biopsy, which is seldom appropriate.

Standard dosage	Acyclovir, 500 mg/m^2 every 8 h (children 12 mo of age or older); 10 mg/kg/d every 8 h (children 3–12 mo of age); 10–20 mg/kg every 8 h (for neonatal HSV in term infants). Duration is 14–21 d.
Contraindications	Hypersensitivity.
Special points	Renal impairment necessitates dose reduction.
Main drug interactions	Possible interaction with zidovudine.
	Ganciclovir may be of benefit when cytomegalovirus is the probable cause.
Main side effects	*Acyclovir*: may cause transient elevation of serum BUN/creatinine.
	Ganciclovir may cause granulocytopenia or thrombocytopenia, requiring dosage reduction or discontinuation.

Prevention
• Infants with perinatal exposure to HSV require isolation if born vaginally or if the interval between rupture of membranes and delivery by caesarian section exceeds 4–6 hours. Close observation and regular cultures (every 24–48 hours, including urine, rectum, mouth, and nasopharynx) are indicated; for positive cultures, acyclovir should be administered. Prophylactic treatment with acyclovir should be considered if the maternal infection appears to be primary (*ie*, first episode).

• A mother with active herpes labialis (cold sores) or stomatitis should wear a disposable surgical mask when touching her newborn until the lesions are crusted and dried; direct contact (*eg*, kissing) is permissible only after the lesions are completely healed.

Treatment aims
To treat herpes simplex encephalitis early: this often implies presumptive treatment of patients with acyclovir if the etiologic agent is uncertain.
To prevent recurrent seizures.
To control raised intracranial pressure.
To provide optimal rehabilitation when necessary.

Prognosis
• The outcome varies with different causative viruses, the age of the patient, and associated underlying disease.
• Death and serious residual disability are frequent with herpes simplex when the diagnosis and treatment are delayed.

Follow-up and management
• Neurological rehabilitation is important for patients with residual disability.
• Rarely, relapses occur with herpes simplex encephalitis.

General references
Connelly BL, Stanberry LR: Herpes simplex virus infections in children. *Curr Opin Pediatr* 1995, 7:19–23.

O'Meara M, Ouvrier R: Viral encephalitis in children. *Curr Opin Pediatr* 1996, 6:11–15.

Diagnosis

Definition

• Encopresis (soiling) is a problem that has serious social implications for a child. The medical issues surrounding this problem are usually not complex but troubling to treat.

Symptoms

Repetitive fecal soiling that occurs without the control of the child: occuring after the child has become toilet trained, usually older than 4 years of age.

Other symptoms of note: whether the child perceives the soiling in advance of it occurring; the pattern of defecation prior to the onset of soiling; the process of toilet training; any emotional or psychological traumas such as child sexual abuse or impending divorce of the parents.

• It is important to know the timing of the onset of the problem as well as its duration.

• Evaluate the impact of the soiling on the child as far as family relationships, peer interaction, and impact on school attendance.

• A complete dietary history is important because dietary manipulation will be needed in the treatment phase.

Signs

• Examine the child for the presence of retained fecal mass; on rectal examination, note the position of the stool.

• Check for signs of lower spinal cord problems in evaluating motor strength and sensation in the lower extremities; check for bladder function; inspect the lumbosacral area for dimples or tufts of hair.

• Also evaluate the child's psychological status by looking for signs of depression, personality disorders, or other symptom complexes.

Investigations

Abdominal radiography: to document the extent and position of the retained stool.

Rectal manometrics, rectal biopsy, or studies of lower spinal cord function: will depend on the findings of the signs and symptoms evaluation, *eg*, constipation since birth will prompt a workup to rule out Hirshsprung's disease.

Complications

• The main complications to this disorder are fecal impaction causing bowel obstruction and toxic megacolon.

• Other complications are related to the severe psychological injury that may occur. It is also important not to overlook the other elements in the differential diagnosis as to do so would delay their proper treatment; this is particularly true for spinal cord tumors.

Differential diagnosis

• Most often the child with encopresis will have concomitant constipation.

• Other elements of the differential include spinal cord tumors, unrecognized Hirschsprung's disease, pelvic mass, unrecognized meningomyelocele, or psychiatric disorder.

• Although there are several elements to the differential diagnosis, usually history and physical examination make clear that the most common scenario by far is that of constipation with overflow "paradoxical" soiling.

Etiology

• The etiology of encopresis is probably multifactorial, including diet, toilet training techniques, genetics, and other behavioral characteristics such as concern for cleanliness. Clearly the issue of bowel motility is an important one. Those with naturally slow motility are probably more at risk.

Epidemiology

• About 1.5% of second-grade students may have this problem.

• Males are much more commonly affected (ratio, 6:1).

• The onset of the condition often begins at school age, when children do not wish to use public facilities and thus begin to withhold stool.

Other information

• Recent studies indicate that some children have a relative insensitivity to their rectal sphincter sensors. Some will contract their external sphincter while trying to defecate. Whether this is cause or effect has yet to be proven.

Treatment

General information

• Education of the child and family is very important, because this is a chronic condition that needs the full participation of the parents and child if the treatment is to be successful.

• Once the diagnosis of encopresis is made, there must be a long-term commitment made on the part of the physician and the family.

Disimpaction: treatment begins with removal of the large fecal mass from the rectum. This can be difficult and painful for the child. At times a child will need to be hospitalized for disimpaction.

Prevention of impaction reoccurrence: this is accomplished by a combination of therapies: stool softeners and dietary and behavioral modifications.

Stool softener administration: may be of the fiber type or the lubricant (mineral oil). Mild stimulants may also be needed, such as senna or bisacodyl.

Dietary changes: include adding roughage and fiber to the diet and decreasing the amounts of refined sugar and dairy products. The child should be encouraged to take more fluids through the day. When mineral oil is being used on a twice a day basis, a multivitamin should be given between the doses.

Behavioral therapy: is aimed at giving the child a time and place to have a regular bowel movement at least twice each day. This is done by selecting a time after a meal and encouraging the child to sit on the toilet, with feet firmly planted, for 15 minutes by a timer, and allowing the bowel movement to occur.

Promotility agents: *eg*, cisapride; some success has been observed in children with chronic constipation.

Treatment aims

To educate the child and family.
To remove impaction.
To keep bowel movements soft while bowel wall tone is reestablished.
To teach child ways to maintain normal bowel patterns for the future.
To remediate any psychological injury.

Prognosis

• Almost 65%–75% will have a lasting improvement in the first 6 mo of treatment.

• For the 25% with continued problems, further investigation may be needed. Patient may also benefit from more intensive psychotherapy or biofeedback techniques.

Follow-up and management

• Close and careful follow-up is very important. This is a chronic condition and, like asthma or diabetes, it must be followed closely and progress monitored. Often after an initial period of success there may be reversal to old habits. There may be need for the child and family to keep a careful diary of intake and toilet habits. A 6-mo period of therapy is often the least possible in order to be successful.

Other information

• In this condition, parent and patient support groups are both educational and decrease the amount of social isolation and stigma that the patients feel.

• For difficult, seemingly intractable cases, specialty services are available at most large children's centers.

General references

Hatch TT: Encopresis and constipation in children. *Pediatr Clin North Am* 1988, **35**:257–280.

Nolan T, Oberklaid F: New concepts in the management of encopresis. *Pediatr Rev* 1993, **14**:447–451.

Levine MD: Encopresis: its potentiation, evaluation, and alleviation. *Pediatr Clin North Am* 1982, **29**:315–330.

Diagnosis

Symptoms

Fever and sweating.

Easy fatiguability, malaise.

Palpitations.

Weight loss and anorexia.

Signs

Fever.

Tachycardia with new (or changing) cardiac murmur(s).

Splenomegaly.

Janeway lesions, splinter hemorrhages, Osler nodes, Roth spots: relatively rare in children.

Embolic phenomena: microscopic to kidney, results in hematuria); macroscopic, may cause vascular occlusion (GI, limbs), stroke, mycotic aneurysm, pulmonary embolism.

Investigations

Laboratory tests

Blood cultures: at least 2–3 over a 24-hour period (not only with temperature spike!) prior to instituting antibiotic therapy.

Acute phase reactants: sedimentation rate (ESR), c-reactive protein (CRP).

Complete blood count: white cell count and differential, anemia, platelet count.

Urinanalysis: hematuria.

Echocardiography: standard transthoracic echocardiography may adequately image a moderate to large valve vegetation, and also demonstrate leaking valves; if suspicion for endocarditis is high, transesophageal echocardiography is more sensitive in detecting small valve vegetations (in adult patients). *Remember:* a negative echocardiogram does not rule out endocarditis!

Complications

Destruction of cardiac valve tissue: can result in aortic, mitral, or tricuspid insufficiency; resultant need for cardiac valve replacement.

Congestive heart failure.

Myocardial abscesses with cardiac arrhythmias and atrioventricular block.

Systemic embolization: potential for stroke or cerebral mycotic aneurysm.

Types

Patients with structural heart disease

• Vegetations occur in areas with a pressure gradient and turbulent blood flow.

1) Valvular heart disease (congenital or acquired): especially aortic and mitral valves.

2) Prosthetic heart valves: all positions.

3) Postoperative patients: postoperative patches, shunts.

4) Ventricular septal defects.

5) Vascular lesions: PDA, aortic aneurysms, aortic coarctation, aortopulmonary shunts

Patients without structural heart disease

1) Intravascular foreign devices: catheters, pacemakers, ventriculoatrial shunts.

2) Immunocompromised hosts (oncology patients, HIV, congenital immune deficiency, neonate).

3) Intravenous drug abusers.

Differential diagnosis

• Endocarditis must be differentiated from other inflammatory conditions of the heart: Kawasaki disease, rheumatic fever, Lyme disease, post-pericardiotomy syndrome, or from transient bacteremia.

Etiology

• Bacteremia can occur with various manipulations: dental, oral, surgical procedures, or may occur spontaneously. In most humans, the bacterial load associated with spontaneous bacteremia is too small to lead to vegetation formation.

• 80–90% of cases are caused by gram-positive streptococci.

alpha-hemolytic *Streptococcus* (*S. viridans*, *S. pyogenes*).

Staphylococci: S. aureus and coagulase-negative *Staphylococcus* organisms.

Rarely (but to be considered in immunocompromised hosts)

Enterococcus, Pneumococcus.

Gram-negative bacteria: *Haemophilus*, enterics, *Pseudomonas, Actinobacillus, Neisseria.*

Candida or other fungal species (*Aspergillus, Histoplasma*).

Anaerobic bacteria ("culture-negative" endocarditis): bacteroides, *Fusobacterium, Clostridium, Propionibacterium, Peptostreptococcus.*

Epidemiology

• Exact incidence is unclear; however, it is estimated at 1 case per 2000 pediatric hospital admissions.

• Even with the advent of antibiotics, incidence of endocarditis may be on the rise in patients with structural heart disease, due to higher survival rates of children with complex heart disease.

• ~20% of all patients with endocarditis are <20 y of age.

• 40% of cases are post-surgical.

• In neonates, incidence is usually related to indwelling catheters without structural heart disease.

• ~5% of cases are "culture-negative" due to prior treatment with antibiotics, to anaerobic bacteria, or to "fastidious" nutritionally deficient organisms.

Treatment

Pharmacologic treatment

Endocarditis prophylaxis (recently revised in 1997 [1]).

• Not required for negligible-risk patients: isolated secundum ASD, surgically repaired ASD, VSD, or PDA 6 mo after surgery, coronary artery bypass grafts, MVP without mitral regurgitation, innocent murmurs, cardiac pacemakers (intravascular, epicardial) and defibrillators.

• Procedures for which prophylaxis is not needed are as follows:

Dental: fluoride treatments, orthodontic appliance adjustment, shedding of primary teeth; **respiratory:** flexible bronchoscopy, tympanostomy tube insertion; **gastrointestinal:** transesophageal echocardiography, endoscopy with or without biopsy; **genitourinary:** (if no infection present) vaginal delivery, cesarean section, circumcision.

• Prophylaxis for patients undergoing dental, oral, respiratory, or esophageal procedures is as follows: (*Note: there is no follow-up dose after the procedure!*)

Standard dosage	Amoxicillin: 50 mg/kg p.o. 1 h prior to procedure; or
	Ampicillin, 50 mg/kg i.m. or i.v 30 min prior to procedure (if patient can not take medication p.o.); or
	Clindamycin, 20 mg/kg i.v. or p.o. 30–60 min prior to procedure (if patient is allergic to penicillin); or
	Cephalexin, 50 mg/kg p.o. 1 h prior to procedure; or
	Azithromycin, 15 mg/kg p.o. 1 h prior to procedure; or
	Clarithromycin, 15 mg/kg p.o. 1 h prior to procedure.

• Prophylaxis for high-risk patients undergoing genitourinary or gastrointestinal (excluding esophageal) procedures is as follows:

Standard dosage	*Ampicillin*: 50 mg/kg i.m. or i.v. and
	Gentamicin, 1.5 mg/kg i.m. or i.v. within 30 min of procedure; then 6 hrs later
	Amoxicillin: 25 mg/kg p.o.

If patient is allergic to penicillin:

Standard dosage	Vancomycin, 20 mg/kg i.v. over 1–2 h prior to procedure and *Gentamicin*: 1.5 mg/kg i.v. or i.m. 30 min prior to procedure.

Endocarditis treatment

• Prolonged antibiotic treatment is required to rid the body of all infecting organisms because they are relatively protected from host defense mechanisms within vegetations. Intravenous therapy is preferred. Bactericidal agents are preferred over bacteriostatic agents, with less relapses.

• For patients with streptococcal endocarditis:

Standard dosage	Penicillin G, 200,000 U/kg/d divided every 4 h for 4 wk, and *Gentamicin*: 7.5 mg/kg/d divided every 8 h (combined for synergy for 2 wk).

If patient is allergic to penicillin:

Standard dosage	*Vancomycin*: 40 mg/kg/d divided every 6 h for 4 wk. MIC >0.5: *vancomycin*: 40 mg/kg/d in divided doses every 6 h.

• For patients with enterococcal or resistant-streptococcal endocarditis:

Standard dosage	*Ampicillin*: 300 mg/kg/d divided every 4 h, and *Gentamicin*: 7.5 mg/kg/d divided every 8 h (combined for synergy for at least 4–6 wk) for a total of 6 wk of therapy.

• For patients with staphylococcal endocarditis:

Standard dosage	Nafcillin or oxacillin, 200 mg/kg/d divided every 4 h for 4–6 wk and *Gentamicin*: 7.5 mg/kg/d divided every 8 h for 5 d.

Treatment aims

To eradicate the infective agent completely from the body
To avoid renal and ototoxicity
To avoid arrhythmic complications
To try to prevent destructive valvular changes

Prognosis

Varies greatly from patient to patient, and depends upon the degree of valve destruction, need for surgical intervention, consequences of embolic events, and efficacy of therapy without relapses.

Follow-up and management

• The key to following patients with endocarditis, both in the hospital and afterwards, is serial physical examinations with close attention to the qualities of the cardiac murmur(s) and evaluation for peripheral embolization.

Surgical intervention

• Surgical intervention must be individualized for each patient. If congestive heart develops, valve replacement may bre needed prior to completing antibiotics. If there is a serious systemic embolus, surgery to remove a vegetation may be indicated. Otherwise, elective valve surgery after antibiotic therapy is complete is preferred.

General references

Dajani A, Taubert K, Wilson W, et al.: Guidelines for the prevention of bacterial endocarditis. *JAMA* 1997, **277**:1794–1801.

Dajani A, Taubert K: Infective endocarditis. In *Moss and Adams' Heart Disease in Infants, Children and Adolescents*, ed. 5. Edited by Emmanouilides G, Allen H, Riemenschneider T, Gutgesell H. Williams and Wilkins: Baltimore; 1995:1541–1553.

Johnson DH, Rosenthal A, Nadas AS: A forty-year review of bacterial endocarditis in infancy and childhood. *Circulation* 1979, **51**:581.

Saiman L, Prince A, Gersony WM: Pediatric infective endocarditis in the modern era. *J Pediatr* 1993, **122**:847–853.

Diagnosis

• Although enuresis or wetting has no serious medical consequences, it is a vexing problem for many parents and children and the source of a great deal of family conflict.

Definition

Primary enuresis: describes the child who never fully gains bladder control.

Secondary enuresis: describes those children who maintain control for more then 6 months and later revert to involuntary voiding.

Symptoms

Involuntary voiding: primary symptom; most often occurs during the night while the child is asleep.

Diurnal enuresis: describes a child who wets both day and night; this pattern of enuresis has more significant pathology associated with it.

• It is important to explore if there is any pattern to the enuresis: whether there are times when the child does not wet, any recent stresses, diet and fluid intake, family history.

• It is also important to determine the reaction of the child and family members to the enuresis. Does it create conflict? Who cleans up? Is there family disruption over these episodes?

Signs

• The child must have a thorough physical examination.

• Make sure there are no neurological findings in the lower extremities to suggest a spinal cord tumor. Check gait, anal tone, and examine the lumbosacral area for abnormalities Check also for pelvic masses and constipation that might be decreasing bladder size by compression effect.

• Examine the urethral orifice and in boys observe their voiding stream.

Investigations

History and physical examination.

Urinalysis: look for the specific gravity to document concentrating ability (*ie*, a specific gravity >1.015). Check the other elements of the urinalysis for blood, protein, and sugar.

• If no specific pathologic processes are found, then more complex studies may be indicated, including voiding studies and structural studies of the urinary tract anatomy.

Complications

The only serious complications that come from enuresis are the social psychological trauma that develop within the family and lessen the child's self-esteem.

Differential diagnosis

Urinary tract infection.
Diabetes mellitus.
Diabetes insipidus.
Hypercalciuria.
Sickle cell anemia or trait.
Constipation.
Pelvic tumor.
Spinal cord tumor.
Urinary tract anomaly, eg, ectopic ureter.
Vulvovaginitis.
Child sexual abuse.
Medications.

Etiology

• There are many factors that may contribute to the cause of enuresis. In about 75% of cases there is a family history. This suggests some genetic influence over a neurolodevelopmental process. Enuresis is sometimes classified as a sleep disorder, as it is believed that at the core of the problem is an inability to gain sufficient arousal to appreciate the sensation of a full bladder.

• Other influences may include stress, sensitivity to caffeine, conditions in which there is a loss of urinary concentrating ability (eg, sickle cell anemia), and others. The 15% per year spontaneous cure rate suggests that some developmental process is a critical element.

Epidemiology

• ~90% of 4-year-old children are dry during the day. Thus diurnal enuresis is a relatively uncommon problem.

• Nocturnal control should be gained in boys by their 6th birthday and in girls by their 5th. Approximately 75% of children are dry during the night by their 4th birthday and 90% by their 8th.

• Males predominate over females, particularly in the category of nightly bed wetting.

• Enuresis is rare during adolescence.

Other information

• For difficult or unusual cases, most pediatric centers have enuresis specialty services that provide multidisciplinary evaluations and treatments.

Treatment

General information

• Because enuresis is a developmental problem, the best strategy for most children is to allow them the time to mature without pressure or social stigmatization.

• Unfortunately, in some cases the watch-and-wait approach is not tolerable, often because of the parental reaction. Sometimes the child may be strongly motivated as well. In such cases there are a variety of therapies available. All treatments are effective because of the spontaneous cure rate that occurs without any therapy. Therapies are pharmocologic and nonpharmacologic.

Pharmacologic treatment

Desmopression or DDAVP nasal spray: one spray each nostril at bedtime and titrate upward at one increased spray per week as needed. This isperhaps the safest and most effective drug. It has a hormonal effect to exceed the child's endogenous level of antidiuretic hormone and thus cause urinary retention overnight. It is safe and effective and may establish a short-term pattern of decreased voiding. It is questionable whether once the medication is stopped that the child can maintain dryness without treatment.

Imipramine: 25 mg given at bedtime or suppertime. This agent apparently works by its anticholinergic action on bladder muscle and perhaps by altering the sleep cycles and allowing the child to sense a full bladder, awake, and void. The major problem with imipramine is that it is a highly toxic agent if accidentally ingested. If there is uncertainty about the family's ability to control this medication from access by younger children, it should not be prescribed.

Oxybutynin: an anticholingergic and antispasmodic agent. This agent is now coming into more widespread use for more complex cases.

Nonpharmacologic treatment

Buzzers, bells, and alarms: work by sensing the first drops of urine and waking the child so that they can retain their urine until they get to the bathroom. These devices seem to work and also may be used to create new habits that the child may then maintain on their own. Alarms may be used alone or in combination with drug therapy.

Other methods involve limiting the child's fluid intake after dinner, avoiding caffeine, bladder-stretching exercises, and decreasing stress levels: if the child voids at a regular time each night, an alarm clock may be set to wake them prior to the time of the void.

• As a child with enuresis grows older, they should be made responsible for some of the clean-up chores. This is not meant to be punitive but to lessen the parents' burden and perhaps their resentment. Children should never be teased or embarrassed with the thought that they are simply lazy or uncooperative. Rewards and star charts do little for a process that has a neurodevelopmental issue at its core. Positive reinforcements should not hasten maturity.

Treatment aims

To educate the family and child.
To make certain there are no underlying disorders.
To allow the child time to develop control.
To support the child and family.
• If necessary, use pharmacologic and nonpharmacologic treatments.

Prognosis

• Overall, the prognosis is excellent with or without treatments.
• In rare cases there may be signs and symptoms that will prompt referral to a specialty center.

Follow-up and management

• When medications are being used, monthly follow-up is suggested.
• All children with this problem need more than routine care, and at least quarterly or semiannual visits should be arranged.

General references

Schmidt BD: Nocturnal enuresis. *Pediatr Rev* 1997, 18:183–190.

Rushton HG: Nocturnal enuresis: epidemiology, evaluation, and currently available treatment options *J Pediatr* 1989, 114:691–696.

Leung AKC, Robson WLM, Halperin ML: Polyuria in children. *Clin Pediatr* 1991, 30:634–640.

Moffatt MEK, Harlos S, Kirshen AJ: Desmopressin acetate and nocturnal enuresis: how much do we know? *Pediatrics* 1993, 92:420–425.

Diagnosis

Symptoms

• Symptoms do not predict the severity of mucosal inflammation.

Heartburn: retrosternal or epigastric burning is the most common symptom; dull ache may resemble angina in older children and adolescents.

Epigastric pain or right upper-quadrant pain: common in all ages.

Retrosternal pain: may resemble chest pain.

Water brash: sour taste in mouth (acid taste).

Odynophagia: painful swallowing; suggests infectious etiology or pill-induced ulcer.

Regurgitation of food, acid, or bitter juice: may be confused with "vomiting" (but without nausea) and is frequently associated with esophagitis.

Dysphagia: stricture or motility disorder.

Globus: sticking sensation in throat.

Respiratory symptoms: *eg*, nocturnal cough or dyspnea, asthma.

Severe crying irritability, poor feeding: occurs in nonverbal infront.

Signs

• Signs are frequently absent.

Heme-positive stools: may represent esophageal mucosal inflammation.

Pulmonary consolidation or bronchospasm: rarely, if aspiration has occurred as a result of regurgitation.

Dental enamel erosion: secondary to chronic acid regurgitation.

Investigations

• Uncomplicated reflux esophagitis often requires no diagnostic testing prior to initiation of therapy.

Radiography: not reliable for showing esophagitis (particularly mild forms) or reflux; extremely useful in assessing esophageal and gastric anatomy (stricture, webs, pyloric stenosis malrotation).

Endoscopy: preferred to radiography because it offers visualization of mucosa and option of obtaining histology; allows determination of severity of etiology and esophagitis. Indicated for dysphagia, complicated recurrent or refractory symptoms.

pH monitoring: for diagnosis of acid reflux, especially in children with unusual symptoms (cough, asthma); for

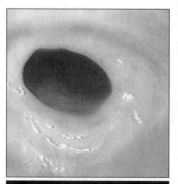

Esophageal stricture secondary to reflux esophagitis.

quantifying reflux to assess effectiveness of treatment or before antireflux surgery.

Manometry: useful to exclude associated motility disorders before antireflux surgery.

Complete blood count: in complicated cases to evaluate for anemia or systemic manifestations of inflammation.

Complications

Stricture.

Barrett's esophagus: rare in children.

Aspiration: leading to night cough, bronchospasm, pneumonia, asthma, hoarseness.

Bleeding: may be life-threatening

Failure to thrive.

Differential diagnosis

Congenital heart disease.

Respiratony disease.

Esophageal motility disorder.

Peptic ulcer disease (*Helicobacter pylori*).

Gallstone disease.

Malrotation, pyloric stenosis.

Etiology

• Esophagitis is mucosal damage most commonly caused by gastroesophageal reflux, which occurs when the lower esophageal sphincter is incompetent or esophageal clearance is impaired.

• Reflux esophagitis is caused by prolonged exposure of esophageal mucosa to gastric contents and is more intense if the mucosa is compromised or if gastric emptying is delayed.

• Reflux symptoms are often erroneously attributed to hiatal hernia, a common condition that is most often asymptomatic.

• Infectious esophagitis due to Candida, herpesvirus, or cytomegalovirus may occur in immunocompromised patients.

• Hiatal hernia is a rare condition that when associated with esophagitis, may be difficult to treat medically.

• Infectious causes: fungal (*Candida*), cytomegalovirus, herpes.

• Eosinophilic esophagitis: numerous esophageal eosinophils may suggest autoimmune or allergic etiology [1].

Epidemiology

• Two thirds of the population may suffer from reflux at some time, but only a small proportion seek medical advice.

• Mechanical and hormonal factors make reflux common during pregnancy.

• Infectious esophagitis is a common component of HIV infections.

• Pill-induced ulcers of the esophagus are most common in bedridden patients with medications such as NSAIDs, tetracyclines, quinidine.

Histologic diagnosis [2]

Basal cell thickness >30%.

Papillary height >60%.

Presence of eosinophils or neutrophils.

Treatment

Diet and lifestyle

• Reducing weight, eating small meals, avoiding certain foods (*eg*, chocolate, coffee, mints, alcohol), and sleeping with the head of the bed raised are crucial measures that decrease reflux [2,3].

• Stopping smoking and avoiding alcohol consumption in adolescent.

• Patients should be advised to remain upright for 2–4 hours after a meal.

• NSAIDs, slow-release potassium chloride, theophylline, nitrates, and calcium blockers (*eg*, nifedipine) may also aggravate symptoms.

Pharmacologic treatment [5]

Antacids

• Antacids may provide reasonable but short-lasting relief; they have little effect on mucosal inflammation.

Standard dosage	0.5–1.0 mL/kg/dose, 3–4 times daily (maximum, 30-mL dose).
Contraindications	Renal failure (magnesium based).
Main drug interactions	Iron, phenytoin, penicillamine, tetrracycline.
Main side effects	Constipation (aluminum based), diarrhea (magnesium based).

Acid antisecretory agents (first-line agents)

• These diminish gastric acid production, thus decreasing exposure of the esophageal mucosa (cinetidine, famotidine). Healing requires 6–8-wk courses with further maintenance therapy as required.

• Proton-pump inhibitors (*eg*, omeprazole, lansoprazole) are more powerful than H_2 antagonists (*eg*, ranitidine) and are favored in severe cases.

Standard dosage	Ranitidine, 2 mg/kg/dose twice daily (maximum, 150 twice daily). Omeprazole, 5–20 mg daily or twice daily. Dose can be titrated against symptoms.
Main drug interactions	*Omeprazole:* warfarin, phenytoin, diazepam.
Main side effects	*Ranitidine:* headache, blood disorders, increased liver enzyme levels. *Omeprazole:* skin reactions, diarrhea, headache, enteric infections are rarely observed.

Motility-enhancing agents

• These are not widely used, with the exception of cisapride, which is as effective as some H_2 antagonists (bethanechol, metodopromide).

Standard dosage	Cisapride, 0.2–0.3 mg/kg/dose 3–4 times daily, 30 min before meals (maximum, 20 mg 3 times daily).
Contraindications	Gastrointestinal hemorrhage or perforation, mechanical bowel obstruction.
Main drug interactions	Anticoagulants: effect possibly enhanced; erythromycin (and like compounds); antifungals.
Main side effects	Diarrhea, abdominal discomfort, headache.

Mucosal-protecting agents

Standard dosage	Sucralfate, 40–80 mg/kg/d in divided doses (maximum, 1 g 4 times daily).
Contraindications	Caution in renal impairment (aluminum toxicity).
Main drug interactions	Decreased bioavailability of tetracycline, phenytoin, cimetidine (avoided by separating administration from sucralfate by 2 h).
Main side effects	Constipation.

Treatment aims

To control symptoms.

To prevent complications, especially for stricture formation.

To prevent behavorial feeding disorders and poor growth.

Other treatments

Antireflux surgery [3]

• Nissen fundoplication and its modifications using a laparoscopic approach are the most popular techniques.

• Surgery is indicated for the following: refractory, debilitating symptoms that are complicated by bleeding, respiratory disease (aspiration, asthma); or severe strictures or esophagitis that are refractory to aggressive medical management.

Prognosis

• Infants (<1 y) will usually improve with medical therapy.

• In older children, this maybe a chronic and relapsing condition, but up to 40% of patients remain in remission.

Follow-up and management

• Some form of treatment may be necessary to maintain remission. Achievement of esophagitis healing may not be necessary; the simple aim of symptom control may be sufficient.

• Long-term treatment and endoscopic surveillance is indicated in patients who have had frequent relapse.

• Identification of Barrett's esophagus is an indication for more careful monitoring for esophageal malignancy. EGD with biopsies are routinely performed every 1–3 y.

Key references

1. Kelly KJ, Lazenby AT, Rowe PC, *et al.:* Eosinophillic esophagitis attributed to gastrointestinal reflux: improvement with an amino acid–based formula. *Gastroenterology* 1995, 109:1503–1512.

2. Orenstein SR: Gastroesophageal reflux. In *Pediatric Gastrointestinal Disease.* Edited by Willie R, Hyams JS. Philadelphia: WB Saunders Co.; 1993:337–369.

3. Fonkalsrud EW, *et al.:* Surgical treatment of the gastroesophageal reflux sundrome in infants and children. *Am J Surg* 1987, 159:11–18.

Diagnosis

Definition

• The term *failure to thrive* (FTT) describes a child who is failing to meet normal standards for growth and development, usually in the first few years of life. The diagnosis requires that the physician look for an explainable cause for the child's growth failure in the child, the family, or the environment.

• Diagnosis begins by taking serial growth measurements of the infant and child. Height, weight, and head circumference should be measured on each well-child visit and they must be plotted on a standard growth curve appropriate for the child's gender, chronological age, and history of birth.

• Children who are below the 5th percentile (two SDs below the mean) or children who are crossing percentile lines (moving from the 90th percentile to the 25th percentile) should be evaluated for FTT.

Signs and symptoms

• The signs and symptoms will depend on the underlying cause of the FTT and the degree of malnutrition the child has sustained.

• The child may appear thin with relatively slender extremities and protuberant abdomen. There will be extra skin folds from loss of subcutaneous tissue and wasted buttocks. The child may keep their hands in their mouth as a form of autostimulation.

• FTT may stem from three etiologic categories: organic, nonorganic, and mixed type.

Organic FTT: there is some physical or physiologic derangement that is causing the growth failure. Often there are other signs and symptoms such has diarrhea, vomiting, or food refusal.

Nonorganic FTT: the problems lies with the family or environmental interaction with the child. With this form there will be an absence of any other symptoms. Other signs may include an apathetic child, flat occiput from being left supine, or signs of neglect such as diaper rash.

Mixed-type FTT: describes children that have a minor medical problem and a family constellation unable to cope with the child's needs.

Investigations

• The most important test is an accurately plotted serial growth curve.

• A count of the child's caloric intake is useful.

• In cases of nonorganic FTT, a change in the child's environment may prove a telling diagnostic test.

Complete blood count, urinalysis, and chemistry panel: first-line laboratory tests.

HIV testing: should be considered if there are other parental risk factors.

• Other laboratory tests should be based on the child's symptom complex.

Complications

• Uninvestigated FTT may fail to lead to important underlying diagnoses.

• Nonorganic FTT is associated with other family problems such as abuse and neglect that have psychological and developmental manifestations.

• There is a low but measurable mortality rate associated with FTT.

Differential diagnosis

• For organic causes of FTT, there is a wide differential, including chronic urinatry tract infection, sinusitis, giardiasis, other parasites, gastroesophageal reflux, food allergy, malabsorption, chronic constipation, lead toxicity, adenoidal hypertrophy, tuberculosis, genetic syndromes, neurologic defects, and HIV infection (common but incomplete list).

• In cases of nonorganic FTT, there may be problem with the parent, with the baby, with the interaction between the specific parent and child, or more pervasive family dysfunction.

• Some suspected FTT cases actually represent intrauterine growth retardation or genetic short stature. Consider the size of the parents and their growth pattern.

• In rare circumstances, there may be inaccurate use of the growth curve or inaccuracies in measurement.

Etiology

• The cause of FTT is lack of adequate caloric intake, increased loss of calories , or abnormally increased requirements to achieve growth.

Epidemiology

• As many as 5%–10% of children may experience some period of growth failure.

• Of the three categories of FTT, 60% are nonorganic, 10%–20% organic, and the remainder mixed.

Other information

• Some cases of FTT are due to child abuse and must be reported to the local child protective service agency.

Treatment

General information

• The first step is try to determine the cause of the FTT. Based on symptoms and signs, carry out studies to determine if there is any organic cause.

• A careful dietary history is helpful in determining cause; if possible, observe a feeding. Having the parent complete a caloric diary for a few weekdays and a few weekend days is helpful.

• When evaluating the child's eating pattern, there are several factors to consider: the proper number of calories, the developmentally appropriate method of eating/feeding, the correct foods, and the proper atmosphere for a healthy mealtime. It is sometimes useful to gain the parents' perceptions of food and eating, as some parental eating disorders may be reflected in the child.

Pharmacologic treatment

• There are no specific pharmacologic agents that are helpful. However, the physician may need to modify standard dietary instructions in order to maximize caloric intake. Foods that are naturally high in calories, supplements, or special formulas may be necessary. Consultation with a nutritionist may add worthwhile and innovative suggestions for dietary manipulation.

Nonpharmacologic treatment

For organic FTT: pursue the underlying diagnosis and correct the problem..

For nonorganic FTT: social work support, home visiting nurse care, or mental health referral may be helpful. Often in helping, supporting, and educating the parent, the result will be weight gain and growth in the infant.

For mixed FTT: a combination of interventions may be needed, both physical and psychosocial.

Hospitalization: may be required if the child is failing to grow significantly, particularly in the first 6–8 months of life, to sort through the possible causes. The use of a multidisciplinary team is most helpful in the treatment of the severely malnourished child.

Treatment aims

To determine cause of FTT.
To correct any underlying diseases.
To reverse nutritional deficiencies.
To support the family.
To establish a pattern of sustained normal growth.

Other treatments

• When nonorganic FTT is suspected, bringing in other family members, day-care providers, or foster parents to assist in the feeding is helpful. If the child can gain weight with alternative caretakers, both the diagnosis is made and the treatment achieved.

Prognosis

• The overall prognosis is good.

• In cases of nonorganic and mixed-type FTT, unless family dysfunction is addressed as well as the child's growth, there may be subsequent issues of developmental delay, educational deficiency, and/or psychological impairment.

• Most case series of children with FTT show a mortality rate of 1%–3%. This is usually due to extreme starvation or concomitant physical abuse.

Follow-up and management

• Close and careful follow-up is extremely important, particularly during the period of brain growth that occurs in the first 6 or 8 mo of life.

General references

Bithony WG, Dubowitz H, Egan H: Failure to thrive/growth deficiency. *Pediatr Rev* 1992, 13:453–460.

Frank DA, Silva M, Needlman R: Failure to thrive: mystery, myth, and method. *Contemp Pediatr* 1993, 114–133.

Ludwig S: Failure to thrive. In *Child Abuse: A Medical Reference*, ed 2. Edited by Ludwig S, Kornberg AE. New York: Churchill Livingstone; 1992:303–319.

Diagnosis

• Fatigue is an unusual and often significant complaint in a child. The natural forces of growth and development always encourage a child to be active and striving for new milestones. An observed pattern of fatigue requires evaluation.

Symptoms

• Children generally develop a pattern of activity that is well recognized by their parents. Although children differ in temperament and amount of physical activity, each child's pattern remains more or less constant. An observed pattern of fatigue at almost any age requires an evaluation.

Activity level: note whether the child tries to engage in normal activities and is unable versus the loss of desire. Does the child show signs of increased respiratory effort as part of the fatigue? Are there psychological factors or issues of family disruption?

Change in appetite and other systemic signs: *eg*, fever, night sweats, and so on, which might point to chronic infection or malignancy.

Changes in personality or in cognitive function: might point to a psychological problem or substance abuse. Who are the child's friends? Review the grades on the most recent and past report cards from school.

Sleep habits: review with the family the child's sleep habits and their pattern of activity. Does the child have any "down time" or is every hour scheduled with school, lesson, and group activities?

Signs

• The patient needs a complete physical examination. Examine the child for pallor and any abnormality in the lymph nodes, liver, or spleen. Does the child appear anemic or have a cardiac murmur or tachycardia?

Neurologic signs: evaluate the child's neurologic examination with attention to cognition, coordination, and muscle strength. Exercise the child in the office to differentiate generalized fatigue from muscle weakness.

Psychological function: look for evidence of depression, anxiety, or signs of posttraumatic stress disorder.

Investigations

• Investigations will depend on the findings of the history and physical examination. A reasonable initial evaluation should include a complete blood count, urinalysis, mononucleosis testing, and liver enzymes.

Muscle enzymes and other neuromuscular studies: if there are specific concerns about muscle strength.

Chest radiography and pulmonary function studies (*eg*, tidal volume, FEV_1: if there appears to be a respiratory or cardiac cause.

Psychological assessment: will need to be explored in depth and consultation with a mental health professional may be necessary. It is important to remember that depression may be both cause and effect of fatigue. A child with hepatitis or mononucleosis or a brain tumor may also be depressed.

Complications

• Complications will depend on the underlying cause of the fatigue.

Differential diagnosis

Infectious/postinfectious
Viral myositis, mononucleosis, hepatitis, tuberculosis, lyme disease, postviral or mononucleosis-like illness.

Endocrine/metabolic
Hypothyroid/hyperthyroid, hypoadrenal, hypokalemia.

Tumor
Leukemia, lymphoma, other tumors.

Allergic
Reactive airway disease, chronic rhinitis, antihistamine-related.

Congenital
Neuromuscular disease, muscular dystrophy.

Other
Sleep disturbance from upper airway obstruction or other causes, psychogenic, drug abuse, anemia, congenital heart disease (including dysrhythmia), chronic fatigue syndrome.

Etiology

• There is no single cause for this complaint. It may relate to muscle weakness, inadequate cardiorespiratory function including anemia, central nervous system disorders, abnormalities of energy production, lack of adequate sleep, or psychological mechanisms that decrease motivation such as depression or substance abuse.

Epidemiology

• The epidemiology of fatigue is unknown. In a recent survey of sleep problems in school-aged children 17% had fatigue complaints. Adolescents will need increased amounts of sleep and may select unhealthy sleep habits if allowed.

• As the age of the child with fatigue increases, the likelihood of an organic pathology decreases. However, an organic pathology should be ruled out in all cases.

Other information

• The final entity in the differential diagnosis listing is a diagnosis of exclusion. It occurs in the adolescent and young adult population and is characterized by fatigue and neurological findings such as loss of attention span, confusion, loss of cognitive function, and memory impairment. This may represent some undescribed form of encephalitis.

Treatment

General treatment

• The treatment of fatigue depends on the underlying cause.

• Treatment may need to be multidisciplinary and include the physician, visiting nurse, mental health specialist, and physical therapist.

• Initial therapy consists of a comprehensive work-up to establish a diagnosis and treatment plan.

• While awaiting a diagnosis, the child should be allowed to set their own level of daytime activity but should have strict guidelines for bedtime. A well-balanced diet should be offered and supplemented with a standard multivitamin.

• For school-aged children, consultation with school officials and the arrangement of extra tutoring may be needed. The child should be encouraged to attend school in order to maintain some academic productivity and to maintain social contacts.

• Specific diagnoses will determine additional therapy, *eg*, tighter control of reactive airway disease or adenoidectomy for upper airway obstruction or iron for anemia that is determined to be iron deficiency.

• There are no drug therapies available or recommended as a general therapy. For some children, antidepressants may be needed. There have been some reports of the beneficial use of beta-blockers for chronic fatigue syndrome.

Treatment aims

To establish a diagnosis.

To support the child and family.

To treat specific disorders.

To return the child to full function.

Prognosis

• Overall, the prognosis is good for most diagnostic possibilities.

• Some conditions may take weeks or months to resolve.

Follow-up and management

• Close physician involvement and family support are helpful.

General references

Ludwig S: Weakness and fatigue. In *Pediatric Primary Care*, ed 2. Edited by Schwartz W, Charney EB, Curry TA, Ludwig S. Chicago: Yearbok; 1990.

Blader JC, Koplewicz HS, Abikoff H, *et al.*: Sleep problems of elementary school children. *Arch Pediatr Adolesc Med* 1997, 151:473–480.

Smith MS, Mitchell J, Corey L, *et al.*: Chronic fatigue in adolescence. *Pediatrics* 1991, 88:195–202.

Diagnosis

Symptoms

• Many children with bacteremia present only with complaints of fever.

• Constitutional symptoms might also be present and may include irritability, lethargy, malaise, poor feeding, decreased urinary output.

• Clinical appearance is variable. Febrile children with bacteremia are likely to appear ill. Clinical appearance can be quantified using McCarthy's infant observation score.

• Other organ system–specific symptoms (*ie*, respiratory distress, stridor, drooling, mottling, meningisms, vomiting, purpuric rash) can be seen in diseases associated with bacteremia.

Signs

Temperature: any measured rectal temperature ≤38.0°C is considered a fever and is potentially a sign of bacteremia.

• The significance of the magnitude of fever differs according to patient age.

• Tachycardia is commonly associated with fever.

• Tachypnea (mild) is also often associated with fever.

Investigations

• The need for laboratory investigations in febrile young children varies according to patient age, appearance, and temperature.

Complications

• Bacteremia can lead to or accompany numerous other organ system infections, including meningitis, osteomyelitis, septic arthritis, pneumonia, pyelonephritis, cellulitis.

• Some children (aged 6 months to 6 years) are prone to seizure activity triggered by high body temperatures (*see* Seizures, acute and febrile).

Age-specific fever guidelines

Patient age, mo	Minumum temperature warranting investigation, °C
<3	>38.0
3–36	
ill-appearing	>38.0
well-appearing	>39.4
>36	individualized

Initial work-up of fever by age

Age, mo	Sex	Temp,	Exam	Initial work-up
<2	M/F	>38.0	Ill/well	CBC, BC, UA, UC, CXR, LP
2–3	M/F	>38.0	Well	CBC, BC, UA, UC
2–3	M/F	>38.0	Ill	CBC, BC, UA, UC, CXR, LP
3–12	M/F	<39.4	Well	UA, UC
3–12	M/F	>39.4	Ill	CBC, BC, UA, UC; CXR, LP as indicated
12–36	M	<39.4	Well	As indicated by H&P
12–36	M	>39.4	Well	CBC, BC
12–36	M/F	>38.0	Ill	CBC, BC; UA,UC; CXR, LP as indicated
12–36	F	<39.4	Well	UA, UC
12–36	F	>39.4	Well	CBC, BC, UA, UC
12–36	F	>38.0	Ill	CBC, BC, UA, UC; CXR, LP as indicated

BC—blood culture; CBC—complete blood count; CXR—chest X-ray; LP—lumbar punctase; UA—urinalysis; UC—urine culture.

Differential diagnosis

• Fever in children is usually a result of infection. Viral infections are much more common than bacterial or other infections.

• Other less common causes of fever include rheumatologic diseases, intoxication, tremors, metabolic diseases, CNS disorders, major trauma, environmental exposures, and inflammatory diseases.

Etiology

• Most of the above disorders will cause other organ-specific or system-specific symptoms in addition to fever that will help to identify the etiology of disease.

• Febrile children younger than 36 mo of age are at increased risk of occult bacteremia. Febrile girls in this age range and febrile boys younger than 1 y are also at increased risk for occult urinary tract infection. Febrile infants less than 2 mo of age are at increased risk of all systemic bacterial infections, regardless of their clinical appearance.

Epidemiology

• Febrile infants younger than 3 mo of age have the highest rate of serious bacterial illness, which is reported to be from 6%–31%.

• Beyond the newborn period, children are at highest risk for bacteremia in the 7–12-mo age range.

• In children older than 3 mo, the prevalence of occult bacteremia increases with increasing temperatures. The chance of having occult bacteremia with temperatures <38.9°C is 7:1000. Children 4–36 mo old with fevers >39.4°C are associated with a 3% risk for bacteremia.

• The bacterial pathogens most likely to be associated with occult bacteremia in febrile infants and young children are those commonly associated with other serious invasive bacterial diseases. *Streptococcus pneumoniae* (60%), *Haemophilus influenzae* type B (20%), *Neisseria meningitidis* (10%), and *Salmonella* species are the most common isolates. Of these, the streptococcal species are least likely (5%) to be associated with invasive infection. Invasive infection associated with *Haemophilus*, *Neisseria*, and *Salmonella* species ranges from 20%–50%.

Treatment

Diet and lifestyle

- The presence of fever alone does not necessitate significant changes in diet or activity. However, increased insensible losses should be anticipated for the child, and attention must be paid to adequate fluid intake.

Pharmacologic treatment

- Treatment of febrile illnesses should be directed toward the etiology of disease.
- Bacterial infections require specific and appropriate antibiotic administration.

Anitpyretics

- Reduction of fever can be accomplished in several ways. Bathing with tepid water is effective; however, antipyretics are the treatment of choice. Aspirin is generally avoided in children due to its possible association with Reye Syndrome. Two types of antipyretics are most commonly utilized for fever reduction—acetaminophen and ibuprofen.

Standard dosage	Acetaminophen, 15 mg/kg every 4–6 h.
	Ibuprofen, 10 mg/kg every 6 h.
Toxic dosage	*Acetaminophen:* >140 mg/kg.
	Ibuprofen: >400 mg/kg.
Symptoms of toxicity	*Acetaminophen:* nausea, vomiting, malaise, hepatic dysfunction (24–48 h later).
	Ibuprofen: gastrointestinal symptoms.

Antibiotics

- The advisability of presumptive use of antibiotics for young children with fever and no apparent source depends mostly on the child's age. Infants younger than one month should receive ampicillin and cefotaxime until culture results are confirmed.

Standard dosage	Ampicillin, 50 mg/kg twice daily (children aged <1 wk), 50 mg/kg four times daily (children aged 1–4 wk).
	Cefotaxime, 50 mg/kg twice daily (children aged <1 wk), 50 mg/kg three times daily (children aged 1–4 wk).

- Infants from 1–3 months of age who require presumptive antibiotic treatment should receive either ampicillin and cefotaxime or ceftriaxone alone.

Standard dosage	*Ampicillin:* 50 mg/kg four times daily (children aged 1–3 mo).
	Cefotaxime: 45 mg/kg 4 time daily (children aged 1–3 mo).
	Ceftriaxone, 50 mg/kg/day, IM (children aged 1–3 mo).

- For febrile children older than 3 months, who are well-appearing but at risk for occult bacteremia, the presumptive use of antibiotics is controversial. Intramuscular ceftriaxone (50mg/kg), has been suggested for this purpose.

Treatment aims

To enhance patient comfort by reducing fever.

To identify and specifically treat the cause of fever.

Prognosis

- The prognosis of febrile disease is related to the etiology of disease causing the fever. Fever rarely causes additional irreversible damage to organ systems. In rare instances of malignant hyperthermia or exceptional heat stroke, fever-related CNS damage can occur.

Follow-up and Management

- The need for follow-up depends upon the primary disease causing the fever. Children at risk for occult bacteremia or occult urinary tract infection should have follow-up within the 36 h arranged with their primary physician. Febrile infants older than one month of age, if selected for home management, should be reexamined by a physician within 24 h of initial evaluation. Any and all bacterial cultures ordered should be checked by the ordering physician until a final report is issued.

General references

Baker MD, Bell LM, Avner JR: Outpatient management without antibiotics of fever in selected infants. *New Engl J Med* 1993, **329:**1437–1441.

Baskin MN, O'Rourke EJ, Fleisher GR: Outpatient treatment of febrile infants 28 to 89 days of age with intramuscular administration of ceftriaxone. *J Pediatr* 1991, **20:**22–27.

Bass JW, Steel RW, Wittler RR, et al.: Antimicrobial treatment of occult bacteremia: a multicenter cooperative study. *Pediatr Infect Dis J* 1993, **12:**466–473.

Jaffe DM, Taviz RR, Davis AT, et al.: Antibiotic administration to treat possible occult bacteremia in febrile children. *New Engl J Med* 1987, **317:**1175–1180.

Foreign body, airway

Diagnosis

Symptoms

History of a distinct coughing or choking episode: occurs in a majority of cases.

Sudden onset of respiratory distress.

Acute or chronic cough.

Hoarseness or aphonia.

• Some patients with small subglottic foreign bodies may be asymptomatic.

Signs

Laryngeal or tracheal foreign bodies

• Total obstruction results in severe respiratory distress with cyanosis, supraclavicular and substernal retractions, aphonia, ineffective cough, and absent or very diminished breath sounds, with or without loss of consciousness.

• Partial obstruction results in stridor, cough, dysphonia, drooling and supraclavicular and/or substernal retractions.

Bronchial foreign bodies

• The classic triad of cough, wheezing, and focally decreased breath sounds occurs in only 30% of patients.

• Respiratory distress is manifested as tachypnea, intercostal retractions, and cough.

• 20% of patients are asymptomatic at presentation.

Investigations

Laryngeal or tracheal foreign bodies

• The diagnosis of total obstruction is made by history and physical examination. As immediate intervention is required; definitive relief of the obstruction must not be delayed by radiographs.

• A partial obstruction may become complete if the patient is forced to move from a position of comfort. If the diagnosis is uncertain, a person skilled in advanced airway management should accompany the patient while radiographs are taken for posteroanterior and lateral chest films and anteroposterior and lateral soft-tissue neck films to visualize the entire airway.

Bronchial foreign bodies

• Inspiratory and expiratory chest radiographs are indicated for the patient with a history of possible bronchial foreign body aspiration. Positive findings include air trapping, atelectasis, consolidation, or mediastinal shift, particularly on the expiratory film. A radiopaque foreign body may be visualized in a minority of cases.

• Infants and young children who are unable to cooperate for inspiratory and expiratory films should have lateral decubitus chest films performed. Bronchial foreign body aspiration is suggested when paradoxical hyperaeration is noted on the lower lung of the decubitus film.

• Patients with normal or equivocal plain films but a very good history of aspiration or focal findings on examination should undergo fluoroscopy. Positive results include mediastinal shift away from the foreign body during respiration.

Complications

Laryngeal or tracheal foreign bodies

• Complete airway obstruction that is not relieved will result in cardiopulmonary arrest with possible death or ensuing neurologic disability.

• Untreated partial airway obstruction may result in complete airway obstruction.

Bronchial foreign bodies

• Delay in diagnosis may cause recurrent pneumonia distal to the obstruction.

Differential diagnosis

Laryngeal or tracheal foreign bodies
Epiglottitis (supraglottitis).
Viral laryngotracheobronchitis (croup).
Bacterial tracheitis.
Retropharyngeal abscess.
Tonsillar/adenoidal enlargement.
Angioedema.
Mechanical or chemical trauma.
Esophageal foreign body.
Bronchial foreign bodies
Asthma/reactive airway disease.
Bronchiolitis.
Pneumonia.

Etiology

• Aspirated airway foreign bodies in children include primarily food substances and children's products.

• In a report on childhood fatal choking by food, 44% were caused by four items—hot dogs (17%), candy (10%), nuts (9%), and grapes (8%).

• 10% of non–food-choking deaths are related to children's products, with 43% caused by toy balloons and 22% by small balls.

• The majority of airway foreign bodies in children lodge in the main or segmental bronchi. Laryngotracheal foreign bodies comprise approximately 10% of these aspirations.

Epidemiology

• Approximately 85% of airway foreign bodies are found in children; only 15% occur in adults.

• Most childhood airway foreign bodies (60%–80%) occur in children younger than 3 y.

• Most series consistently reveal a male:female ratio of 2:1.

• Foreign body aspiration is the most common cause of accidental death in children less than 1 y.

• Nearly 3000 people die each year in the US due to aspiration of foreign bodies where it is the sixth leading cause of accidental death. Children account for ~300 of these deaths each year.

Treatment

Diet and lifestyle management
• Accident prevention must be emphasized with parents of infants and children. Small objects must be kept from children, and risky foods should be avoided or cut into small pieces.

The Consumer Product Safety Commission has limited small parts in children's toys.

Pharmacologic treatment
• Pharmacologic therapy is not indicated for patients with foreign bodies of the airway.

Other treatment options

Supraglottic foreign bodies with complete airway obstruction
• For children aged <1 year, basic life support consists of repeated series of five intrascapular back blows followed by five chest thrusts.

• For children aged >1 year, basic life support consists of repetitive abdominal thrusts (the Heimlich maneuver).

• Direct visualization and extraction. When basic life support measures are unsuccessful, perform direct laryngoscopy and remove the foreign body with Magill forceps. Blind finger sweeps of the oral cavity are contraindicated since the foreign body could be pushed back into the airway causing further obstruction.

• If both of the above are unsuccessful, attempt vigorous bag valve mask ventilation followed by intubation or needle cricothyroidotomy if needed. Prepare patient for immediate bronchoscopy.

Supraglottic foreign bodies with partial airway obstruction
• Allow the patient to maintain a position of comfort while avoiding noxious stimuli.

• Provide supplemental oxygen and perform noninvasive monitoring by pulse oximetry.

• Arrange for controlled airway evaluation in the operating room with rigid bronchoscopy for foreign body removal.

Infraglottic foreign bodies
• Have the patient remain npo and monitor oxygen saturation.

• Bronchoscopy, which has a 98% success rate, is indicated for the following groups of patients: 1) those with plain films suggestive of a foreign body; 2) those with fluoroscopy suggestive of a foreign body; and 3) those with an excellent ingestion history or new onset of focal sign/symptom complex (wheezing, decreased breath sounds and cough), regardless of radiographic studies.

• Observation with follow-up in 2–3 days is warranted in the following groups of patients: 1) those with no symptoms or signs and normal radiographs, and 2) those with normal fluoroscopy and a low index of suspicion for foreign body aspiration.

• Thoracotomy is rarely needed for patients with lower respiratory tract foreign bodies.

Treatment aims
To prevent cardiopulmonary arrest, death, or neurologic disability from complete airway obstruction.
To prevent inflammation and granulation tissue formation associated with subsequent atelectasis or pneumonia, necessitating complete or partial lobectomy in bronchial foreign bodies.

Prognosis
• Complete airway obstruction is rapidly fatal unless prompt measures to relieve obstruction are initiated; immediate therapy has an excellent prognosis.
• Approximately 50% of bronchial foreign bodies have a delay in diagnosis; these patients are more likely to experience pneumonia or difficult bronchoscopic removal.

Follow-up and management
• Laryngeal or tracheal foreign bodies cause airway edema, secondary bacterial infection or post-obstructive pulmonary edema.
• Bronchial foreign bodies may cause pneumonia or wheezing.
• Hospital admission for respiratory observation is warranted after definitive therapy.
• Treatment with steroids, antibiotics or inhaled beta-agonists should be considered on an individual case basis.

General references
Halvorson DJ, et al. Management of subglottic foreign bodies. Ann Otol Rhinol Laryngol 1996, 105:541–544.

Kelly SM, Marsh BR: Airway foreign bodies. Chest Surg Clin N Am 1996, 6:253–276.

Landwirth J, Tepas JJ, Todres ID, et al.: Pediatric Basic Life Support. In Textbook of Pediatric Advanced Life Support. Edited by Chameides L, Hazinski MF. American Heart Association/American Academy of Pediatrics: Dallas; 1993.

Respiratory Distress. In Advanced Pediatric Life Support. American Academy of Pediatrics/American College of Emergency Physicians: Elk Grove Village, Illinois; 1993.

Westfal R. Foreign body airway obstruction: when the Heimlich maneuver fails. Am J Emerg Med 1997, 15:103–105.

Foreign body, gastrointestinal

Diagnosis

Types of foreign bodies [1]

Coins: the most commonly ingested object in children. Coins approximately 24 mm or less (*eg*, quarter) almost always pass spontaneously through the gastrointestinal tract. Parents should be instructed to screen all stools for the object. Radiographs should be taken every 7 to 10 days to determine the object's location. If the object does not pass spontaneously within 4 to 6 weeks, it should be removed endoscopically.

Disk (button) batteries: urgent radiographic evaluation should be performed. Esophageal impaction requires immediate removal. Once in the stomach, repeat abdominal radiography should be performed within 3 days. Removal is indicated if the battery remains in the gastric cavity.

Sharp/elongated objects: objects longer than 5 cm (for small infants >3 cm) or wider than 2 cm are unlikely to pass through the stomach. Sharp objects cause up to 35% of intestinal perforations; long straight pins, bones, toothpicks, and glass carry higher risk. Screws, thumbtacks, small nails, and safety pins can be managed conservatively. The same conservative rules for coins apply.

Food: esophageal impaction of food must be removed within 24 hours (meat and hot dogs most common offenders). Food impaction suggests an underlying anatomic disorder. Treatment with meat tenderizer *should be avoided*.

Radiolucent objects: glass, wood, and plastic objects pose major problems. Investigation with contrast studies need to be considered in all symptomatic patients and when large or elongated objects are ingested in asymptomatic patients.

Symptoms

• Up to 40% of children with esophageal foreign bodies are asymptomatic.

Drooling, vomiting, abdominal pain, dysphagia, odynophagia: common symptoms with obstructing objects.

Respiratory symptoms: cough, stridor, wheezing, chest pain, choking, abnormal respirations.

Hypogastric pain, pain on defecation, rectal bleeding: may be associated with a colonic foreign body either placed by the child or secondary to an ingested foreign body lodged in the colon.

Signs

Increased salivation: suggestive of esophageal impaction.

Neck mass: suggestive of proximal esophageal perforation.

Inspiratory stridor: suggestive of airway involvement.

Fever, peritoneal signs: suggestive of gastrointestinal perforation.

Investigations

Blood tests: lead levels should be obtained for all objects that remain in the gastrointestinal tract and contain lead as lead toxicity can occur.

Chest/abdominal radiography: plain radiographs provide information on the location of all radiodense objects. Objects lodged in the esophagus will appear "flat" on an anteroposterior view (on "edge" on a lateral view); the opposite is true of tracheal objects (anteroposterior view "edge;" lateral view "flat"). Plain radiographs can be used to follow the gastrointestinal progression of ingested objects. [2]

Radiographic contrast studies: thin barium can be used to visualize radiolucent objects in the esophagus. Gastrograffin should not be used when esophageal foreign bodies are suspected because aspirated gastrograffin can cause pulmonary edema. A normal barium upper gastrointestinal series should be performed when questioning the location of foreign objects in the stomach and small intestine.

Epidemiology

• Peak incidence of childhood ingestion occurs between 6 mo and 3 y of age.

• Children with neurologic impairment or developmental delay at increased risk.

• ~80%–90% of all ingested object will spontaneously pass through the gastrointestinal system within 4–7 d.

• Approximately 10% to 20% will require endoscopy for removal; less than 1% will need surgical removal.

• Coins comprise more than 90% of all ingested foreign objects.

Complications

Intestinal obstruction, perforation, or stricture.

Esophageal pouch.

Aspiration pneumonia.

Mediastinitis.

Esophageal-aortic or tracheoesophageal fistula.

Abscess.

Emergent care required

• Esophageal foreign bodies require removal within 24 h secondary to the risk of perforation; esophageal disk button batteries obligate immediate endoscopic removal.

• Gastric button batteries require urgent removal if still present in the stomach after 3 d.

• Symptoms of vomiting, abdominal pain, pulmonary symptoms or dysphagia in association with foreign body ingestion necessitate immediate removal.

Gastrointestinal sites of obstruction

Esophagus: aortic arch, lower esophageal sphincter.

Stomach: pylorus.

Small intestine: ligament of Treitz, ileocecal valve.

Large intestine: sigmoid colon, rectum.

Treatment

Diet and lifestyle

Prevention relies on careful observation of infants and toddlers. Older children should be frequently reminded not to place objects in their mouth.

Pharmacologic treatment

Intravenous glucagon: hormone that induces smooth muscle relaxation. It is particularly effective for distal esophageal object secondary to its effect on lower esophageal sphincter relaxation. Dose, 0.05 mg/kg [3].

Enzymatic dissolution (meat tenderizer): the use of digestive enzymes (*eg*, papain, Adolph's meat tenderizer) for esophageal food impactions is not recommended secondary to potential esophageal mucosal injury and possible perforation.

Nonpharmacologic treatment

Endoscopy: all gastrointestinal foreign bodies should be removed under direct endoscopic vision. If an esophageal object is difficult to remove it may be pushed into the gastric cavity. Sharp objects should be removed with the sharp end "trailing." General endotracheal anesthesia should be performed to prevent possible aspiration of the foreign body during removal. An endoscopic overtube is useful when removing sharp objects [4].

Nonstandard methods of removal

Foley catheter: some investigators recommend esophageal coin removal via the use of a Foley catheter. The procedure is performed under flouroscopy in an immobilized patient by an experienced physician. The risks of this procedure include aspiration and esophageal perforation. The increased availability of endoscopy has replaced this procedure.

Laparotomy: indicated when an object causes intestinal obstruction or perforation.

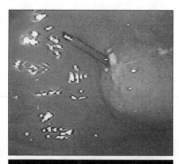

Nail perforating the stomach with accompanying abscess.

Treatment aims

Removal of the gastrointestinal object.

Prognosis

• On removal, the prognosis is good.

Follow-up and management

• Once the object has been removed or is passed spontaneously, no follow-up is required unless mucosal injury or a complication has occurred.

Key references

1. Webb WA: Management of foreign bodies of the upper gastrointestinal tract. *Gastroenterology* 1988, **94:**204–216.

2. Hodge D, Tecklenburg F, Fleisher G: Coin ingestion: does every child need a radiograph. *Ann Emerg Med* 1985, **14:**105–108.

3. Friedland GW: The treatment of acute esophageal food impaction. *Radiology* 1983, **149:**601–602.

4. Rosch W, Classen M: Fiberendoscopic foreign body removal from the upper gastrointestinal tract. *Endoscopy* 1972, **4:**193–197.

Diagnosis

Symptoms

Developmental delay.

Signs

Dysmorphic features: macrocephaly (in childhood), long face, large ears, macroorchidism (after age 8); however, some affected individuals do not have any dysmorphic features.

• Both developmental delay and dysmorphism are more common in affected males than females. The phenotype (appearance) and degree of neurological involvement of affected (heterozygous) females is extremely variable, and some individuals are intellectually normal. Fragile X syndrome should be investigated in all males who have unexplained developmental delay, especially if there is a family history of mental retardation.

Investigations

• DNA-based molecular analysis of the number of fragile X trinucleotide repeats is required. Neither a standard karyotype nor cytogenetic methods of diagnosis alone are reliable for diagnosis.

Complications

• Autistic features are present in the majority of individuals. Other behavioral problems include attention deficit hyperactivity disorder and gaze aversion. Strabismus and mitral valve prolapse may occur.

Differential diagnosis

Fragile X syndrome should be considered in individuals with developmental delay or mental retardation of unknown etiology, especially if they are males. A family history consistent with X-linked mental retardation is also suggestive. The presence of behavioral problems may also be suggestive for fragile X syndrome. However, there are other forms of nonspecific mental retardation which are X-linked and for which the molecular basis is unknown. It must be remembered that the facial and other abnormalities associated with fragile X syndrome that are detectable on physical examination are not present in all patients, and these features may often become more prominent with age.

Etiology

• The gene on the X chromosome (Xq27.3), FMR1, has a variable number of trinucleotide CGG repeats. Normal individuals have less than approximately 50 repeats. Individuals with 50–200 repeats have a premutation and normal phenotypes. Individuals with greater than 200 repeats have the full mutation. The exact number of repeats differentiating between normal, premutation, and full mutation depends on the laboratory performing the test. Essentially all males with the full mutation show clinical effects. Expansion of the repeat sequences occurs only in female meiosis in the germ line. Thus, a woman with a premutation may have expansion to a full mutations and have affected children. However, a man with a premutation ("transmitting male") is not at risk of having affected children, although all of his daughters will inherit the premutation. Prenatal diagnosis is reliable.

Epidemiology

• Fragile X syndrome affects 1:1250–5000 males and 1:1600–5000 females. It is the most frequent cause of mental retardation that follows a mendelian inheritance pattern.

Treatment

General information

• At the present time, there is no specific pharmacologic therapy that has consistently shown to be beneficial for individuals with Fragile X syndrome. Medical management should include appropriate genetic counseling, and the implications for other family members should be explained. The pediatrician should be alerted to problems in several areas that occur more frequently in children with Fragile X syndrome. Ophthalmologic abnormalities include strabismus and myopia; ptosis and nystagmus are occasionally present. A thorough assessment for connective tissue abnormalities should be carried out. This may include hyperextensibility of joints (including the hip), flat feet, inguinal hernias, and scoliosis. Mitral valve prolapse occurs with an increased frequency, and referral to a cardiologist should be done if a murmur or click is present. A careful history for seizures should be taken. Recurrent otitis media is associated, and audiologic examination should be performed as indicated.

• Behavior problems are frequent, and treatment may be helpful for some individuals. Attention deficit–hyperactivity disorder commonly occurs, and this may improve with age. Head banging and hand biting may also occur.

• The names of support groups and services for Fragile X syndrome should be supplied to the family. Children should be referred for appropriate intervention so that speech, occupational, and physical therapy can be instituted as indicated.

Prognosis/natural history

• Mental retardation in males varies from profound to mild, with the majority having an IQ in the 30–55 range. Speech and language are usually most severely affected. Approximately 50% of females with a full mutation (see Etiology) show some degree of cognitive deficit.

General references

American Academy of Pediatrics Committee on Genetics: Health supervision for children with fragile X syndrome. *Pediatrics* 1996, **98:**297–300.

Hagerman RJ, Jackson C, Amiri K, *et al.*: Girls with fragile X syndrome: physical and neurocognitive status and outcome. *Pediatrics* 1992, **89:**395–400.

Lachiewicz AM, Dawson DV: Do young boys with fragile X syndrome have macroorchidism? *Pediatrics* 1994, **93:**992–995.

Sutherland GR, Gedeon A, Kornman L, *et al.*: Prenatal diagnosis of fragile X syndrome by direct detection of the unstable DNA sequence. *N Engl J Med* 1991, **325:**1720–1722.

Diagnosis

Symptoms

Hematemesis: fresh red blood or darker altered blood that may resemble ground coffee.

Melena: passage of black, sticky, foul-smelling stool.

Rectal bleeding (hematochezia): passage of fresh red blood or darker red "maroon" from rectum; may be unaltered blood, blood mixed into the stool, blood clots, or bloody diarrhea.

Collapse, loss of consciousness, angina, shortness of breath, malaise, headache: symptoms of hypotension or anemia secondary to catastrophic blood loss.

Signs

Tachycardia: earliest sign of shock.

Hypotension: especially postural.

Splenomegaly, spider nevi, palmar erythema: stigmata of chronic liver disease (varices should be considered).

Abdominal tenderness: unusual (consider perforated ulcer).

Findings of telangiectasia: Osler–Weber–Rendu syndrome, or liver disease.

Investigations

Apt test: newborns with hematemesis may have swallowed maternal blood from breast feeding [1].

Hemoglobin and hematocrit analysis: time needed for hemodilution, so initial hemoglobin may not reflect severity of bleeding.

Platelet count: raised with recent bleeding or iron deficiency, may be low in liver or HIV-related disease or in patients with splenomegaly.

Prothrombin time, partial thromboplastin time: elevated in patients with liver disease or easy bruising.

Urea (BUN) measurement: concentration often elevated with bleeding and may rise further in hypotensive patients.

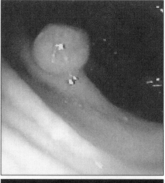

Juvenile polyp.

Fiberoptic endoscopy: visible vessel in peptic ulcer indicates 50% chance of further hemorrhage and increased risk of death; large varices and cherry-red spots may predict increased risk of further bleeding; endoscopy superior to barium studies in making diagnosis in most situations.

Colonoscopy: useful for hemtochezia (polyp, colitis, hemorrhoids).

99m Tc-labeled erythrocyte scanning: may detect bleeding rate of 1 mL/min and is used to locate site of bleeding distal to the ligament of Treitz.

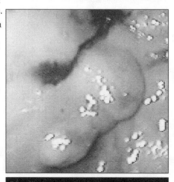

Bleeding gastric varices.

Tc pertechnate scanning: useful for Meckel's diverticulum because isotope taken up by ectopic gastric mucosa in diverticulum.

Angiography: occasionally useful for severe recurrent bleeding (needs bleeding rate of >5 mL/min); presence of barium may compromise angiography.

Differential diagnosis

Hematemesis: nose bleeds and hemoptysis, with subsequently swallowed blood.

Melena: ingestion of iron, bismuth-containing preparations, producing black stool; foods (licorice, blueberries).

Hematochezia: fruit juices, foods.

Etiology

History of previous bleeding, ulcer, or GI disease (in <50% of patients).

Hematemesis preceded by retching (suggesting Mallory–Weiss tear).

Liver disease, coagulopathy, amyloidosis.

Family history of bleeding.

Previous surgery for peptic ulcer or arterial bypass grafts.

Drugs can cause esophageal and gastric erosion.

Causes of upper GI bleeding

Gastric erosions, duodenal ulcer, gastric ulcer, varices, esophagitis, erosive duodenitis, Mallory–Weiss tear, esophageal ulcer, polyp.

Reflux esophagitis and hiatal hernia.

Helicobacter pylori and AIDS-related disease.

Causes of lower GI bleeding

Hemorrhoids, polyps, inflammatory bowel disease, drug-induced ulcer or solitary rectal ulcer.

Meckel's diverticulum, intestinal duplication cyst, intussusception, hemangioma, volvulus.

Hemolytic uremic syndrome, Henoch-Schönlein purpura.

• Anal fissures are the most usual cause of lower GI bleeding. Bright blood unmixed with stool often seen only on toilet paper; this is rarely a cause of major bleeding. In infants: milk-protein allergy, necrotizing enterocolitis, Hirschprung's enterocolitis.

Epidemiology

• The incidence of GI bleeding in children is unknown; it accounts for <5% of visits to a gastroenturologist.

Complications

Recurrent or continued bleeding.

Exsanguination.

Aspiration (upper GI bleeding).

Treatment

Diet and lifestyle

• Patients should avoid aspirin and other NSAIDs and should not smoke.

• Patients must not eat just before endoscopy or surgery; at other times, no evidence suggests that starving or feeding patients confers benefit.

Pharmacologic treatment

For peptic ulcer

• There is little evidence that drug treatment affects outcome from bleeding peptic ulcer; omeprazole (bleeding peptic ulcers) or octreotide (bleeding varices) may reduce the risk of recurrent bleeding when added to endoscopic management.

• Treatment by long-term H2 blockade or eradication of *Helicobacter pylori* may reduce the incidence of readmission with peptic ulcer bleeding.

For bleeding varices

• Drug treatments are probably ineffective in the long-term treatment of bleeding varices. Some clinicians claim that a somatostatin analogue (octreotide) or propanolol may improve outcome.

• Intravenous vasopressin is used in the acute management of bleeding esophageal varices. Given by continuous infusion, side effects include hypoatremia, vasoconstriction, bradycardia, and arrythmia.

Nonpharmacologic treatment

Transfusion

Whole blood or packed cells; not for patients with minor bleeding or who are at low risk for further bleeding; nasogastric tube should be placed to determine presence of upper GI bleeding; hematochezia may represent rapid transit from upper source.

For peptic ulcer

Endoscopic treatment (laser, monopolar, bipolar, heater probe, and injection of adrenaline alone, adrenaline and a sclerosant, or alcohol): can reduce rebleeding rate, need for surgery, and mortality; repeat endoscopic treatment may be preferable to surgery in elderly patients [3–5].

Surgery: in patients with continued or recurrent bleeding in hospital; best done before repeated episodes of hypotension have impaired chances of recovery.

For bleeding varices

Endoscopic variceal injection sclerotherapy, using sclerosants such as mono-ethanolamine, alcohol, sodium tetradecyl sulfate, or sodium morrhuate: has been shown to reduce the incidence of further bleeding and to reduce mortality in patients with recent bleeding from esophageal varices, and it can stop bleeding from varices.

Endoscopic variceal band ligation: less invasive than surgery, has lower complication rate than endoscopic sclerotherapy (experimental in children) [3].

Balloon tamponade: stops bleeding in 85% of patients, but bleeding recurs in 21%–60% and survival not improved; complications include esophageal rupture and aspiration pneumonia, with lethal complications of 10%.

Percutaneous transhepatic cannulation of portal vein: with injection of sclerosant or obliterative substance, *eg*, Gelfoam, thrombin, cyanoacrylate.

Transjugular intrahepatic portacaval shunt: for patients who have recurrent variceal bleeding despite sclerotherapy or ligation therapy.

Surgery: for the few patients who do not respond to endoscopic treatment; options include portosystemic shunt, esophageal transection, devascularization, or hepatic transplantation [6].

For colonic polyps: colonoscopy with electrocautery by snare technique or by hot biopsy forceps. Polyps should be sent for histology.

Treatment aims

To reduce mortality, need for urgent surgery, and rebleeding rate.

Prognosis

• Complications occur more frequently with upper GI bleeding.

• The risk of death is <1% in the majority of children who present with GI bleeding.

• Patients with esophageal varices and lower disease usually require liver transplantation within 5 y.

• Bleeding due to Mallory–Weiss tear, esophagitis, gastritis, and duodenitis has excellent prognosis.

Follow-up and management

• Ulcer patients with major bleeding should have follow-up endoscopy to check healing and eradication of *H. pylori.*

• Patients with second major bleed should be considered for surgery.

• Patients with bleeding varices need repeat endoscopy and sclerotherapy until varices are eradicated.

Complications of treatment

After surgery: pneumonia, renal or cardiac failure, further bleeding.

Endoscopy for bleeding peptic ulcer: precipitation of acute bleeding, perforation, infarction of stomach or duodenum (with injection).

Endoscopy for bleeding varices: esophageal ulceration, perforation, septicemia, distant thrombosis, pleural effusion, aspiration.

Colonoscopy: perforation, hemorrhage.

Key references

1. Apt L, Downey WS: "Melena" neonatorum: the swallowed blood syndrome: a simple test for the differentiation of adult and fetal hemoglobin in bloody stools. *J Pediatr* 1955, **47:**6–12.

2. Sherman NJ, Clatworthy HW: Gastrointestinal bleeding in neonates: a study of 94 cases. *Surgery* 1967, **62:**614–619.

3. Laine L, el-Newihi HM, Migikovsky B, et al.: Endoscopic ligation compared with sclerotherapy for the treatment of bleeding esophageal varices. *Ann Intern Med* 1993, **119:**1–7.

Gaucher disease

Diagnosis

Symptoms

- **Type 1:** hepatomegaly, painless splenomegaly, acute bone pain (Gaucher bone crisis), and poor growth and development in childhood; children may have a history of frequent nose bleeds and bruising; symptoms can occur at any age and vary within the same family; most patients have no symptoms from lung or heart involvement.

- **Type 2 (acute neuronopathic):** onset is in first few months of life with a history of developmental arrest, then regression; symptoms may be inattentiveness, failure to reach for objects, inability to roll over, and loss of head control; early bulbar involvement causes poor sucking and swallowing reflexes. Generalized spasticity is severe and associated with head retraction and tonic arching of the back, resembling opisthotonus; seizures are generally late manifestations; massive enlargement of liver and spleen may be noted, but without the severe hypersplenism seen in type 1 disease; progression is rapid, culminating in death within several months from respiratory complications.

- **Type 3 (subacute neuronopathic):** prominent neurological abnormalities and relatively mild visceral involvement; presentation is usually mid- to late childhood with myoclonus, dementia, and ataxia; a typical feature is early development of an isolated horizontal supranuclear gaze palsy; vertical movements are generally intact; tonic–clonic seizures and progressive spasticity are followed by neurological degeneration in the second and third decades of life; spleen and liver are usually enlarged, but not to the extent seen in type 3b or severe type 1; skeletal manifestations are similar to type 1.

- **Type 3b:** subtle neurological abnormalities, but with severe visceral disease. Patients may be initially thought to have type 1 disease; however, presentation is usually at 2 to 3 years and the degree of hepatosplenomegaly is greater and more rapidly progressive; failure to thrive is often severe and may be accompanied by ascites, peripheral edema, easy bruising, nose bleeds, and other evidence of coagulopathy; portal hypertension, bleeding from esophageal varices, and other evidence of cirrhosis may be prominent.

Signs

- Anemia, low leukocyte and platelet counts are seen on routine CBCs. Elevations of total acid phosphatase and angiotensin-converting enzyme are common.

- Bone deterioration in types 1 and 3 can cause discomfort. Erlenmeyer flask deformities of the distal femur are a common feature. Osteopenia, osteonecrosis, osteosclerosis, cortical thinning, demineralization, and joint degeneration may be noted on bone MRI. Encroachment of these cells in the marrow space may result in aseptic necrosis of bone. Proximal areas of the long bones are usually affected before distal areas. The femur should be evaluated first.

Investigations

Glucocerebrosidase activity: markedly decreased in leukocytes, fibroblasts, tissues.

Molecular genetic analysis to determine genotype.

Complete blood count: leukocytes, hemoglobin, hematocrit, platelet count.

Total acid phosphatase.

Radiologic: bone MRI of femur and hip (also any other symptomatic bone or joint area).

MRI or CT to determine liver and spleen volume.

DEXA: bone densitometry.

Complications

- Type 1 disease has both visceral and bone complications.
- Type 2 disease has cardiorespiratory problems.
- Type 3 disease may manifest ocular–motor degeneration as well as bone and visceral complications (*see* type 1).

Differential diagnosis

Type 1: Distinguish from other conditions presenting with hepatosplenomegaly including infections, infestations, neoplasias, reticuloendothelioses, hemoglobinopathies, and storage diseases. Leukemia, thalassemia, von Willebrand factor deficiency, factor IX deficiency, factor XI deficiency are often misdiagnosed in individuals presenting initially with hematological abnormalities. Patients with bone pain initially may be thought to have septic osteomyelitis. Limping due to avascular necrosis of the hip occurs in Legg–Calvé–Perthes disease.

Type 2: Must be differentiated from other early-onset neurodegenerative storage disorders.

Type 3: Conditions featuring myoclonus resembling this type include benign juvenile myoclonic epilepsy, neuronal ceroid lipofuscinosis, sialidosis, late-onset GM_1 and GM_2 gangliosidosis, Niemann-Pick disease types C and type D, MERRF syndrome, Univerricht–Lundborg disease, Lafora disease, dentatorubral-pallidoluysian atrophy.

Etiology

- Patients are deficient in glucocerebrosidase. Resulting in accumulation in the lysosomes of reticuloendothelial cells to produce the characteristic Gaucher cells. Areas most affected are spleen, liver, bone marrow, and lung.
- Progressive and inherited in an autosomal recessive manner. The principal difference among the types is the presence and progression of neurologic complications. Type 1 is the most common and has a chronic, nonneuronopathic course. Type 2 disease is the acute neuronopathic or infantile form. Type 3 is referred to as the subacute neuronopathic or juvenile form.
- Gaucher disease is caused by mutations in the gene encoding the lysosomal enzyme glucocerebrosidase, resulting in an unstable enzyme with little or no enzymatic activity in the lysosome.

Epidemiology

Type 1 disease: in Ashkenazic Jewish population, disease incidence is ~1:500–1:1000. In non-Jewish population, incidence is ~1:60,000 to 1:200,000.

Type 2 disease: incidence is 1:100,000

Type 3 disease: incidence is 1:50,000.

Treatment

General information
• Patients diagnosed with Gaucher disease should be referred to a multispecialty comprehensive Gaucher treatment center for evaluation and treatment.

• Macrophage-directed exogenous enzyme replacement therapy, using imiglucerase, is available for treatment of patients with type 1 Gaucher disease. For exogenous enzyme to be effective, it must reach the lysosome in the macrophage. The discovery that macrophage receptors recognized mannose as the terminal sugar residue on the glycoprotein's oligosaccharide chain provided the rational for macrophage-targeted enzyme replacement therapy. The carbohydrate portion of glucocerebrosidase is modified to expose the mannose terminal, facilitating the recognition and uptake of glucocerebrosidase into macrophages. Recombinant enzyme and imiglucerase are used for injection. Treatment should be started on patients with moderate to severe signs and symptoms of the disease. Dosage is based on the severity of disease.

• Splenectomy should only be considered in patients with mechanical cardiopulmonary compromise in whom enzyme replacement therapy has not decreased the size of the organs sufficiently to facilitate medical management.

• Bone disease may require orthopedic procedures to relieve pain and promote better use of affected joints. These procedures should be considered along with enzyme replacement therapy to achieve optimal outcome, especially in patients with cortical thinning.

• Patients with bone crisis should be admitted to hospital for intravenous hydration and administration of analgesics for pain control. Blood cultures and bone scans should be done to ensure that there is no osteomyelitis.

Lifestyle management
• Patients with severe bone disease or who have grossly enlarged liver and spleen should avoid activities that could result in pathologic fractures of bone or rupture of organ. Patients with early satiety may benefit from small, frequent meals.

Support group
The National Gaucher Foundation, 11140 Rockville Pike, Rockville, MD 20852-3106. tel: 800-925-8885; fax: 301-816-1516; website: www.gaucherdisease.org. There are also many local chapters in large metropolitan areas.

General references

Beutler E, Grabowski GA: Gaucher disease. In *The Metabolic and Molecular Bases of Inherited Disease*, vol II. Edited by Scriber CR, Beaudet AL, Sly WS, Valle D. New York: McGraw-Hill; 1995:2641–2670.

Grabowski GA: Gaucher disease, enzymology, genetics, and treatment. *Adv Hum Genet* 1993, 21:377.

Beutler E: Gaucher disease [review article]. *N Engl J Med* 1991, 325:1354–1360.

Kaplan P, Mazur A, Manor O, et al.: Acceleration of retarded growth in children with Gaucher disease after treatment with alglucerase. *J Pediatr* 1996, 129:149–153.

Stowens DW, Teitelbaum SL, Kahn, et al.: Skeletal complications of Gaucher disease. *Medicine (Baltimore)* 1985, 64:310–322.

Beutler E, Saven A: The misuse of marrow examination in the diagnosis of Gaucher disease. *Blood* 1990, 76:646–648.

Shafit-Zagardo B, Devine EA, Smith M, et al.: Assignment of the gene for acid beta-glucosidase to human chromosome 1. *Am J Hum Genet* 1981, 33:564–575.

Theophilus B, Latham T, Grabowski GA, Smith FA: Gaucher disease: molecular heterogeneity and phenotype-genotype correlations. *Am J Hum Genet* 1989, 45:212–225.

Barton NW, Brady RO, Dambrosia JM, et al.: Replacement therapy for inherited enzyme deficiency-macrophage-targeted glucocerebrosidase for Gaucher disease. *N Engl J Med* 1991, 324:1464–1470.

Ming JE, Mazur AT, Kaplan P: Gaucher disease and Niemann-Pick disease. In *Pediatric Gastroenterology*. Edited by Liacouras C, Altschuler S, in press.

Diagnosis

Definition
Acute onset of hematuria, oliguria, edema, hypertension, and azotemia.
Follows a pharyngitis or impetigo.

Symptoms and signs
Hematuria: painless, cola-colored.
Fatigue: general malaise, abdominal pain.
Edema: mainly periorbital.
Hypertension: mild to severe.
Ascites and/or pleural effusions.
Urine: output decreased or normal.

Investigations
Urinalysis: crenated erythrocytes, erythrocyte casts.
Urine dipstick: positive for blood and protein.
Serum creatinine and BUN: increased.
Serum albumin: may be decreased.
Serum potassium: may reach life-threatening levels.
Hemoglobin: slightly decreased.
Throat culture for β-hemolytic *Streptococcus*.
Positive Streptozyme test.
Positive antistreptolysin O titer (ASOT).
Complement (C3): markedly decreased.
Renal biopsy: indicated if atypical presentation or course; or if C3 is low after 8 weeks.
Renal imaging studies: not routinely indicated.

Complications
Acute renal failure.
Hypertension: can be severe.
Seizures.
Chronic renal failure: almost never occurs in acute poststreptococcal glomerulonephritis.

Differential diagnosis
IgA nephropathy: negative serologies for antecedent streptococcal infection; normal C3 concentration.

Henoch-Schönlein purpura: typical purpuric-urticarial rash on extensor surfaces; arthritis; abdominal pain, melena; testicular swelling; normal C3 concentration.

Antineutrophil cytoplasmic antibody (ANCA)–positive glomerulonephritis: rapidly progressive course; may have pulmonary infiltrates, sinusitis, arthritis; ANCA positive; normal C3; kidney biopsy indicated.

Goodpasture syndrome (antiglomerular basement membrane [GBM] antibody disease): extremely uncommon in children; rapidly progressive course; hemoptysis; pulmonary infiltrates; normal C3; positive serum anti-GBM antibodies; kidney biopsy indicated.

Membranoproliferative glomerulonephritis (MPGN): usually insidious onset; nephrotic syndrome with nephritic components; low C3; serum nephritic factors; kidney biopsy indicated.

Systemic lupus: can occasionally present with acute nephritic symptoms and signs (usually butterfly rash, arthritis, fever, anemia, thrombocytopenia, leukopenia, serositis); low C3, positive antineutrophil antibodies, DNA binding; kidney biopsy indicated if there is proteinuria.

Postinfectious glomerulonephritis: causes include hepatitis B, C; infective endocarditis; *Mycoplasma pneumoniae*.

Alport syndrome: onset rarely acute; positive family history; sensorineural hearing deficit; X-linked inheritance..

Etiology
Antecedent infection with β-hemolytic streptococcal pharyngitis or impetigo. Immunologically mediated with hypocomplementemia and glomerular deposits of C3 and IgG.

Epidemiology
Incidence is decreasing.
Peak ages 5–15 y.
Occurs mainly in winter, spring.

Treatment

Diet and lifestyle

Bed rest as needed by the patient.

Restrict salt (1 g/d) to reduce edema and hypertension.

Restict potassium intake.

Treat hyperkalemia (*see* Renal failure, acute).

Dialysis if oligoanuric, hyperkalemic, fluid overloaded.

Pharmacologic treatment

Hyperkalemia: exchange resin, insulin plus glucose.

Diuretics: fluid overload—furosemide if mild; dialysis if severe.

Hypertension: furosemide if not oliguric; hydralazine or nifedipine.

Antibiotics: not indicated for renal disease.

Course

Onset of diuresis in a week.

C3 normalizes in 6–8 weeks.

Gross hematuria rapidly resolves.

Proteinuria may persist for months.

Microscopic hematuria may persist for up to 2 years.

Treatment aims

To avoid, treat hyperkalemia.

To treat hypertension.

Prognosis

Excellent outcome.

Relapses are rare.

Follow-up and management

Most patients can be treated at home. Indications for admission to hospital: oliguria, hypertension, hyperkalemia, elevated serum creatinine.

General references

Andreoli SP: Chronic glomerulonephritis in childhood: membranoproliferative glomerulonephritis, Henoch-Schölein purpura nephritis, and IgA nephropathey. *Pediatr Clin North Am* 1995, **42:**1487–1503.

Austin HA, Boumpas DT: Treatment of lupus nephritis. *Sem Nephrol* 1996, **16:**527–535.

Fish AJ, Herdman RC, Michael AF, et al.: Epidemic acute glomerulonephritis associated with type 49 streptococcal pyoderma: II. Correlative study of light, immunofluorescent and electron microscopic findings. *Am J Med* 1970, 48:28–39.

Hogan SL, Nachman PH, Wilkman AS, et al.: Prognostic markers in patients with antineutrophil cytoplasmic autoantibody-associated microscopic polyangiitis and glomerulonephritis. *J Am Soc Nephrol* 1996, **7:**23–32.

Kaplan EL, Anthony BF, Chapman SS, Wannamaker LW: Epidemic acute glomerulonephritis associated with type 49 streptococcal pyoderma: I. Clinical and laboratory findings. *Am J Med* 1970, 48:9–27.

Kashtan CE: Alport syndrom. *Kidney Int* 1997, **58(suppl):**S69–S71

Potter EV, Siegal AC, Simon NM, et al.: Streptococcal infections and epidemic acute glomerulonephritis in South Trinidad. *J Pediatr* 1968, 72:871–884.

Roy S III, Stapleton FB: Changing perspectives in children hospitalized with poststreptococcal acute glomerulonephritis. *Pediatr Nephrol* 1990, 4:585–588.

Diagnosis

Symptoms

Fever: recurrent or prolonged.
"Swollen glands": lymphadenopathy.
Oropharyngeal, gingival pain.
Skin infection.
Headache, sinus pain.
Eye pain, discharge.
Cough, shortness of breath.
Sputum production.
Chest pain.

Abdominal pain, vomiting, nausea.
Diarrhea: chronic.
Rectal pain.
Bone pain.
Swollen, tender joints.
Flank pain.
Hesitancy or frequency of urination.
Failure to thrive, growth delay.

Signs

Sinus tenderness.
Mouth ulcers, gingivitis.
Folliculitis, impetigo, cutaneous granulomata, abscesses, or other superficial skin infections.
Lymphadenopathy, -adenitis.
Pneumonia, pleural effusion, consolidation.

Hepatomegaly, splenomegaly.
Abdominal mass, tenderness.
Perirectal abscess.
Bone tenderness, swelling.
Arthritis.
Flank tenderness.
Growth failure.

Investigations

Complete history (including detailed family history) and physical examination.

Culture site of infection: because the primary defect is the phagocyte's failure to produce hydrogen peroxide (H_2O_2), the most common infecting organisms are those that do not provide an alternate source of H_2O_2. These produce catalase, an enzyme that degrades H_2O_2. The most common pathogen is *Staphylococcus aureus* and others include *Klebsiella* spp, *Serratia marcescens*, *Escherichia coli*, *Aspergillus* spp, *Burholderia cepacia* (formerly *Pseudomonas cepacia*), *Candida albicans*, *Salmonella* spp, other enteric bacteria, *Nocardia* spp, *Mycobacteria spp*, and even *Pneumocystis carinii*.

Imaging studies to localize infection sites.

Biopsy as appropriate.

Complete blood count with differential and platelet count; ESR; CH_{50}, C3, C4 levels.

Quantitative immunoglobulins: IgG, IgA, IgM, IgE.

Antibody response (IgG) to immunizations: protein (tetanus, diphtheria) and polysaccharide (pneumococcus) antigens.

Screen for phagocyte metabolic defect using Nitroblue tetrazolium (NBT) test.

Specialized studies: to identify the specific defect in the NADPH oxidase complex (protein by Western blot, messenger RNA by Northern blot, and gene mutation by cDNA or genomic sequencing).

Bacterial killing assay.

Chemotaxis assay: in vitro.

Myeloperoxidase stain.

Flow cytometric analyses of CD11b/CD18 and Sialyl–Lewis X antigen (CD15s).

Baseline and acute pulmonary function assessments.

Complications

Sepsis; gastric outlet obstruction: other sites possible; malabsorption; pulmonary abscess, emphysema; restrictive lung disease; obstructive uropathy: hydronephrosis, hydroureter, pyelonephritis, cystitis; anemia of chronic disease; growth failure.

Differential diagnosis

Glucose-6-phosphate dehydrogenase (G6PD) deficiency: X-linked, rare disorder causing decrease in NADPH substrate for oxidase function if deficiency is severe (5%–10% of normal); associated with anemia.
Disorders of glutathione metabolism: severe deficiencies of glutathione reductase or glutathione synthase enzymes.
Myeloperoxidase deficiency.
Leukocyte adhesion deficiency -1 and -2.
Specific granule deficiency.
Chediak–Higashi syndrome.
Hyperimmunoglobulin E syndrome.
Neutrophil actin dysfunction.
Neutropenia.
Complement disorders.

Etiology

• Chronic granulomatous disease (CGD) is caused by mutations involving any one of the genes encoding a component of the NADPH oxidase complex found in phagocytes. Stimulated by ingestion of a pathogen, phagocyte NADPH oxidase becomes activated and reduces molecular oxygen to form superoxide anion and its derivatives H_2O_2 and hypochlorous acid, which provide critical antimicrobial function. Mutations have been documented in each of the four integral components of the NADPH oxidase complex:

1. p91-phox gene, X-linked (Xp21.1), ~60% of patients
2. p47-phox gene, autosomal recessive (chromosome 7), ~35% of cases
3. p22-phox gene, autosomal recessive (chromosome 16), rare
4. p67-phox gene, autosomal recessive (chromosome 1), rare

Epidemiology

• This genetically heterogenous disorder affects 1:750,000–1,000,000 individuals. Presentation is most often in childhood, although the diagnosis may be made in adulthood. CGD is an immunodeficiency disorder that results most commonly in more indolent types of infection in which inflammation is not always prominent until significant progression has occurred.

Treatment

Lifestyle management

• Patients must adapt to chronic disease, long-term medication, life-threatening infection.

• Active lifestyle is encouraged in combination with prophylactic measures and modest limitations on activity.

Preventive measures

• All routine immunizations (including live-virus) and influenza vaccine should be administered yearly.

• Superficial wounds should receive prompt cleansing, H_2O_2 treatment, dressing, and follow-up inspection.

• Reduce rectal infections by avoiding constipation and soaking early lesions.

• Patients should employ active oral hygiene to prevent gingivitis and periodontitis.

• Minimize exposure to inhalant mold spores. Environmental air should not include irritants or allergens that provoke chronic lung inflammation.

• Minimize use of oral and topical corticosteroids, except as essential (*eg*, asthma or gastric outlet obstruction).

Pharmacologic treatment

Prophylactic antibiotics

Daily trimethoprim–sulfamethoxazole or dicloxacillin.

Selective use of antifungals: *eg*, itraconazole for *Aspergillus*.

Aggressive treatment of infections

Parenteral antibiotics: early, appropriate application.

Granulocyte transfusions: may be useful for poorly responsive infections; intralesional transfusions have been successfully applied in hepatic abscess management (combined with interferon-γ).

Prophylactic recombinant human interferon-γ.

Other treatment options

• Consider surgical drainage or resection.

Special consideration

• Allogenic bone marrow transplantations in selected cases in which medical aggressive management fails to decrease the frequency of severe infections.

• A rare, null, Kell red blood cell phenotype is linked to the X chromosome and is occasionally found in CGD patients. Before transfusion, Kell phenotyping should be performed.

Treatment aims
To prevent infection.
To identify infection early.
To aggressively treat infection.
To preserve organ function.
• Genetic counseling and family support for chronic disease issues are recommended.

Prognosis
• With current treatment modalities, many patients reach adulthood.

Follow-up and management
Routine monitoring of infection and complications of disease and treatment.

Other information
• Prenatal diagnosis has been achieved using NBT testing of fetal neutrophils. Current DNA techniques allow presumptive diagnosis by restriction fragment length polymorphism analysis in informative families (deletion identified). Analysis of the specific mutation in fetal DNA obtained from chronic villus sampling or amniocentesis is possible in cases in which the responsible mutation has been identified in an affected family member or known carrier. Carrier detection is possible using the NBT test or flow cytometric methods in X-linked (not autosomal) cases, because two populations of cells can be detected (abnormal and normal). The ratio of normal to abnormal cells can vary widely since random X-inactivation may range from 10%–90%.

General references

Abramson SL: Phagocyte deficiencies. In *Clinical Immunology: Principles and Practice*. Edited by Rich RR. Mosby: St. Louis; 1996:677–693.

Hopkins PJ, Bemiller LS, Curnette JT: Chronic granulomatous disease: diagnosis and classification at the molecular level. *Clin Lab Med* 1992, 12:277–304.

Quie PG, Millo EL, Roberts RL, Noya FJD: Disorders of the polymorphonuclear phagocytic system. In *Immunologic Disorders of Infants and Children*, ed 4. Edited by Steihm ER. WB Saunders: Philadelphia; 1996:443–468.

Diagnosis

Symptoms

Height above the 95th percentile or increase in growth rate: the child is not necessarily tall but increasing in height percentiles is of concern.

Symptoms of hormone excess (hyperthyroidism, precocious puberty, virilization, galactorrhea).

Lax, hyperestensible joints, visual difficulties.

Facial or skin rashes.

Learning problems or neurologic symptoms, including hydrocephalus.

Signs

Height above 95th percentile or growth rate greater than 1.5 SD of mean velocity for age and gender, resulting in height increasing in percentiles.

Marfan syndrome or homocystinuria: hyperestensible joints, arachnodactyly, aortic regurgitation murmur, subluxated lens (inferior in homocystinuria and superiorly in Marfan syndrome); facial rash in homocystinuria; dominant inheritance in Marfan syndrome.

Large head, developmental delay in cerebral gigantism (Sotos' syndrome).

Macrocephaly, enlarging hands, feet, jaws, tongue, and nose: in pituitary gigantism.

Galactorrhea: occasionally.

Large café-au-lait spots: suggesting association of pituitary growth hormone producing adenoma and McCune–Albright syndrome.

Other signs of hormone excess: such as hyperthyroidism or precocious puberty or virilizing adenoma.

Investigations

Bone age radiography: normal bone age suggests either constitutional familial tall stature or genetic syndromes (Marfan, homocystinuria). Advancement of bone age is seen in excessive hormone production but only modestly so in pituitary gigantism. The bone age is advanced in cerebral gigantism.

Ophthalmologic examination: to detect subluxated lens.

Insulin growth factor-1 (somatomedin-C): is increased substantially in pituitary growth hormone excess.

Biochemical studies: elevation of urinary and serum homocysteine and lack of cystine in homocystinuria; thyroid function, androgens, and gonadotropins in other conditions suggestive of hormone excess.

Complications

• Marfan syndrome is associated with sudden death due to aortic aneurysm.

• Homocystinuria and Sotos' syndrome is associated with developmental delay.

• Pituitary gigantism is associated with hypogonadism, visual loss, and heart failure.

Differential diagnosis

Familial tall stature.
Syndromic conditions: Marfan, Sotos', and homocystinuria.
Excessive hormone production.

Etiology

Familial tall stature, Marfan syndrome, and homocystinuria: genetically determined.
Sotos' syndrome: not known.
Excessive hormone production: pituitary adenoma in growth hormone excess.

Epidemiology

Familial tall stature: 3% of the population.
• The syndromic conditions are relatively rare and pituitary gigantism is extremely rare.

Treatment

Diet and lifestyle
No changes are necessary.

Pharmacologic treatment
• Occasionally, medical treatment to induce precocious puberty to decrease final height is necessary. This is especially true in children with Marfan syndrome with orthopedic problems. It is necessary to use gonadal steroid treatment before age 8 in girls and 9 in boys.

Standard dosage   *Estrogen therapy*: conjugated estrogens, 0.3 mg daily to be increased to 0.625 mg daily.

Testosterone therapy: testosterone esters, 50 mg i.m. every 4 weeks, increasing to 100 mg at 6 months, then increasing to 150 mg and 200 mg until epiphyseal fusion occurs.

Special points   *Estrogen*: if menstrual bleeding begins, cycle with 20 μg of ethinyl estradiol daily in 21-day cycles with 10 progesterone daily the last 7 days of the 21-day cycle.

Somatostatin analogues: used to treat pituitary growth hormone–producing adenoma as adjunctive therapy to surgery.

Treatment aims
Reduction of excessive height.

Prognosis
Dependent on cause of tall stature; the induction of precocious puberty has both psychological and hormonal risks.

Follow-up and management
• Children with medical conditions such as Marfan syndrome, homocystinuria, and hormone excess need appropriate medical surveillance (eg, cardiac and orthopedic care in Marfan patients).

Other treatments
• Pituitary gigantism needs surgical or irradiation therapy.

General references

Blizzard RM, Johanson A: Disorders of growth. In *The Diagnosis and Treatment of Endocrine Disorders in Childhood and Adolescence*. Edited by Kappy M, Blizzard RM, Migeon CJ. Springfield, IL: Charles C. Thomas; 1994:424–433.

Diagnosis

Symptoms

Decrease in growth rate: the child is not necessarily short (< 5th percentile) but decreasing in height percentiles.

Symptoms may reflect chronic illness: gastrointestinal, renal, anorexia or central nervous system disorder (headache, vertigo, visual disturbance).

Symptoms may reflect hypothyroidism or hypoglycemia of growth hormone deficiency.

Signs

Height less than fifth percentile or growth rate less than 1.5 SD of mean growth velocity for age and gender, resulting in height decreasing in percentiles.

Signs of chronic illness may be present: weight loss, abdominal tenderness, neurologic findings.

Syndromic features may be present: *eg,* Turner's syndrome, Noonan's syndrome, Russell-Silver syndrome, Seckel's dwarfism).

Limb length to height ratio and sitting height to height ratio should be determined to evaluate for possible chondrodystrophies.

Investigations

Bone age: a bone age compatible to chronologic age indicates genetic short stature (both normal familial as well as genetic or chromosomal abnormalities). A bone age retarded for chronologic age indicates either healthy (familial) constitutional delay of growth or the possibility of a systemic illness causing growth failure.

Complete blood count, biochemical profile, erythrocyte sedimentation rate: to screen for systemic illnesses and inflammatory diseases.

Thyroid function tests: to evaluate for both central and primary hypothyroidism.

Growth factors: insulin growth factor-1 (IGF-1) or somatomedin-C is a sensitive indicator of pituitary growth hormone function but is not specific for growth hormone deficiency and is low in the very young, malnourished and chronically ill. IGF binding protein-3 (IGFBP-3) also reflects pituitary growth hormone function and is not as likely to be perturbed by non–growth hormone deficient systemic illnesses, such as malnutrition, inflammatory bowel disease. The finding of low serum concentrations of both IGF-1 and IGFBP-3 is suggestive of growth hormone deficiency.

Karyotyping: in girls to rule out Turner's syndrome.

Head MRI: in patients with growth hormone deficiency is needed to evaluate the possibility of a central nervous system lesion.

Complications

• Growth failure often indicates an underlying illness and may reflect serious consequences if undetected, such as chronic renal failure.

Differential diagnosis

Familial short stature.

Constitutional delay of growth and development.

Syndromic syndromes.

Systemic illness or hormone deficiency.

Etiology

• Familial short stature and many syndromic conditions, such as chondrodystrophies, are genetic or chromosomally determined.

• Constitutional delay is a normal variant.

• Growth hormone deficiency may be genetic, due to congenital anomalies (e.g., septo-optic dysplasia) or due to brain tumors or tumor treatment.

Epidemiology

• Five percent of the pediatric population is short by statistical definition.

• Turner's syndrome occurs in 1:2000 live female births and in 1:100 girls less than third percentile.

• Growth hormone deficiency is estimated at 1:4000 children.

Treatment

Lifestyle
• Many causes of short stature and growth failure cannot be treated. These children need to recognize that their worth is not dependent on their size. Short children should be encouraged to develop interests in which success is not dependent on size.

Pharmacological treatment
• Growth hormone is indicated to treat children with growth hormone deficiency and Turner's syndrome.
• Growth hormone is also used to treat the growth failure due to chronic renal failure.
• Growth hormone has not been beneficial in familial short stature and most syndromic conditions with short stature.

Standard dosage   Growth hormone, 0.02–0.05 μg/kg s.c. The higher doses are reserved for Turner syndrome.

Treatment aims
To treat the systemic illness causing the growth failure.
• In growth hormone deficiency, growth hormone is important not only for restoring normal growth but normal body composition as well (increasing lean body mass and bone density).

Prognosis
Dependent on cause of growth failure.
• The prognosis for growth hormone deficiency and hypothyroidism is excellent.
• Improved adult height in Turner's syndrome is excellent but infertility is likely.
• The prognosis in other syndromic conditions and serious chronic illnesses is more variable.

Follow-up and management
• Children being treated for growth failure need to be followed at 3–6-mo intervals to ascertain improvement in growth velocity. At each interval, height and weight changes must be recorded. Puberty, which can decrease the amount of time for "catch-up" growth, need to be noted and perhaps suppressed if necessary.
• Bone age radiography should be obtained at 6-month to yearly intervals.
• Appropriate biochemical studies, including growth factors and thyroid function tests, should be obtained at 6-month to yearly intervals.

Other treatments
• Leg-lengthening surgical procedures have been used with success in achroplasia and other chondrodystrophies.

General references
Furlanetto RW, Lawson Wilkins Pediatric Endocrine Society Therapeutics Committee: Guidelines for the use of growth hormone in children with short stature. *J Pediatr* 1995, **127**:857–867.

Mahoney CP: Evaluating the child with short stature. *Pediatr Clin North Am* 1987, **34**:825–849.

Diagnosis

Definition

Typical diarrhea-associated hemolytic uremic syndrome (D+HUS): prodrome of acute bloody diarrhea, rapid onset of acute hemolytic anemia, thrombocytopenia, and acute renal injury.

Acute onset of hemolytic anemia with fragmented erythrocytes.

Thrombobocytopenia.

Acute renal injury.

Symptoms

Gastroenteritis.

Bloody diarrhea.

Increasing pallor.

Dehydration and/or edema.

Oliguria, anuria, gross hematuria.

Seizures.

Signs

Pallor, petechiae.

Dehydration.

Edema.

Hypertension.

Tender abdomen, hepatomegaly rectal prolapse, anal excoriation.

Investigations

Urine analysis: protein, blood, cysts, specific gravity.

Serum sodium, potassium, chloride, bicarbonate, calcium, phosphate, creatinine, BUN.

Hemoglobin, leukocyte and platelet count.

Stool cultures for *Escherichia coli* 0157:H7.

Kidney biopsy rarely indicated.

Complications

Anemia, thrombocytopenia.

Acute renal failure.

Seizures, hemiplegia, coma.

Anal excoriation, rectal prolapse, bowel gangrene.

Pancreatitis, diabetes mellitus.

Chronic renal failure.

Differential diagnosis

Acute renal failure: shock, sepsis, nephrotoxins.

Atypical non–diarrhea-associated HUS (D-HUS): onset insidious, often progressive, may relapse, poor outcome.

Thrombotic thrombocytopenic purpura (TTP): rare in children, onset insidious, asynchronous manifestations, neurologic features predominate, no bloody diarrhea, poorer prognosis.

Etiology

D+HUS: *E. coli* 0157:H7 contamination of ground beef, milk.

Atypical D-HUS: autosomal recessive inheritance, autosomal dominant inheritance, *Streptococcus pneumoniae*, HIV, cyclosporin A.

TTP: Unknown.

Epidemiology

Mainly infants, children.

Blacks infrequently affected.

Sporadic cases and epidemics.

Causes and associations of hemolytic uremic syndromes		
Infections	**Inherited**	**Drugs**
Escherichia coli 0157:H7	Autosomal recessive; dominant	Cyclosporin A
Shigella dysenteriae	Cobalamin C defect	Mitomycin C
Aeromonas hydrophilia		Oral contraceptives
Streptococcus		Quinine
pneumoniae		"Crack" cocaine
HIV		Pregnancy-associated HUS
		Transplant-associated HUS
		Cancer-associated HUS
		Systemic lupus–associated TMA
		Systemic sclerosis

Treatment

Diet

Sodium and fluid restriction if edematous.

Potassium restriction.

Provide adequate calories orally or intravenously.

Pharmacologic treatment

Phosphate binders: calcium citrate preferred.

Sodium bicarbonate: for metabolic acidosis.

Hypertension: calcium channel blockers.

Try angiotensin-converting enzyme inhibitors but monitor serum creatinine and potassium.

Nonpharmacologic treatment

Educate child and family.

Psychosocial support during acute dialysis.

Surgical treatment of surgical intestinal complications.

Peritoneal dialysis, hemodialysis: anuria >24 hours.

Blood transfusions: use slowly, sparingly, if hemoglobin under 6 g/dL.

Platelet infusions: for surgery, active bleeding.

Precautions

Check contacts for *E. coli* 0157:H7.

Prevent person-to-person spread.

Notify public health agencies.

Treatment aims

To manage fluid and electrolyte disturbances.

To control blood pressure.

To provide adequate calories.

To support with dialysis until renal function recovers.

Prognosis

Death in acute stage: 5%–10%.

Recurrences are extremely uncommon.

Chronic hypertension, proteinuria, moderate renal insufficiency: 10%–30%.

End-stage renal failure: less than 5%.

Insulin-dependent diabetes mellitus: 2% to 3%.

Good prognostic signs in postacute phase: normal blood pressure, urinalysis, and serum creatinine.

Follow-up and management

• If there is proteinuria, hypertension, and/or elevated serum creatinine, monitor serum creatinine, electrolytes, calcium, phosphate, intact parathyroid hormone, hemoglobin, height and weight, and blood pressure at regular intervals.

General references

Arbus GS: Association of verotoxin-producing E. coli and verotoxin with hemolytic uremic syndrome. *Kidney Int* 1997, **58:**S91–96.

Kaplan BS: The hemolytic uremic syndromes (HUS). *AKF Nephrology Letter* 1992, **9:**29–36.

Kaplan BS, Trompeter R, Moake J, eds.: *Hemolytic Uremic Syndrome/Thrombotic Thrombocytopenic Purpura.* New York: Marcel Decker; 1992:29–38.

Schulman SL, Kaplan BS: Management of patients with hemolytic uremic syndrome demonstrating severe azotemia but not anuria. *Pediatr Nephrol* 1996, **10:**671–674.

Siegler RL: Spectrum of extrarenal involvement in postdiarrheal hemolytic-uremic syndrome. *J Pediatr* 1994, **125:**511–518.

Siegler RL: The hemolytic uremic syndrome. *Pediatr Clin North Am* 1995, **42:**1505–1529.

Hemophilia and von Willebrand's disease

Diagnosis

Signs (hemophilia)

Swollen, painful warm joint; unexpected bleeding after surgery: acute.

Excessive bruising.

Crippling joint deformity: chronic.

von Willebrand's disease: bruises, rarely petechiae.

Hemophilia

Episodic spontaneous hemorrhage bold into joints and other tissues.

Deep-tissue hematoma: particularly after trauma or surgery.

Excessive bleeding after circumcision.

von Willebrand's disease

Bruising.

Epistaxis and menorrhagia.

Excessive bleeding after dental extraction or surgery.

Investigations

Hemophilia

Activated partial thromboplastin time measurement: prolonged.

Hemophilia A: low factor VIII:C; hemophilia B, low factor IX; and hemophilia C, low factor XI assays.

Coagulation factor activity measurement: correlated with disease severity in hemophilia A and B (normal range, 50–150 U/dL): Less than 1% indicates severe disease, manifest as spontaneous bleeding episodes, potential for joint deformity.

• One percent to 5% indicates moderate disease; five percent to 20% indicates mild disease. Mild and moderate patients have posttraumatic or postsurgical bleeding.

von Willebrand's disease

Bleeding time measurement: prolonged (variable); activated partial thromboplastin time: prolonged (variable).

Factor VIII clotting activity, von Willebrand's factor (vWF) antigen, and vWF activity measurement: low values.

Analysis of vWF multimeric structure determines subtype of von Willebrand's disease (type 1, 2, or 3).

• Determining subtype is important for deciding treatment.

Complications

Transfusion-transmitted disease

Hepatitis A: has been a recent problem with a solvent detergent–sterilized product; all patients with bleeding disorders should be vaccinated.

Hepatitis B: although all blood donors are tested for hepatitis B virus, sterilization processes for clotting factor concentrate cannot be regarded as 100% safe; vaccination is mandatory in patients with bleeding disorders.

Hepatitis C: all patients treated by unsterilized clotting factor concentrates have been infected (sterilization introduced in 1985); some patients progress to chronic liver disease; treatment with interferon may normalize transaminases.

HIV infection: occurred in patients receiving concentrates between 1979 and 1985.

Inhibitor

Neutralizing antibodies: IgG antibodies may develop after infusion of concentrates. Patients with high-titer inhibitors may benefit from induction of immune tolerance.

Chronic arthropathy

Chronic disabling arthritis: caused by recurrent hemarthroses.

Other bleeding: serious bleeding may occur with or without a history of trauma in severe hemophilia; headache may herald an intracranial bleed, abdominal pain may be an ileopsoas bleed.

Differential diagnosis

Other clotting factor deficiencies or platelet function disorders.

Etiology

Causes of hemophilia

Quantitative deficiency of clotting factors.

Factor VIII: hemophilia A (most common).

Factor IX: hemophilia B.

Factor XI: hemophilia C.

Causes of von Willebrand's disease

Quantitative or qualitative deficiency of vWF, which is an adhesive protein for primary platelet hemostasis (and carrier protein for factor VIII).

Genetics

Hemophilia A and B: X-linked (men affected, but some women carriers may need concentrate for surgery or trauma).

von Willebrand's disease: autosomal-dominant.

Hemophilia C (severe disease): autosomal-recessive or compound heterozygote.

Epidemiology

• One in 10,000 men are affected by hemophilia A; hemophilia A is four times more common than hemophilia B.

• Hemophilia C is common in Ashkenazi Jews; it may occur in any ethnic group.

• von Willebrand's disease is the most common inherited bleeding disorder if all grades of severity are considered; clinically significant disease occurs in ~125:1,000,000.

Carrier detection and antenatal diagnosis

Carrier status and presence of the disorders in fetuses can be detected by the following:

Restriction fragment length polymorphisms.

Variable-number repeat sequences.

Direct mutational analysis.

Fetal sexing and choriocentesis (for carriers without a molecular marker).

Treatment

Diet and lifestyle
• Patients should avoid contact sports, but regular exercise, *eg*, swimming, should be encouraged.

Pharmacologic treatment
• Intramuscular injections must be avoided in patients with bleeding disorders.
• Aspirin or nonsteroidal anti-inflammatory drugs that impair platelet function must also be avoided.

Indications
For hemophilia A: factor VIII concentrate or for moderate and mild disease, DDAVP (desmopressin).
For hemophilia B: factor IX concentrate.
For hemophilia C: factor IX concentrate.
For von Willebrand's disease: factor VIII concentrate that contains vWF or DDAVP.

Clotting factor preparations
• For severe hemophiliacs, factor concentrates can be given "on demand" to stop an established bleeding episode or prophylactically to prevent bleeding episodes.
• Recombinant concentrates of factor VIII and IX are licensed in US.
• Concentrates extracted from plasma by conventional separation include very high purity products (>100 U/mg), high purity and intermediate purity (<50 U/mg); Humate P and Alphanate are plasma-derived products that contain vWF.
• The units of clotting factor needed (x) can be calculated by the following equation: x=(rise in clotting factor required [%] $\times$ weight [kg]) / K (where $K = 1.5$ for factor VIII, 1 for factor IX, and 2 for factor XI).
• Approximate levels for hemostasis are as follows:
15–20 units clotting factor/dL for minor spontaneous hemarthroses and hematomas.
20–40 units clotting factor/dL for severe hemarthroses and hematomas, minor surgery.
80–100 units clotting factor/dL plasma for major surgery.

DDAVP
• DDAVP releases factor VIII:C and vWF from endothelial cells.
• DDAVP can be used to treat minor bleeding episodes or to prevent surgical bleeding in patients with mild hemophilia and von Willebrand's disease.
• It is not indicated for severe hemophilia or severe and certain variant types of von Willebrand's disease.

Standard dosage	DDAVP, 0.3 µg/kg in 100 mL normal saline solution i.v. infusion over 20 minutes, or intranasal DDAVP (1–2 metered dose inhalations).
Contraindications	Vascular disease.
Special points	Response should be monitored using factor assays.
Main drug interactions	None.
Main side effects	Hyponatremia and seizures, coronary occlusion (in patients >60 years).

Tranexamic acid and aminocaproic acid
• Tranexamic acid, an inhibitor or fibrinolysis, reduces blood loss, particularly in mucosal bleeding, *eg*, oral surgery, epistaxis, and tonsillectomy.

Standard dosage	Tranexamic acid, 25 mg/kg three times daily.
	Epsilon aminocaproic acid, 400 mg/kg/day divided in four doses (maximum, 24g/day) for 5 days.
Contraindications	Hematuria, risk of "clot colic."
Special points	Dose should be reduced in patients with renal impairment.

Treatment aims
To prevent spontaneous bleeds and to make surgery safe.

Prognosis
With the advent of virally safe blood products and home-treatment programs, many severely hemophiliac patients can lead a relatively normal life.
Mild disease, whether hemophilia or von Willebrand's disease, may impinge little unless an injury occurs or surgery is planned.

Follow-up and management
All patients with bleeding disorders should be registered and regularly reviewed at a designated hemophilia center; regular review and access to treatment are of paramount importance for the successful long-term management of these patients.
Patients with severe hemophilia are taught self-infusion, to treat bleeding episodes or perform prophylaxis at home. Education and follow-up are key for successful home treatment.

General references

Kasper CK, Lusher JM, and the Transfusion Practices Committee: Recent evolution of clotting factor concentrates for hemophilia A and B. *Transfusion* 1993, **33**:422–434.

Vermylen J, Briet E: Factor VIII preparations: need for prospective pharmacovigilance. *Lancet* 19xx, **343**:693–694.

Troisi CL, Hollinger FB, Hoots WK, et al.: A multicenter study of viral hepatitis in a United States hemophiliac population. *Blood* 1993, **81**:412–418.

Goerdert JJ, et al.: A prospective study of human immunodeficiency virus type 1 infection and the development of AIDS in subjects with hemophilia. *N Engl J Med* 1989, **321**:1141–1148.

Bolton-Maggs PHB, et al.: Production and therapeutic use of a factor XI concentrate from plasma. *Thromb Haemost* 1992, **67**:314–319.

Nilsson IM, Berntorp E, Lofgrist T, Pettersson J: Twenty-five years' experience of prophylactic treatment in severe hemophilia A and B. *J Int Med* 1992, **232**:25–32.

Diagnosis

Symptoms

• In most patients, symptoms occur 24–48 h after infection (usually upper respiratory tract infection) or drug ingestion (antibiotics).

Florid palpable purpuric skin rash: predominantly on lower legs but also on buttocks and arms (cardinal symptom).

Cramping abdominal pains: in 60%–70% of patients

Joint pains: in 60%–70%.

Blood in urine or stool: in 20%–30%.

Symptoms of intestinal obstruction: due to intussusception, in <5% of young children.

Fever and toxicity: if severe.

Signs

Rash: "papular purpura" lesions that do not blanch on pressure, some forming a necrotic center that may vesiculate, usually on buttocks and extremities (lower>>upper); usually painless; may persist or recur for up to 2 months.

Joint involvement: mild to moderate symmetrical arthropathy in 60%–70%; some periarticular swelling; a few patients also have edema of hands and feet.

Gut involvement: cramping abdominal pain, and some rebound tenderness in 60%; frank blood in stool in 10%–20%; obstructive symptoms (intussusception) or perforation.

Renal involvement: 50% of patients develop nephritis.

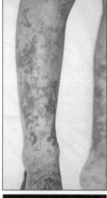

Pretibial and lower leg purpuric lesions in a 7-year-old boy.

Investigations

Skin biopsy: may show cutaneous necrotizing venulitis but does not indicate cause.

History: may be positive for recent infective episodes or drug ingestion (antibiotic).

Full blood count: may show mild polymorphonuclear leukocytosis and normal platelet count.

Stool and urine analysis: regularly during and after rash, with formal microscopy if positive; 30% of patients show evidence of erythrocytes, raised protein concentration, and casts on urinalysis.

Formal renal investigations, including biopsy: if findings indicate renal disease that is not progressively improving as the disease resolves.

Complications

• In children, this condition is often thought of as "harmless."

Secondary infection of vasculitic lesions.

Glomerulonephritis, IgA nephropathy: in ~50% of patients.

Renal failure: 1%–2% of these progress to renal failure.

Gastrointestinal or surgical problems: eg, intussusception or perforation in young children; of the 60%–70% of patients with gastrointestinal complications, a few develop intramural hematomata, associated with intussusception, infarction, or gut perforation; protein-losing enteropathy.

Renal problems: eg, immunoglobulin nephropathy in older children and adults.

Treatment

Diet and lifestyle
- Other than bed rest during the acute phase, observe for severe abdominal pain.

Pharmacologic treatment
- Treatment is symptomatic and does not alter the course or outcome of the condition or its complications.
- Local treatment of the rash, if needed, should be designed to prevent secondary infection.
- Nonsteroidal anti-inflammatory drugs (NSAIDs) can help the joint symptoms.
- Steroids have no effect on renal abnormalities but may rapidly ameliorate significant gastrointestinal symptoms.

For pain relief
Standard dosage	NSAIDs, *eg,* naproxen, 10–15 mg/kg/d divided in 2 doses for 5–10 d.
Contraindications	Active peptic ulceration, abdominal pain, or renal insufficiency.
Special points	Asthma may be exacerbated.
Main drug interactions	Oral anticoagulants.
Main side effects	Gastrointestinal disturbances, discomfort, nausea, or ulceration.

For joint abnormalities
Standard dosage	Corticosteroids, (*eg,* prednisone) 1 mg/kg/day for 5–10 d.
Contraindications	Active peptic ulceration.
Special points	Possible adrenal suppression with use more than 3 weeks.
Main drug interactions	NSAIDs, oral anticoagulants.
Main side effects	Cushing's syndrome, growth retardation in children, osteoporosis.

Treatment aims
To prevent secondary infection in vasculitic skin lesions.
To relieve symptoms of joint or abdominal pain.

Other treatments
- Antihypertensive therapy may be needed in the 5%–10% of patients who develop renal insufficiency.

Prognosis
- The prognosis of the rash alone is good.
- Crops of lesions may recur within 4–8 wk.
- Spontaneous remission is the norm.
- Relapses of the rash alone often occur in adults.
- Generally, 5%–10% of patients develop renal failure insufficiency.

Follow-up and management
- Renal function or urinary sediment must be monitored for evidence of renal involvement for approximately 3 mo after the rash has cleared, then as indicated based on presence of sediment.
- If renal involvement is detected, full renal investigation, including biopsy may be needed.

General references

Blanco R, Martínez-Taboada V, Rodríguez-Valverde V, *et al.*: Henoch–Schönlein purpura in adulthood and childhood. *Arthritis Rheum* 1997, **40**:859–864.

Koskimies O, Mir S, Rapola J, Vilska J: Henoch–Schönlein nephritis: long-term prognosis of unselected patients. *Arch Dis Child* 1981, **56**:482–484.

Rosenblum ND, Wrater HS: Steroid effects on the course of abdominal pain in children with HSP. *Pediatrics* 1987, **79**:1018–1021.

Diagnosis

Symptoms
• Acute hepatitis is often asymptomatic.

Constitutional symptoms
Malaise, headache, myalgias, arthralgias, anorexia, nausea, right upper-quadrant discomfort, fevers, and gastrointestinal flu-like symptoms.

Later symptoms
Jaundice, pruritus, acholic (pale) stools, dark urine.

Signs
Jaundice, tender hepatomegaly, splenomegaly, vasculitis.

Stigmata of chronic liver disease: absent in uncomplicated acute hepatitis.

Fetor hepaticus, hepatic encephalopathy, or asterixis: signs of severe disease.

Rash, arthralgia: rare presentation of hepatitis B when associated with fever and lymphadenitis (Gronotti–Crosti syndrome).

Investigations [1]
Biochemical assays: elevated serum transaminases (most sensitive indicators of hepatocellular injury); increase in alkaline phosphatase (indicative of biliary tract disease, although in children can be elevated secondary to bone activity).

• Direct hyperbilirubinemia (>30% of total bilirubin) peaks 5–7 days after beginning of jaundice.

Prothrombin time: if elevated, fulminant hepatic failure should be watched for; underlying chronic liver disease should be considered.

Serum glucose: hypoglycemia significant complication of severe hepatitis.

Virology tests: *Hepatitis A:* check for IgM antibody (indicates acute infection; IgG antibody present for life and suggests previous infection).

Hepatitis B: check for IgM antibody (develops early in illness) and surface antigen (present in most symptomatic patients but may be eliminated quickly). Presence of HBV DNA and hepatitis B e antigen markers of acute disease and active viral replication.

Hepatitis C: antibody may take several months to convert, although most patients become positive within 3 months and only indicates exposure (viral assay using polymerase chain reaction is positive early and indicates infection).

Hepatitis D: sought by detection of antibody; superinfection with hepatitis D virus in a chronic hepatitis B virus carrier (IgM anticore negative) may be differentiated from coinfection by hepatitis B (IgM anticore to hepatitis B positive).

Hepatitis E: enzyme-linked immunosorbent assay (very rare) [4].

Cytomegalovirus (CMV) and Epstein-Barr virus (EBV): should be sought when viral cause suspected and other serological tests negative.

Liver biopsy: may be indicated in rare circumstances when diagnostic confusion exists or when underlying liver damage is suspected.

Complications
Fulminant liver failure: 1% of hepatitis A.

Progression to chronic hepatitis: may occur with hepatitis B (over 50% infected neonates, 20% of children, and 10% of adults); hepatitis C; hepatitis D associated with hepatitis B.

Aplastic anemia, vasculitis, cryoglobulinemia: rarely, in cases of hepatitis B or C.

Guillain–Barrè syndrome: hepatitis A.

Nephrotic syndrome: hepatitis B.

Hepatocellular carcinoma: hepatitis B (chronic disease); hepatitis C (less common).

Differential diagnosis
Infections: EBV, CMV, herpes, adenovirus, coxsackievirus, reovirus, echovirus, rubella arbovirus. leptospirosis, toxoplasmosis, tuberculosis.
Hepatitis viruses: A–E, non-A, non-B.
Neisseria gonorrhoeae perihepatitis (Fitz–Hugh–Curtis syndrome).
Wilson's disease.
Medications.

Etiology and epidemiology
Hepatitis viruses
A: fecal–oral transmission; infection associated with foreign travel, consumption of shellfish, overcrowding, poor sanitation practices, contaminated food and water, sexual contacts, and day-care centers.

B: parenteral transmission; vertical transmission in newborns; i.v. drug users at risk; no identifiable risk factors in 50%.

C: 20%–40% of all acute hepatitis in the US; associated with i.v. drug use and transfusion; transmitted vertically and sexually; no identifiable risk factors in 50% [2].

D: transmitted predominantly by i.v. drug use; occurs only with concomitant hepatitis B infection [3].

E: fecal–oral transmission; in developing countries (in epidemics, pregnant women are most vulnerable).

Non-A, non-B: unidentifiable viral agent; cause of posttransfusion hepatitis not caused by hepatitis B or C.

• Epstein–Barr virus [4].

• Cytomegalovirus (particularly in immunosuppressed patients).

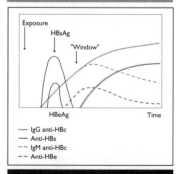

Exposure
HBsAg
"Window"
HBeAg
Time

— IgG anti-HBc
— Anti-HBs
-- IgM anti-HBc
-- Anti-HBe

Serological diagnosis of acute hepatitis B (HB) infection. HBeAg—HBe antigen; HBsAg—HB surface antigen.

Treatment

Diet and lifestyle

• Dietary changes have no proven benefit.

• Rest is recommended; many patients are unable to return to school for weeks and, even after return, may need time before normal function fully returns.

• Patients must understand the routes by which the hepatitis infection has been acquired and may, therefore, be transmitted. This may place short-term restrictions on attendance in day-care centers and school, and for adolescent sexual activity.

• Hospitalization is indicated for vomiting and dehydration, mental status changes, or bleeding from coagulopathy.

Hepatitis B: 10%–15% of chronic carriers spontaneously become HBV surface antigen negative.

Prevention

• Instituting infection control measures (improved sanitation, hand washing, education).

• Improved screening of blood products.

• Rapid diagnosis and treatment for outbreaks in day-care centers or for institutionalized children.

Pharmacologic treatment

Passive immunization

Hepatitis A: pooled immune serum globulin effective in diminishing clinical symptoms, although typically disease is self-limited. Prophylaxis with immunoglobulin recommended for household contacts or others with intimate exposure to index case. Routine administration is not indicated for school contacts but should be given to everyone in non–toilet-trained trained day-care centers. Dose, 0.02 mL/kg.

Hepatitis B: Hepatitis B immune globulin (HBIG) should be administered immediately after exposure from accidental needle puncture exposure to other infected bodily fluid, perinatal exposure of neonate born to infected mother, sexual exposure, or household contact. Dose, 0.06 mL/kg.

Active immunization [4]

Hepatitis A vaccine: not available in all countries.

Hepatitis B vaccine: requires three doses of vaccine.

Now recommended to be given to all children by the American Academy of Pediatrics. Should be started in newborn period.

Interferon

• Synthetically synthesized proteins that act as antiviral, immunomodulating and antireplicating agents. Should be considered in all patients with biopsy-proven chronic hepatitis B. Interferon has also been shown to have some effect in reversing chronic hepatitis C in children.

• Interferon should be given to all patients with posttransplantation HBV infection.

Liver transplantation

• The persistence of viral hepatitis occurs in the majority of patients who undergo liver transplantation for viral hepatitis. Immunoprophylaxis and interferon therapy should be considered in all patients.

Treatment aims

To palliate symptoms.

To prevent infection and spread of disease.

To observe for progression to fulminant hepatic failure.

Prognosis

• Acute hepatitis is often a debilitating illness, but recovery is usual, although patients may experience fatigue for several months before full recovery.

• Hepatitis A is almost always a self-limiting disease with rapid recovery.

• Over 40% of patients infected by hepatitis C virus and ~10% infected by hepatitis B become carriers; for the latter, chronic infection is less common after a severe, acute illness.

• Hepatocellular carcinoma is related to chronic hepatitis B, C, and D.

• Prognosis of chronic hepatitis D is poor.

Follow-up and management

• Patients with acute hepatitis A, B, or E should be followed until the liver function tests have returned to normal and the patient has made a full symptomatic recovery.

• Patients with hepatitis B should also be followed until hepatitis B surface antigen is eliminated; persistence of hepatitis Be antigen or HBV DNA beyond 6 wk suggests that a carrier state may be evolving.

• In the present state of uncertainty about the prognosis of patients with hepatitis C, they should be followed every 6–12 months unless evidence for persistent hepatitis C is lacking, *ie,* disappearance of hepatitis C virus antibody or RNA.

Key references

1. Krugman S: Viral hepatitis: A, B, C, D, and E infection. *Pediatr Rev* 1992, **13:**203–212.

2. Alter MJ: Hepatitis C: a sleeping giant? *Am J Med* 1991, **91:**1125–1155.

3. Hoofnagle JH: Type D (delta) hepatitis. *JAMA* 1989, **261:**1321–1325.

4. Centers for Disease Control: Protection against viral hepatitis: recommendations of the Immunization Practices Advisory Committee (ACIP). *MMWR Morb Mortal Wkly Rep* 1990, **39(no. RR-2):**19–21.

Diagnosis

Symptoms

Persistence or relapse of symptoms of acute hepatitis >3 months from onset.

Chronic malaise, anorexia, weight loss; jaundice; easy bruising; encephalopathy; growth failure.

Signs [1]

Small, hard, nodular liver; ascites; edema; muscle wasting; splenomegaly; testicular atrophy, gynecomastia in men; palmar erythema, spider telangiectasia; caput medusae; clubbing of nailbeds; GI bleeding; anemia.

Investigations

Liver function tests: show chronic hepatocellular disease; ALT, GGTP, and AST typically elevated to a greater degree than alkaline phosphatase; elevation in bilirubin variable.

Coagulation screening: impaired hepatic synthetic function causes prolonged prothrombin time and low albumin.

Ophthalmic evaluation: can determine viral etiology or metabolic disease.

Serum protein analysis: immunoglobulins elevated in chronic liver disease but particularly prominent in autoimmune hepatitis (especially IgG).

α_1-**antitrypsin level and PI typing.**

Autoantibody analysis: antinuclear antibody, double-stranded DNA, smooth-muscle antibody, anti–liver–kidney microsomal antibody, and soluble liver antigens are often positive in autoimmune diseases.

Sweat chloride evaluation.

Serum ferritin: elevated in hemochromatosis.

Hepatitis A serology: only in fulminant liver failure.

Hepatitis B serology: interpreted as follows:
Immune, postvaccination: sAb+, sAg–, cAb–, eAg–, eAb–, DNA–.
Immune, past exposure to hepatitis B virus: sAb+, sAg–, cAb+, eAg–, eAb+, DNA–.
Infected, carrier: sAb–, sAg+, cAb+, eAg–, eAb+, DNA–.
Infected, high risk of transmission: sAb–, sAg+, cAb+, eAg+, eAb–, DNA+.

Hepatitis C serology: interpreted as follows:
Positive, active disease: ELISA+, RIBA+ (2–4 bands), ALT increased, RNA+.
False-positive: ELISA+, RIBA– or indeterminate (1 band), ALT normal, RNA–.

Hepatitis D serology: +IgM and +IgG δ-Ab.

Ceruloplasmin: decreased and 24-hour urine copper increased in Wilson's disease; presence of Kayser–Fleischer rings in eyes.

Liver ultrasonography or CT: often normal but may show small liver with splenomegaly and portal hypertension.

Liver biopsy for histology: shows the following:
Hepatitis B/D virus: inflammatory cells spreading into parenchyma from enlarged portal tracts; hepatitis B sAg on immunohistochemistry; hepatitis D infection increases severity and can be detected by immunohistochemistry.
Hepatitis C virus: usually mild chronic hepatitis with lobular component, prominent lymphoid follicles in portal tracts, acidophil body formation, focal hepatocellular necrosis; no immunohistochemical staining currently available.
Autoimmune disease: periportal inflammatory infiltrate and piecemeal necrosis; negative to hepatitis B/D staining on immunohistochemistry.
Primary sclerosing cholangitis: onion-skinned appearance near bile ducts [2].
Wilson's disease: abnormal mitochondria on electron microscopy.
Metabolic disease: storage material and abnormal hepatocytes.

Endoscopic retrograde cholangiopancreatography (ERCP): indicated for bile duct disorders.

Leukocyte enzyme activity.

Differential diagnosis

Autoimmune chronic active hepatitis.
Wilson's disease.
α_1-Antitrypsin deficiency.
Drug-induced hepatitis (acetaminophen, antibiotics, halothane, valproic acid, carbamazepine, estrogen.
Hepatitis associated with inflammatory bowel disease.
Cystic fibrosis.
Metabolic liver disease: galactosemia, tyrosinemia
Chronic viral hepatitis.
Bile duct lesions.
Bile acid synthetic disorders.
Bile acid synthetic disorders.
Storage disorders: Gaucher and glycogen storage disease, Niemann-Pick syndrome.
Toxins: environmental.

Definition

Hepatic dysfunction (*ie*, abnormal liver enzyme levels, often with progression to abnormal synthetic function) of at least 3-months' duration secondary to inflammation of the hepatic parenchyma [1].

Associated systemic disorders

Skin: urticaria, acne, lupus erythematosus, vitiligo.
Joints: arthralgia, arthritis.
Renal: renal tubular acidosis, glomerulonephritis.
Pulmonary: pleural effusion; pulmonary arteriovenous malformation.
Endocrine: thyroiditis; amenorrhea.
Ocular: iridocyclitis.
Hematologic: hemolytic anemia.

Complications

Liver failure: can occur in all types of chronic liver disease manifested by coagulopathy, rising conjugated hyperbilirubinemia, hypoalbuminemia, hypoglycemia, and encephalopathy.
Variceal bleeding, ascites: secondary to portal hypertension.
Hepatocellular carcinoma: increased in cirrhosis patients.
Spontaneous bacterial peritonitis: in patients with ascites.
Hepatorenal syndrome: functional renal failure in patients w/chronic liver disease.
Gallstones.

Treatment

Diet and lifestyle

• Fat-soluble vitamin supplementation and vitamins A, E, D, K.

Sodium restriction: not more than 5 mEq/day in children 1–4 years of age; not more than 20 mEq/day in children 5–11 years of age.

Tyrosinemia: restrict phenylalanine and tyrosine from diet.

Hereditary fructose intolerance: removal of dietary fructose and sucrose.

Wilson's disease: supplement zinc and remove dietary copper.

Pharmacologic treatment

For hepatitis B virus infection

• Treatment is indicated for patients who have histological evidence of chronic hepatitis and are positive for hepatitis B e antigen or virus DNA [2]; 40%–50% of patients with hepatitis B virus can have meaningful remission.

Standard dosage	Interferon-α, 10 MU s.c. 3 times a week for 4–6 mo [3]. Alternative regimens also available.
Contraindications	Hypersensitivity, evidence of liver failure (eg, ascites, varices, thrombocytopenia).
Main side effects	*Induction:* low-grade fever, malaise, arthralgia, myalgia, headache, anorexia, nausea, vomiting, diarrhea. *Maintenance:* fatigue, anorexia, weight loss, alopecia, depression, neutropenia, thrombocytopenia, exacerbation of autoimmune disease, induction of thyroid disease, myalgia.

For hepatitis C virus infection

• Treatment is indicated for patients with histological evidence of hepatitis and are positive for recombinant immunoblot assay (2–4 bands) or virus RNA by the polymerase chain reaction (PCR).

• Remission persists in only 20% of patients after treatment is stopped.

Standard dosage	*Hepatitis B:* Interferon-α, 3 MU s.c. 3 times weekly for 4–12 mo [4]. *Hepatitis C:* Interferon-α, 3 times weekly for 4–12 mo.
Contraindications	Hypersensitivity, evidence of liver failure (eg, ascites, varices, thrombocytopenia).

For autoimmune disease

• Treatment is indicated for patients with raised transaminase and IgG, histological evidence of chronic hepatitis, and serologic test results consistent with autoimmune hepatitis (eg, ANA, SMA, LKM antibodies).

Standard dosage	Prednisone, 20–60 mg initially, reduced gradually (depending on clinical response); 5–10 mg daily maintenance dose may be needed. Azathioprine, 25–75 mg orally daily as adjunct.
Contraindications	Systemic infection; previous serious reaction to corticosteroids (eg, psychosis).
Main side effects	*Steroids:* osteoporosis, proximal myopathy, skin thinning, cataracts, diabetes mellitus, weight gain, amenorrhea, depression, hypertension. *Azathioprine:* pancreatitis, bone marrow suppression.

For Wilson's disease

• Without treatment, Wilson's disease is fatal.

Standard dosage	D-penicillemine; 250 mg, 3–4 times per day, for life.
Contraindications	Hypersensitivity.
Main side effects	Fever, rash, lymphadenopathy, and pancytopenia.

Treatment aims

To induce and thus prevent progression to cirrhosis.
To eliminate active replication of viruses.
To treat underlying disease process.
To provide supportive care.

Surgical treatment

Orthotopic liver transplantation: liver transplantation is a treatment option for all patients with end-stage liver disease from chronic hepatitis; the 5-y survival rate is 50%–70% depending on the cause. For HBV patients, recurrence of HBV accompanied by aggressive progression of liver disease is common; patients with recurrent HBV disease may require regular hepatitis B immune globulin infusions or lumivadine.

Follow-up and management

• During interferon-α treatment, patients must be monitored closely for leukopenia and thrombocytopenia.

• Thyroid function must be checked because autoimmune disease can be exacerbated.

• Patients on long-term corticosteroid treatment should be monitored for steroid side effects and should have annual bone densitometry to check for osteoporosis.

• Patients who have progressed to cirrhosis are at risk of hepatocellular carcinoma; some investigators advocate surveillance with alpha fetoprotein and ultrasound evaluations every 6 months.

Key references

1. Hardy SC, Kleinman RE: Cirrhosis and chronic liver failure. In *Liver Disease in Children.* Edited by Suchy EJ. St. Louis: Mosby; 1994:214–248.
2. Saracco G, Rizetto M: A practical guide to the use of interferons in the management of hepatitis virus infections. *Drugs* 1997, **53**:74–85.
3. Wilschanski M, *et al.*:Primary sclerosing cholangitis in 32 children: clinical, laboratory, and radiographic features with survival analysis. *Hepatology* 1995, **22**:1415–1422.
4. Morris AA, Turnbull DM: Metabolic disorders in children. *Curr Opin Neurol* 1994, **7**:535–541.

Hepatosplenomegaly

Diagnosis

Symptoms

Increased bruising: may indicate vitamin K deficiency secondary to liver disease.

Splenomegaly associated with GI bleeding: suggests portal hypertension.

Right upper quadrant pain: occurs with hepatitis and hepatic congestion.

Fever, lethargy, fatigue: can occur secondary to infections but are nondiagnostic.

Signs

Palpable, large mass under right costal margin extending to midline: hepatomegaly; liver span should be determined as the liver may extend below costal margin secondary to inspiration or to a low-lying diaphragm (normal liver span, 5–9 cm in midclavicular line) [1].

Palpable mass under left costal margin: splenomegaly; should be elicited by performing examination with the patient lying on their right side and palpating from the lower quadrant to the upper quadrant.

Jaundice: conjugated hyperbilirubinemia in infants and young children.

Associated with hepatomegaly

Recurrent pneumonia: cystic fibrosis.

Neurologic abnormalities and Kayser–Fleischer rings (eyes): Wilson's disease.

Papilledema: hypervitaminosis A.

Nodular, hard liver: suggests cirrhosis or neoplasm.

Large, soft, spongy liver: suggests infiltration.

Cystic kidneys: congenital hepatic fibrosis.

Neutropenia, abscess: glycogen storage disease.

Urinary tract infection in newborns: galactosemia.

Associated with splenomegaly

Lymphadenopathy: suggests infection, infiltrative disease, or malignancy.

Isolated splenomegaly: portal/splenic vein abnormality; Gaucher disease; Niemann–Pick disease.

Investigations

Complete blood count (differential): may indicate leukemia (blasts or depression of cell lines), infection (atypical lymphocytes), hemolytic anemia, or hemoglobinopathy; leukopenia and thrombocytopenia secondary to splenomegaly.

Chemistry panel: evaluation of liver enzymes.

Albumin, prothrombin time, bilirubin: reflects hepatic syntheic dysfunction.

Abdominal ultrasound: helpful in determining portal hypertension, splenic anatomy, portal/splenic vein flow.

Abdominal CT scan: performed whenever splenic injury is suspected.

Liver–spleen scan: highlights the reticuloendothelial system of the liver and spleen to provide structural information and anatomic detail.

Percutaneous liver biopsy: small-core needle biopsy of the liver that provides tissue for culture and histology.

Complications

Splenic rupture: an enlarged spleen is at risk for rupture and bleeding, especially following blunt abdominal trauma.

Ascites: progressive cirrhosis with increased portal hypertension and hypoalbuminemia often causes ascites; spontaneous bacterial peritonitis occurs more frequently in these patients [2].

Esophageal varices/hemorrhoids: diseases that produce secondary portal hypertension may lead to potentially life-threatening GI bleeding from esophageal/gastric varices or rectal hemorrhoids.

Differential diagnosis of hepatomegaly [3]

Infectious: hepatitis viruses; sepsis.

Metabolic: glycogen storage disease; Niemann–Pick disease; alpha$_1$-antitrypsin deficiency; Wilson's disease; tyrosinemia; galactosemia; hereditary fructose intolerance; iron storage disorders.

Anatomic: biliary atresia, primary sclerosing cholangitis; Budd–Chiari syndrome.

Malignant: hepatoblastoma; histiocytosis.

Congestion: constrictive pericarditis; right-sided heart disease.

Autoimmune: chronic active hepatitis; lupus erythematosus, AIDS.

Drugs: halothane; acetaminophen; phenytoin; valproic acid.

Toxins: arsenic, mushrooms, carbon tetrachloride.

Other: cystic fibrosis; Zellweger syndrome.

Differential diagnosis of splenomegaly [4]

Infections: sepsis, viral (cytomegalovirus, Epstein–Barr virus, herpes); fungal (histoplasmosis); bacterial; rickettsial; protozoan (malaria, Rocky Mountain spotted fever).

Hematologic: autoimmune hemolytic anemia, sickle-cell disease, thalassemia, hereditary spherocytosis/elliptocytosis.

Neoplastic: leukemia, lymphoma, neuroblastoma, histiocytosis X.

Metabolic: Gaucher's disease, Niemann–Pick disease, gangliosidoses, porphyria, amyloidosis.

Congenital hepatic fibrosis.

Splenic cyst, hamartoma, hamatoma, torsion.

Portal vein cavernous transformation.

Vacular (portal hypertension): portal vein thrombosis, Budd–Chiari syndrome, splenic artery abnormality.

Serum sickness.

Beckwith–Wiedemann syndrome.

Epidemiology

• A palpable spleen more than 1 cm below the left costal margin constitutes splenomegaly; however, the spleen is palpable in 30% of newborns and in 15% of infants younger than 6 mo of age.

• The liver is palpable in more than 90% of infants younger than 1 y and up to 50% of children 10 y.

Treatment

Diet and lifestyle

• Patients with chronic liver disease should be prescribed a salt-restricted diet and be provided with adequate calories to ensure continued growth and development.

• Children with splenomegaly or coagulopathy secondary to chronic liver disease should be advised to avoid all contact sports. Spleen guards should be fitted for children with splenomegaly participating in noncontact sports.

Pharmacologic treatment

• The management of hepatomegaly and splenomegaly is based on etiology.

For acute bleeding from esophageal varices

Standard dosage: Vasopressin, continuous infusion of 0.1–0.4 U/min.

Contraindications: Hypersensitivity, renal disease.

Main drug interactions: Epinephrine, heparin, alcohol.

Main side effects: Sweating, hypertension, arrhythmia, vasoconstriction, tremor, hyponatremia, water intoxication, nausea, vomiting.

Gene therapy

• Diseases caused by abnormal genes or enzymes may be successfully treated with gene enzyme replacement therapy. Experimental work is being conducted on α_1-antitrypsin deficiency, cystic fibrosis, Niemann–Pick disease, and other metabolic and storage disorders.

Nonpharmacologic treatment

For hemetemesis secondary to variceal bleeding.

Gastrointestinal endoscopy: has vastly improved the control of esophageal varices. Injection sclerotherapy or banding agents during acute bleeding episode and prophylactically has been demonstrated to significantly reduce the risk of bleeding.

Sengstaken–Blakemore tube: used to control profuse variceal esophageal/gastric bleeding or bleeding that cannot be controlled via endoscopy.

For portal hypertension

Transjugular intrahepatic portosystemic shunt (TIPS): catheter placed via the jugular vein to form a tract between the portal vein and hepatic vein in order to shunt blood flow from the portal vessels and decrease portal hypertension[5].

Surgical portosystemic shunt: surgical procedure using human or mechanical grafts to shunt blood flow from the portal system. In children, surgical shunting has decreased in practice secondary to increased incidence of encephalopathy, thrombosis, and greater difficulty of performing subsequent liver transplantation.

Orthotopic liver transplantation

• Liver transplantation has become an effective treatment choice for the majority of diseases that cause hepatosplenomegaly and for the complications that occur secondary to these diseases.

For traumatic splenic injury

• Observation in a pediatric intensive care unit with frequent vital signs and aggressive fluid replacement. Repeated complete blood counts should be performed in order to diagnose late splenic hemorrhage. Serial CT scans are often useful as is a liver-spleen nuclide study. Although every effort should be made to preserve the spleen, surgery may be required.

Treatment aims

• Treatment aims depend on the etiology.
To provide supportive care.
To prevent gastrointestinal hemorrhage.
To decrease symptoms and to prevent complications whenever possible.

Prognosis

• Patients with infectious and drug- or toxin-induced hepatosplenomegaly often improve spontaneously; many patients with viral hepatitis require antiviral treatment. A significant percentage (2%–15%) develop cirrhosis and liver failure.

• Abnormalities of the portal or splenic vein improve with time, as collateral vessels can form to decrease the complications of portal hypertension.

• Presently, the remaining causes of hepatosplenomegaly often lead to a shortened life span unless orthotopic liver transplantation is performed.

Follow-up and management

• Patients with hepatosplenomegaly require persistent routine follow-up.

• Most causes of hepatomegaly do not have a definitive treatment, but they can be effectively managed medically.

• Patients with isolated splenomegaly should be followed up for gastrointestinal bleeding.

Key references

1. Lawson EE, Grand RJ, Neff RK, Cohen LF: Clinical estimation of liver span in infants and children. *Am J Dis Child* 1978, **132:**474–476.

2. Almadal TP, Skinhoj P: Spontaneous bacterial peritonitis in cirrhosis. *Scand J Gastroenterol* 1987, **22:**295–300.

3. Treem WR: Large liver. In: *Principles and Practice of Clinical Pediatrics.* Edited by Schwartz MW, Curry TA, Charney EB, Ludwig S. Chicago: Year Book Publishers; 1987:238–245.

4. Altschuler SM: Large spleen. In: *Principles and Practice of Clinical Pediatrics.* Edited by Schwartz MW, Curry TA, Charney EB, Ludwig S. Chicago: Year Book Publishers; 1987:246–250.

5. Zemel G, et al.: Percutaneous transjugular portosystemic shunt. *JAMA* 1991, **266:**390–393.

Diagnosis

History
• Consider testing asymptomatic children with the following parental risk factors:

Intravenous drug use; noninjectable drug use; sexually transmitted diseases, especially syphilis; bisexuality; transfusions received before 1986.

Symptoms
Frequent sinopulmonary infections or recurrent pneumonia/invasive bacterial disease; severe acute pneumonia (eg, *Pneumocystis carinii* pneumonia [PCP]); recurrent or resistant thrush, especially after 12 months of age; congenital syphilis; sexually transmitted diseases in an adolescent; progressive encephalopathy, loss of developmental milestones; immune thrombocytopenic purpura or thrombocytopenia; failure to thrive; recurrent or chronic diarrhea; recurrent or chronic enlargement of parotid gland; recurrent invasive bacterial disease (pneumonia, bacteremia, meningitis).

Signs
• Physical examination may be normal in the first few months of life; 90% will have some physical findings by age 2. Most common findings are:

Adenopathy, generalized; hepatosplenomegaly; failure to thrive; recurrent or resistant thrush, especially after 1 year of age; recurrent or chronic parotitis.

Investigations (for children over 18 months)
Enzyme-linked immunosorbent assay (ELISA) antibody screen: repeatedly reactive result indicates HIV infection.

Western blot analysis: performed after ELISA screen, is diagnostic of HIV infection.

• For children under 18 months of age, positive HIV ELISA and Western blot antibody tests confirm maternal infection.

HIV blood culture and/or polymerase chain reaction (PCR) DNA testing: most reliable way of diagnosing HIV infection in infancy. Both tests have sensitivities and specificities of better than 95% when performed after 4 weeks of age.

Elevated IgG levels: are the first observed immune abnormality noted in HIV-infected infants, generally reaching twice the normal values by 9 months of age.

CD4+ counts: are obtained at diagnosis, and every 1–3 months.

Complications
Pneumocystis carinii pneumonia: the most common AIDS diagnosis in children; with a peak age of 3–9 months.

Lymphocytic interstitial pneumonitis (LIP): frequently asymptomatic, LIP can lead to slow onset of chronic respiratory symptoms.

Recurrent invasive bacterial infections: pneumococcal bacteremia is the most common invasive bacterial disease. Bacterial pneumonia, sinusitis, and otitis media are very common among infected children.

Progressive encephalopathy: generally diagnosed between 9 and 18 months of age, the hallmark is progressive loss of developmental milestones or neurologic dysfunction. Cerebral atrophy is noted on neuroimaging.

Disseminated *Mycobacterium avium-intracellulare*: occurs in children usually >5 years of age, with severe immunodeficiency (CD4+ <100/mm^3). Symptoms include prolonged fevers, abdominal pain, anorexia, and diarrhea.

Candida esophagitis: seen in older children with severe immunodeficiency

Disseminated cytomegalovirus (CMV) disease: retinitis less common in HIV-infected children than adults; also pulmonary disease, colitis, hepatitis.

HIV-related cancers: non-Hodgkin's lymphoma most common cancer.

Cardiomyopathy, hepatitis, renal disease, thrombocytopenia immune thrombocytopenic purpura.

Differential diagnosis
Neoplastic disease: lymphoma, leukemia, histiocytosis X.

Infectious: congenital/perinatal CMV, toxoplasmosis, congenital syphilis, acquired Epstein-Barr virus.

Congenital immunodeficiency syndromes: Wiskott-Aldrich syndrome, chronic granulomatous disease.

Etiology
• HIV-I and HIV-2 are single-stranded RNA retroviruses, capable of infecting human cells and incorporating their viral genome into host-cell DNA. For most infected individuals, a long clinically asymptomatic period (5–15 y in adults, frequently shorter in children), is followed by the development of generalized nonspecific signs and symptoms (weight loss, adenopathy, hepatosplenomegaly) and mild clinical immunodeficiency. After progressive immunologic deterioration, patients are left severely immunodeficient and susceptible to opportunistic infections and cancers that represent the clinical syndrome known as AIDS.

Epidemiology
• HIV infection is transmitted via sexual contact, exposure to infected blood, breast milk, and perinatally, either *in utero* or during labor/delivery.

• HIV is not believed to be transmitted by bites; sharing utensils, bathrooms, bathtubs; exposure to urine, feces, vomitus; casual contact in the home, school, or daycare center.

• In many cities, AIDS is the leading cause of death for adults 25–44 y of age and is among the leading cause of death in children 1–5 y of age.

• In the U.S., 1.5–2:1000 pregnant women are HIV-infected at the time of delivery. In inner-city areas, rates as high as 40:1000 pregnant women have been reported.

• More than 90% of new pediatric infections are perinatally acquired.

• The risk of an HIV-infected mother giving birth to an infected infant is ~25%.

Treatment

General treatment

• Antiretroviral therapy–specific therapy delays progression of illness, promotes improved growth and neurologic outcome, and improves survival. The present standard of care includes combinations of at least two, and usually three, antiviral agents. As this is a rapidly changing field, clinicians are urged to refer infected children to the nearest tertiary center offering HIV-related specialty care for consultation regarding new drug treatment protocols.

Other treatments

• Other treatments involve immune enhancement: passive, vaccine therapy, immune modulators..

Passive: Recent studies suggest that monthly infusions of gamma-globulin (400 mg/kg) does decrease febrile episodes and pneumococcal bacteremia. The children that benefit the most are those with CD4 counts above 200/mm^3 and not on antibiotic therapy for PCP or otitis prophylaxis.

Vaccine therapy: experimental vaccines to boost anti-HIV immune responses are under study. The vaccines are composed of single components of the viral envelope or core proteins.

Immune modulators: also under active study. Both interleukin-2 (shown to increase CD4 counts in adults) and interferon gamma (designed to prevent secondary bacterial infections) are currently undergoing trials in National Institutes of Health–sponsored protocols.

Prophylaxis

• The drug of choice is trimethoprim-sulfamethoxazole, 150 mg/m^2/day, 3 days per week. One of the cornerstones of therapy for HIV-infected children is prophylaxis against opportunistic infections, the most important of which is PCP. All exposed or at-risk children should receive PCP prophylaxis until HIV infection is definitively ruled out. All HIV infected infants should receive PCP prophylaxis until 12 months of age; for older infants, prophylaxis is based on age adjusted CD4$^+$ counts.

• Absolute CD4$^+$ counts are elevated in childhood, with normal median values of over 3000/mm^3 in the first year of life, then gradually decline with age, values comparable to adult levels (800–1000/mm^3) by age 7. Quantitative PCR assays now allow for measurement of viral activity (viral load), with results reported in number of viral copies per milliliter. Viral load is best indicator of long-term prognosis and short-term response to antiviral therapy.

Immunizations

• HIV-infected children receive the standard series of DaPT, HIB, and hepatitis B vaccines. Inactivated poliovirus vaccine should always be substituted for oral polio vaccine. Although a live virus MMR (measles-mumps-rubella) is given, except in children with severely depressed CD4$^+$ counts. Yearly influenzae A/B immunization is also recommended, as is pneumococcal vaccine at age 2.

Prognosis

Bimodal survival curve: 25% of perinatally infected infants develop early symptomatic disease, with an AIDS diagnosis by 1–2 y, and frequently succumb by 3 y. The remaining 75% have late onset of symptoms, usually after 5 y, and the median survival of this group is now 8–12 y.

Prevention

• HIV infection is almost completely preventable.

• Educational efforts, aimed at achieving behavior change is a most important part of HIV-directed work.

• It is now possible to significantly decrease the risk to newborns of maternally transmitted HIV.. Prenatal zidovudine therapy, followed by continuous i.v. zidovudine therapy during labor, and treatment of the infant for the first 6 weeks of life has been shown to decrease the risk of HIV infection in the infant from 25% to 8%.

• All pregnant women should receive counseling about the benefits of HIV testing, including the possibility of preventing fetal/infant infection, and should be offered HIV testing at the first prenatal visit.

General references

American Academy of Pediatrics, Committee on Pediatric AIDS: Evaluation and medical treatment of the HIV-exposed infant. *Pediatrics* 1997, **99**:909–917.

Carpenter CC, Fischl MA, Hammer SM; Antiretronial therapy for HIV infection in 1997. *JAMA* 1997, **277**:1962–1969.

Lane HC, Davy Jr RT; Diagnosis of HIV infection. *Immunol Allergy Clin North Am.* 1995, **15**:367–384.

Diagnosis

Symptoms

- The usual presentation is a lymph node mass noticed by the patient or parents.
- Fluctuation in size is not unusual.
- Approximately 25% of patients have other symptoms.

"B" symptoms: unexplained fever > 38°C, loss of > 10% body weight in 6 months, night sweats.

Pruritis: may lead to extensive excoriation from scratching.

Anorexia, lethargy.

Signs

Palpable lympadenopathy: careful examination and measurement of all node-bearing areas essential; assessment of spleen size essential.

Extranodal involvement: *eg*, bone marrow, liver, central nervous system; in ~10% of patients.

Infrequently involves bones or pulmonary parenchyma.

Investigations

- Initially, a good biopsy specimen must be carefully examined to make the diagnosis. Reed-Sternberg cells are the hallmark of Hodgkin's disease and the putative malignant cell. "Malignant" effusions are often reactive without tumor cells.
- Investigation is then systematic to "stage" the disease.

Full blood count: possible neutrophilia, eosinophilia, lymphopenia, leukoerythroblastic picture if bone marrow is involved. May be consistent with anemia of chronic inflammation or poor iron utilization.

Erythrocyte sedimentation rate (ESR) measurement: sometimes raised; can be useful disease marker and prognostic feature.

Liver function tests: abnormalities associated with liver involvement.

Lactate dehydrogenase measurement: useful disease marker and prognostic feature.

Chest radiography: to look for nodal and pulmonary disease, evaluate for mediastinal mass.

CT of chest and abdomen: to detect nodes; poor at detecting small nodules of hepatic and splenic disease.

Gallium scanning: Increased gallium uptake in two thirds of HD patients; useful for monitoring for disease persistence or recurrence.

Lymphangiography: in centers with expertise, lymphangiography is better than CT for assessing retroperitoneal nodes; however, this is seldom done in children.

Bone marrow examination: rarely reveals unsuspected bone marrow involvement. Multisite bone marrow aspirates and biopsies are necessary for completeness.

Staging laparotomy: controversial now; in theory, might detect unsuspected splenic disease and change treatment plan. Reserved for those patients receiving radiation therapy (RT) only; patients receiving systemic chemotherapy (with or without RT) may not require this.

Complications

- Infection related to underlying defect in cell-mediated immunity: herpes zoster seen in 20% and tuberculosis not unusual.
- *Pneumocystis carinii* prophylaxis is required.

Differential diagnosis

Non-Hodgkin's lymphoma.
Local infections, Epstein–Barr virus (EBV), toxoplasma, cytomegalovirus, cat-scratch disease, Mycobacterium, dilantin hypersensitivity syndrome.

Etiology

- The origin of the Reed–Sternberg cell, the putative malignant cell, is still debated; cell-surface marker CD15 is usually expressed; T- or B-lymphocyte markers are also sometimes expressed.
- Recent evidence implicates EBV in the cause of some cases of Hodgkin's disease; the EBV genome has been found incorporated into DNA in Reed-Sternberg cells, and serological evidence links EBV with Hodgkin's disease.

Epidemiology

- Hodgkin's disease has a first peak at 15–40 y, although it does occur throughout childhood.
- Male patients are more frequently affected than female patients.
- The incidence is higher in whites.

Classification

Based on the Rye system: pathologic classification includes nodular sclerosing (>80% of patients), lymphocyte predominant, mixed cellularity, and lymphocyte depleted.

- Pathology is no longer of prognostic significance given current treatment strategies.

Staging

- Hodgkin's disease appears to start unifocally and to spread to adjacent lymph nodes in an orderly fashion. Staging (based on the Ann Arbor scheme) is important for rational planning of treatment.

Stage I: involvement of single lymph node region.

Stage II: two or more lymph node regions on same side of diaphragm.

Stage III: lymph-node involvement on both sides of diaphragm, including spleen.

Stage IV: diffuse involvement of extranodal sites.

Suffix A: no systemic symptoms.

Suffix B: "B" symptoms as described earlier.

Treatment

Diet and lifestyle
• Some patients continue a normal lifestyle during chemotherapy; others feel quite unwell. This mainly reflects stage of disease and the intensity of treatment necessitated.

• Adequate nutrition should be maintained throughout therapy.

Pharmacologic treatment
• Hodgkin's disease is a chemo- and radiosensitive disease.

• Treatment decision depends on accurate staging and should also take into account current clinical trials. Current pediatric protocols involve limiting the amount of RT due to late effects. Primary treatment involves chemotherapy with or without low-dose involved-field RT.

Chemotherapy
• Several standard drug combinations are used, *eg*, COPP (cyclophosphamide, vincristine, procarbazine, prednisone), ABVD (doxorubicin, bleomycin, vinblastine, dacarbazine), and others; often in combination therapies over four to six cycles.

• Precise details of treatment should always be determined by an experienced oncologist, and preferably at a cancer center with pediatric experience.

• Good intravenous access is needed because some drugs, particularly vinca alkaloids and anthracyclines, are vesicant.

• Admission to the hospital is not usually required for treatment, although treatment should commence as soon as practical after initial diagnosis and staging.

Radiotherapy
• Older patients with low-stage disease may be cured with radiotherapy alone, which is preferable in certain select situations.

• Radiotherapy is usually given to an extended field beyond the area of overt nodal disease over 1 month. Dosing and timing depend on the adjuvant therapy given and the particular protocol used.

Treatment after relapse
• Relapse after initial treatment may still be compatible with long-term survival.

• Patients who relapse after RT can be "salvaged" with chemotherapy.

• The longer the duration of first remission, the greater is the chance of obtaining a second remission on standard treatment.

• Increasing dose intensity of treatment is of benefit in Hodgkin's disease; approximately 50% of patients resistant to standard treatment can still achieve long-term survival with high-dose chemotherapy regimens (including etoposide, cytarabine, and others), and autologous hematopoietic stem cell support.

Complications of treatment
Skin reactions and pneumonitis after RT: especially at higher doses.

Radiotherapy: impaired growth of soft tissues and bone (second neoplasms).

Myelosuppression, emesis, hair loss, and neurotoxicity after chemotherapy.

Impaired cardiac function (anthracyclines).

Second malignancy: lung cancer; acute myeloid leukemia (approximately 1%), peak incidence 4–11 years after initial treatment; breast cancer in women receiving RT to breast tissue.

Impaired fertility after chemotherapy.

Pulmonary fibrosis (from RT and/or chemotherapeutic agents such as bleomycin).

Treatment aims
To cure the disease with minimal toxicity from the treatment. This is critical when discussing management of children due to issues of growth and development.

Prognosis
• The overall survival at 5 y is approximately 90% (65% for stage IV patients).

• Poor prognostic features include the following:

Presence of B symptoms.

Stage III or IV disease at presentation.

ESR >40 mm/h.

Lactic dehydrogenase > normal.

Mass >10 cm.

Failure to obtain complete remission after adequate first-line treatment.

Follow-up and management
• Regular review during treatment is essential to detect complications and assess response.

• Full blood count is mandatory before administration of each cycle of treatment.

• After treatment is finished, full restaging is needed.

• Follow-up interval may gradually lengthen but should be continued indefinitely to detect complications of treatment or relapse. Depending on therapy, risk of second malignant neoplasm may be significant. Patient education (eg, breast self-examination for women) is critical.

General references
Collins RH, Jr.: The pathogenesis of Hodgkin's disease. *Blood Rev* 1990, 4:61–68.

Longo DL: The case against routine use of radiation therapy in advanced stage Hodgkin's disease. *Cancer Invest* 1996, 14:353–360.

Mauch PM: Controversies in the management of early stage Hodgkin's disease. *Blood* 1994, 83:318–329.

Prosoritz LR, Wu JJ, Yahalom J: The case for adjuvant radiation therapy in advanced Hodgkin's disease. *Cancer Invest* 1996, 14:361–370.

Yuen AR, Horning SJ: Hodgkin's disease: management of first relapse. *Oncology* 1996,

Hyperimmunoglobulinemia E syndrome

Diagnosis

Symptoms

Rash: itch, scale, infection (superficial or deep).

Coarse facial appearance.

Fever: recurrent.

Headache, purulent nasal discharge.

Cough, chest pain, sputum production, hemoptysis.

Joint or bone pain.

Unexplained bone fractures.

Gingival, oropharyngeal pain.

Signs

Coarse facies, broad nasal bridge, prominent nose: progress with age.

Atypical eczematoid dermatitis: papular and pruritic, often pustular and lichenified; prominent on face, neck, and ears but may occur on flexural surfaces of upper and lower extremities.

Skin infections: superficial to pustular, including soft tissue.

"Cold" abscesses: lymphadenitis without substantial inflammatory signs is common.

Lung, ear, sinus, eye, oral mucosa, and gingiva infections: common.

Bone, joint, viscera, and blood infections: less common.

Keratoconjunctivitis with corneal scarring.

Growth retardation.

Investigations

Complete history (including detailed family history for immunodeficiency) and physical examination.

Culture infection site: *Staphylococcus aureus* predominant organism isolated but *Haemophilius influenza*, pneumococcal, group A streptococcal, gram-negative, and fungal infections also occur.

Imaging studies: to localize infection sites.

Biopsy: as appropriate.

Complete blood count with differential and platelet count.

Erythrocyte sedimentation rate.

Quantitative immunoglobulins: IgG, IgA, IgM, IgE.

Total serum hemolytic complement (CH_{50}).

Nitroblue tetrazolium (NBT) test.

Immunologic abnormalities

Extremely elevated IgE: >2000 IU/mL.

Eosinophilia: in blood, sputum, and tissue biopsy sections.

Anergy: in delayed hypersensitivity testing.

Research findings: variable abnormalities in granulocyte locomotion (chemotaxis); elevated IgD concentrations; impaired antibody responses to proteins and polysaccharides; defective regulation of IgE synthesis.

Normal immunologic functions

Normal complement component production and function.

Normal neutrophil phagocytosis, metabolism and killing; normal phagocytic cell production and circulation.

Near normal serum IgG, IgA, and IgM concentrations.

Normal T-cell proliferative responses *in vitro*.

Baseline and acute pulmonary function assessments.

Complications

Recalcitrant infections: multiple but distinctive sites, especially lung and skin.

Persistent pneumatoceles: progressive parenchymal destruction.

Bronchiectasis.

Pulmonary hemorrhage: may be life threatening.

Scoliosis.

Growth retardation.

Osteopenia: idiopathic fractures (rare).

Differential diagnosis

Atopic dermatitis (eczema).

Chronic granulomatous disease.

Other neutrophil defects.

Leukocyte adherence deficiency.

Specific granule deficiency.

Chédiak–Higashi syndrome.

Myeloperoxidase deficiency.

Wiskott–Aldrich syndrome.

Complement deficiency (especially early components).

Di George syndrome (although phenotypically quite different, rare cases have elevated serum IgE levels).

Etiology

Unknown; no definitive defect identified (possible regulatory T-cell defect).

Occasionally familial occurrence; pattern suggests autosomal-dominant inheritance with incomplete penetrance.

Epidemiology

Rare disorder.

Other information

• Distinguish from eczema by pronounced increase in total IgE, atypical rash (less pruritus, pustular character, distribution), facial appearance, and general absence of other chronic allergic stigmata seen in eczema.

• Distinguish from chronic granulomatous disease by occurrence of catalase-negative infective organisms; predominance of pneumatoceles; and low incidence of osteomyelitis, urinary tract infections, diarrhea, and intestinal obstruction.

• Whereas Wiskott-Aldrich patients show increased susceptibility to infection, a pruritic eczematoid dermatitis, and elevated serum IgE levels, this disorder can be distinguished by genetic characteristics (autosomal-recessive, male-affecting), thrombocytopenia, distinctively small platelet size, and a characteristic decrease in expression of T-cell membrane CD43.

156

Treatment

Lifestyle management
• Patients must adapt to chronic disease, chronic medication, and life-threatening infection.

Pharmacologic treatment
Continuous antistaphylococcal antibiotic therapy: co-trimoxazole, dicloxacillin, erythromycin.

Skin care: emollients; topical steroids, intermittent for inflammatory component; topical antibacterials (impetigo); topical antifungals (candidiasis, tinea); antihistamines (pruritus).

Immunizations: routine, pneumococcus, influenza A, varicella.

Nonpharmacologic treatment
Pulmonary care: bronchodilators and chest percussion and drainage as appropriate.

Treatment of specific infections and their complications: including surgical management.

Experimental treatment: plasmapheresis, i.v. immunoglobulin, interferon-γ, other immunostimulants.

Treatment aims
To prevention infection.
To identify and aggressively treat infection early.
To preservation of lung function.
To attend to cosmetic problems.
• Genetic counseling and family support for chronic disease issues is recommended.

Prognosis
Fair, if aggressive treatment and continuity of care available.

Follow-up and management
• Monitor infection, complications of disease, and treatment.

General references
Buckley R: Disorders of the IgE system. In *Immunologic Disorders in Infants and Children*, ed 4. Edited by Stiehm ER. WB Saunders Co.: Philadelphia; 1996.

Quie PG, Mills EL, Robert RL, Noya FJD: Disorders of the polymorphonuclear phagocytic system. In *Immunologic Disorders in Infants and Children*, ed 4. Edited by Stiehm ER. WB Saunders Co.: Philadelphia; 1996.

Roberts RL, Stiehm ER: Hyperimmunoglobulin E syndrome (Job syndrome). In *Current Therapy in Allergy, Immunology and Rheumatology*, ed 5. Edited by Lichtenstein CM, Fauci A. Mosby: St. Louis; 1996.

Diagnosis

Symptoms

Acute reactions (single or multiple episodes)
Dyspnea, cough, and chest pain.

Fever, chills, malaise.

Weight loss, hemoptysis: rare.

Subacute presentations (progressive onset over weeks)
Dyspnea: can be severe (cyanosis possible).

Cough: usually dry but later productive.

Weight loss usually evident.

Chronic form (insidious onset due to continuous response to allergen)
Fatigue and weight loss may be presenting complaints.

Dyspnea: present, patient is often unaware due to very gradual onset.

Signs

Acute reactions
Appear acutely ill with fever, tachypnea, and tachycardia.

Auscultation of lung fields: usually diffuse, fine, crackly rales (especially at the bases); rhonchi and/or wheeze possible; occasionally clear lung fields.

Chronic form
Tachypnea.

Auscultation of lung fields: decreased breath sounds; increased inspiratory to expiratory phase ratio occasionally when an obstructive component coexists.

Investigations

Detailed clinical history and assessment of chronic environmental exposures.

Complete blood count with differential: eosinophilia absent.

Erythrocyte sedimentation rate: normal to moderate increase.

Immunologic: quantitative immunoglobulins, total serum hemolytic complement (CH_{50}), C3, C4, and energy testing are all normal.

Arterial blood gas assessment (hypoxemia).

Airway hyperreactivity (measured by methacholine challenge) may be present.

Document presence of precipitating antibody to suspected allergen.

Skin testing: is not useful.

Bronchoalveolar lavage: research tool.

Bronchoprovocation with suspected allergen (must monitor for 24 hours) or "Site challenge" (revisit to suspected exposure site).

Environmental assessment for allergens: specialized technology.

Pulmonary function testing
Acute episodes: are restrictive with minimal obstruction; reversible with time.

Chronic forms: restrictive findings; may respond to corticosteroids; obstructive component possible (bronchitis obliterans).

Chest radiograph
Acute forms: both interstitial and alveolar filling processes.

Chronic forms: tendency for interstitial/nodular pattern; volume loss.

Complications

Cor pulmonale, respiratory failure, bronchitis obliterans, irreversible obstructive lung disease: can be fatal during any phase of disease.

Differential diagnosis
Pulmonary mycotoxicosis (toxic pneumonitis from massive inhalation of fungi).

Recurrent infectious pneumonia (especially viral and mycoplasmal).

Sarcoidosis.

Vasculitides.

Cryptogenic fibrosing alveolitis.

Histiocytosis.

Pulmonary hemosiderosis.

Pulmonary eosinophilia.

Asthma.

Allergic bronchopulmonary aspergillosis.

Pneumoconiosis.

Etiology
• Hypersensitivity pneumonitis ("extrinsic allergic alveolitis") is an immunologically mediated disease in which the predominant mechanism of lung injury involves cell-mediated (T-cell) mechanism(s).

Examples of causative allergens
Bacteria
Thermophilic actinomycetes–contaminated air-conditioning and humidifier systems.

Contaminated hay or grains.

Moldy sugar cane.

Mushroom compost.

Bacillus subtilis–contaminated walls.

Streptomyces albus–contaminated fertilizer.

Fungi
Moldy grain, tobacco, compost (Aspergillus spp).

Cephalosporium–contaminated sewer water and air-conditioning system.

Moldy cork (Penicillium).

Pullularia–contaminated sauna water.

Puffball spores in moldy dwellings.

Moldy maple bark (Cryptostroma).

Insects
Sitophilus granorius–infested flour (wheat weevil).

Animal proteins
Serum proteins from urine (parrot, parakeet, dove, pigeon), droppings (pigeon), feathers (duck, chicken, turkey, pigeon), or pelts (rat, gerbil, other animals).

Organic chemicals
Workers who handle isocyanates.

Other
Pyrethrum insecticide.

Amebae-contaminated water (in humidifiers).

Treatment

Lifestyle management
• Adjust environment to avoid specific trigger and any related allergens.

Pharmacologic treatment
• Administer systemic glucocorticoid for 10–14 days to manage acute or subacute presentations; chronic form may require prolonged, alternate day administration.

• Institute basic respiratory support depending on clinical status:

Oxygen.

Cough suppressant.

Bronchodilator.

Antipyretics.

Treatment aims
To avoid allergen exposure.

To reverse acute symptoms.

To identify pulmonary function abnormalities and monitor improvement.

To identify concurrent pulmonary inflammatory disease (eg, asthma).

Prognosis
Excellent if allergen exposure can be eliminated; occasionally, patients with chronic disease have poorly reversible disease and, rarely, continued progression despite allergen avoidance.

Follow-up and management.
• Monitor pulmonary function.
• Manage side-effects of treatment.
• Monitor environmental exposures.

Other treatment options
• Inhaled glucocorticoids are not sufficient to reverse the inflammatory process, and the addition of this modality will not permit continued exposure to allergen.

General references
Fink JN: Hypersensitivity pneumonitis. In *Allergy*, ed 2. Edited by Kaplan AP. Philadelphia: WB Saunders Co.; 1997:531–541.

Pfaff JK, Taussig LM: Pulmonary disorders. In *Immunologic Disorders in Infants and Children*, ed 4. Edited by Stiehm ER. Philadelphia: WB Saunders Co.; 1996:659–696.

Diagnosis

Symptoms
- Many patients can be asymptomatic.

Headache, blurry vision, epistaxis, chest pain: are generalized symptoms associated with hypertension.

Drooling, inability to close eyes: Bell's palsy.

Flushing, palpitations: associated with pheochromocytoma.

Weight gain or loss: renal insufficiency, acute glomerulonephritis.

Rash: systemic lupus erythematosus, Henoch-Schönlein purpura.

Signs
Unusual body habitus: thin, obese, growth failure, virilized, stigmata of Turner or Williams syndrome.

Skin lesions: café-au-lait spots, neurofibromas, rashes.

Moon facies: Cushing's syndrome.

Hypertensive retinopathy: rare in children.

Congestive heart failure: crackles, gallop, hepatomegaly, jugular venous distention.

Abdominal mass: tumor or obstruction.

Abdominal bruit: renal artery stenosis.

Ambiguous or virilized genitalia: adrenal etiology.

Investigations
Blood pressures: should be obtained using an appropriate-sized cuff; the inflatable bladder should encircle the arm and cover 75% of the upper arm; several measurements should be obtained in a relaxed setting; normative data by age and gender should be reviewed before labeling patients as hypertensive.

Lower-extremity BP less than upper-extremity BP: coarctation of the aorta.

Urinalysis: for hematuria, proteinuria, and casts in glomerulonephritis.

Serum electolytes, renal function studies, uric acid, and cholesterol: to assess renal function, other risk factors, and potential adrenal dysfunction.

Echocardiogram: the most sensitive measurement of end-organ changes in hypertensive children.

Renal ultrasound: to visualize anatomic anomalies and scarring.

The following studies should be considered if the history and physical examination suggest a secondary cause.

Voiding cystourethrogram/DMSA renal scan: to identify vesicoureteral reflux and reflux nephropathy.

24-hour urine for catecholamines and metanephrines, MIBG scan: for pheochromocytoma.

Plasma renin activity (peripheral), renal vein renin activity, magnetic resonance arteriography, and renal arteriography: although the first three studies can be considered for screening, the latter is the "gold standard" in diagnosing renal artery stenosis.

Complications
Congestive heart failure.
Renal failure.
Encephalopathy.
Retinopathy.

Differential diagnosis
Inappropriate cuff size.
"White coat" hypertension.

Etiology
- Secondary causes of hypertension are more common the younger the child and the greater the blood pressure.
- Secondary causes include renal parenchymal disease, cystic kidney disease, reflux nephropathy; renal artery stenosis secondary to fibromuscular dysplasia, neurofibromatosis, Williams syndrome; coarctation of the aorta; pheochromocytoma, hyperthyroidism, hyperaldosteronism; corticosteroids, sympathomimetics, oral contraceptives.

Epidemiology
- The prevalence of hypertension in children has been reported from 1.2% to 13%, although less than 1% require medication.
- The rate of hypertension in black adults is greater than in whites, although differences in children are not seen until after age 12.

Treatment

Diet and lifestyle

• Mild primary hypertension can be managed without medication. Emphasis should be placed on weight reduction (assuming the patient is obese), increased exercise, and some degree of sodium restriction. Smoking should be discouraged.

• Adolescents with well-controlled hypertension may participate in competitive athletics if they do not have end-organ involvement.

Pharmacologic treatment

• Medications should be considered if nonpharmacologic therapy has failed or if end-organ changes are present.

Angiotensin-converting enzyme inhibitors

Standard dosage	Captopril, 1–6 mg/kg divided 3 times daily, 0.1–0.5 mg/kg divided 2 times daily.
Contraindications	Bilateral renal artery stenosis, pregnancy.
Main drug interactions	Hyperkalemia when given with potassium-sparing diuretics; less antihypertensive effect when given with nonsteroidal anti-inflammatory drugs.
Main side effects	Angioedema is rare, but can be very serious; cough, renal insufficiency.

Calcium channel blockers

Standard dosage	Nifedipine, 0.25–0.5 mg/kg (maximum, 20 mg) every 2 h as needed orally or sublingually; several long-acting forms are available (isradipine, amlodipine).
Contraindications	None.
Main drug interactions	Verapamil and beta-blockers can have an additive effect and cause bradycardia.
Main side effects	Flushing, headache, tachycardia, edema.

β-Blockers

Standard dosage	Propranolol, 0.5–1 mg/kg/d divided 2 or 3 times daily; gradually increase to 1–5 mg/kg/d; long-acting forms are available (atenolol).
Contraindications	Reactive airway disease, heart block, heart failure.
Special points	Use with caution in diabetics as beta-blockers may interfere with the usual responses seen with hypoglycemia.
Main drug interactions	Phenobarbital and rifampin increase drug clearance, cimetidine decreases drug clearance.
Main side effects	Exercise intolerance, nightmares.

Thiazide diuretics

Standard dosage	Chlorothiazide, 10–20 mg/kg/d. Hydrochlorothiazide, 1–2 mg/kg/d.
Contraindications	Anuria, hypersensitivity to thiazide or sulfonamide derivatives.
Main drug interactions	Introduce at a low dose when patients are already taking other hypertensive medications, particularly angiotensin-converting enzyme inhibitors.
Main side effects	Hypokalemia.

Other hypertensive agents

Direct vasodilators (hydralazine, minoxidil), α-blockers (prazosin, doxazosin), and centrally acting agents (clonidine) can also be considered but are not usually first-line agents for hypertension in children.

Treatment aims

To reduce blood pressure to levels that diminish the risk of associated organ involvement.

To maximize compliance by using long-acting agents and monotherapy, if possible.

To monitor for and address adverse effects, should they arise.

Other treatments

• Some forms of secondary hypertension require surgical correction, such as coarctation of the aorta and some forms of renovascular hypertension.

• Percutaneous transluminal angioplasty can be considered in some cases of renovascular hypertension.

Prognosis

• The patient's prognosis depends on the underlying cause of the hypertension.

Follow-up and management

• Patients should be followed up for life.

• In cases of mild hypertension, medication tapering can be considered.

General references

Dillon MJ, Ingelfinger JR: Pharmacologic treatment of hypertension. In *Pediatric Nephrology*, ed 3. Edited by Holliday MA, Barratt TM, Avner ED. Baltimore: Williams & Wilkins; 1994:1165–1174.

Ingelfinger JR, Dillon MJ: Evaluation of secondary hypertension. In *Pediatric Nephrology*, ed 3. Edited by Holliday MA, Barratt TM, Avner ED: Baltimore: Williams and Wilkins; 1994:1146–1164.

Rocchini AP: Childhood hypertension. *Pediatr Clin North Am* 1993, **40**:1–212.

Task Force on Blood Pressure Control in Children: Report of the Second Task Force on Blood Pressure Control in Children. *Pediatrics* 1987, **79**:1–25.

Yetman RJ, Bonilla-Felix MA, Portman RJ: Primary hypertension in children and adolescents. In *Pediatric Nephrology*, ed 3. Edited by Holliday MA, Barratt TM, Avner ED. Baltimore: Williams & Wilkins; 1994:1117–1145.

Diagnosis

Symptoms

Hyperactivity; often mistaken for attention deficit disorder.

Weight loss, polyphagia.

Anxious, palpitations, shortness of breath, weakness.

Heat intolerance, sweating.

Staring.

Signs

Increased systolic blood pressure, tachycardia.

Goiter with or without nodules, often with bruit.

Exophthalmos, tremors, and proximal muscle weakness.

Investigations

Thyroid function tests: T4 is generally elevated; total T3 is almost always elevated; thyroid-stimulating hormone (TSH) is suppressed and is the best indicator of thyroid hormone excess; a normal TSH suggests the possibility of familial dysalbuninemic hyperthyroxinemia, familial thyroxine-binding globulin excess, or familial thyroxine resistance.

[123]Thyroid uptake and scan: will demonstrate a rapid elevated uptake and enlarged thyroid gland; a single hyperfunctioning nodule will depress radioactive iodine uptake in the rest of the gland; in subacute and chronic thyroiditis (Hashimoto thyroiditis hyperthyroidism or "Hashi-toxicosis"), the uptake is low.

Anti-TSH receptor antibodies or thyroid-stimulating immunoglobulins: will be elevated in Graves' disease.

Antithyroglobulin, antimicrosomal, and antiperoxidase antibodies: can be elevated in Graves' disease as well as chronic lymphocytic thyroiditis.

Complications

Excessive growth with advancement of bone age.

Cardiac high-output failure is unlikely in children.

Differential diagnosis

Factitious thyroxine ingestion.

Attention deficit disorder.

Familial thyroxine resistance.

Familial dysalbuminemic hyperthyroxinemia.

Etiology

Autoimmune: Graves' disease.

Autoimmune: toxic phase of Hashimoto's thyroiditis.

Postviral: subacute thyroiditis.

Hyperfunctioning nodule.

Neonatal Graves' secondary to maternal transfer of thyroid-stimulating antibodies.

Epidemiology

Most common in second to fourth decade of life.

Four to five times more frequent in females.

Treatment

Lifestyle
• Avoid frequent use of sympathomimetic drugs and significant iodide ingestion.

Pharmacological treatment
Thionamide drugs (propylthiouracil and methimazole) comprise first line of treatment.

Standard dosage
Propylthiouracil, 300 mg, or methimazole, 30 mg is the usual starting dose (the dose of propylthiouracil is 10 times greater than methimazole) but may need to be higher in older and larger children then titrate down after controlling hyperthyroidism.

Propranolol, 20–60 mg/d during the first 6–12 wk of treatment, is often useful to ameliorate the symptoms.

Special points
Some groups add L-thyroxine when the patient is biochemically hypothyroid on the initial higher dose of thionamide. Other groups titrate the dose down to 100–150 mg of propythiouracil (10–15 mg methimazole) and then add L-thyroxine if the patient remains hypothyroid.

Other treatments
• In those children who are nonresponsive or noncompliant with medical therapy, radioablation is the second line of therapy.

• As a third option, especially in very large thyroid glands, subtotal thyroidectomy is extremely effective. In nodular hyperthyroidism, subtotal thyroidectomy is the first line of treatment.

Treatment aims
To restore the patient to a normal metabolic state.

• The relief of clinical symptoms and signs, coupled with normal biochemical studies of thyroid function, are the goals of therapy.

Prognosis
• Restoration of the child to normal thyroid metabolic function can be achieved with treatment (medical, surgical, or with radioablation and use of L-thyroxine to treat iatrogenic hypothyroidism) in greater than 90% of patients.

• In children, remission occurs in 25%–40$ of patients in 2 y and approximately another 25% each following 2 y. Approximately 80% of patients will be in remission in 8 y. Relapses occur in 3%–30% of patients, however.

Follow-up and management
• Patients should be followed at 6–8-wk intervals both clinically and biochemically until a euthyroid state is achieved. Once a maintenance program is achieved, the patients can be followed at 3-mo intervals.

• Discontinuation of pharmacologic therapy can be attempted after 2 y of stability and if levels of thyroid-stimulating antibodies are found to be low.

General references
Alter CA, Moshang T: Diagnostic dilemma: the goiter. *Pediatr Clin North Am* 1991, **38**:567–578.

Foley TP: Thyrotoxicosis in childhood. *Pediatr Ann* 1992, **21**:43–49.

Lippe B, Landau EM, Kaplan SA: Hyperthyroidism in children treated with long term medical therapy: twenty-five percent remission every 2 years. *J Clin Endocrinol Metab* 1987, **65**:1241–1245.

Diagnosis

Symptoms

Sweating, shakiness, anxiety, blurry vision: due to sympathetic adrenergic responses to low blood glucose concentrations.

Dizziness, lethargy, confusion: due to impaired cerebral function resulting from low blood glucose concentrations.

Signs

Pallor, diaphoresis, tachycardia, occasional hypothermia (adrenergic).

Altered behavior, lethargy, irritability, coma, seizure (neuroglycopenic).

Investigations

For all cases

• Blood glucose must be confirmed by laboratory measurement unless cause is already known; however, emergency treatment can begin based on blood glucose meter strip test.

• Blood glucose <40 mg/dL is appropriate criteria for symptomatic hypoglycemia at any age (including newborn infants).

For all unexplained cases

• In addition to blood glucose, obtain the following pretreatment "critical" samples:

Serum bicarbonate.

Urine ketones by dipstick.

Chemistry panel, blood ammonia.

Plasma levels of β-hydroxybutyrate and free fatty acids.

Plasma hormone levels, including insulin, C peptide, growth hormone, cortisol.

• Preserve 1–3 mL plasma for free and total carnitine, acylcarnitine profile, and other tests as may become needed.

• Preserve 5 mL acute urine for organic acid profile, and so on.

• Further workup of unexplained cases may require formal provocative fasting study with sequential measurements of fuels and hormone levels: if hyperinsulinism suspected, give i.v. glucagon, 1 mg, when glucose falls < 50 mg/dL and monitor rise in glucose at 10-minute intervals for 30–45 minutes.

Complications

Seizure.

Permanent brain damage and developmental retardation.

Death.

Differential diagnosis

Other causes of coma or acute, life-threatening episode in infancy, including sepsis, asphyxia, seizure, poisoning, inborn errors of metabolism.

Etiology

Excess insulin action in diabetic patients.

Normal infant ("ketotic hypoglycemia")

Metabolic defects

Glycogen/gluconeogenic disorders.

Glucose-6-phosphatase deficiency.

Glycogen debrancher deficiency.

Liver phosphorylase and phosphorylase kinase deficiency.

Fructose-1,6-diphosphatase deficiency.

Pyruvate carboxylase deficiency.

Fatty acid oxidation disorders (>10 known).

Hormone disorders

Hyperinsulinism.

Congenital hyperinsulinism (autosomal recessive, autosomal dominant, or hyperinsulinism/hyperammonemia syndrome).

Islet adenoma.

Small for gestational age or asphyxiated neonate.

Infant of diabetic mother.

Pituitary deficiency

Isolated growth hormone or growth hormone plus adrenal insufficiency.

Adrenal insufficiency

Tumor hypoglycemia

Insulin growth factor-2 production or excessive glucose utilization.

Drugs/intoxications

Surreptitious insulin administration, oral hypoglycemics, alcohol.

Epidemiology

Neonates: may occur transiently in >10%–25% of infants not fed immediately at delivery.

• Incidence of most genetic disorders is approximately 1:20,000.

Treatment

Diet and lifestyle

- For acute treatment, give i.v. glucose to quickly correct hypoglycemia.
- Adjust feeding frequency to match fasting tolerance.
- For glycogen storage disease 1 (GSD 1), consider use of continuous intragastric feeding.
- Consider use of home glucose meters, urine dipsticks.

Pharmacologic treatment

Standard dosage: *Acute treatment*: intravenous glucose as 10% dextrose, 3—5 mL/kg, push then continue at maintenance or as needed to maintain blood glucose >60 mg/dL.

Glucagon, 1 mg i.v., i.m., s.q. for insulin-induced hypoglycemia.

Diazoxide, 10 mg/kg/d p.o. in 23 divided doses.

Octreotide, 2—30 µg/kg/d divided into 3–4 doses s.q. or continous infusion.

Treatment aims

To maintain blood glucose >60 mg/dL.

To prevent permanent brain damage.

To maintain optimal growth and development.

Prognosis

Depends on etiology.

Late complications of poor growth, hepatic tumors, renal failure in GSD 1.

Late cardiomyopathy in some forms of GSD 3, severe fatty acid oxidation defects.

Follow-up and management

Referral to pediatric endocrine/metabolic specialist.

Home glucose monitoring.

Chronic conditions: periodic reevaluation to assess control of hypoglycemia.

General references

Finegold DN: Hypoglycemia. In *Pediatric Endocrinology*. Edited by Sperling MA. Philadelphia: WB Saunders: 1996:571–593.

Katz LL, Stanley CA: Disorders of glucose and other sugars. In *Intensive Care of the Fetus and Neonate*. Edited by Spitzer A. City: Publisher; 1995.

Stanley CA: Carnitine disorders. *Adv Pediatr* 1995, **42:**209–242.

Stanley CA: Hyperinsulinism in infants and children. *Pediatr Clin N Am* 1997, **44:**363–374.

Hypothyroidism, acquired

Diagnosis

Symptoms

Poor growth with continued gain.

Constipation, cold intolerance, itchy skin.

Lethargy and easy fatiguability.

Signs

Short stature.

Hypothermia, decreased pulse pressure and bradycardia.

Dry skin, increased vellous hair and carotinemic, sallow complexion.

Delayed relaxation phase of deep tendon reflexes.

May have signs of early puberty.

May or may not have goiter.

Investigations

Thyroid function tests: T4 will be low and thyroid-stimulating hormone (TSH) concentrations elevated in acquired hypothyroidism. TSH levels are normal in patients with secondary hypothyroidism.

Antithyroid antibodies: the presence of antithyroglobulin, antimicrosomal or antiperoxidase antibodies will be elevated in patients with hypothyroidism secondary to chronic lymphocytic thyroiditis, which is the most common cause of acquired hypothyroidism.

Head MRI: necessary in those patients with secondary hypothyroidism.

Thyroid radiouptake and scan: will show diminished or patchy uptake.

Fine-needle aspiration: nodular goiters should be aspirated for pathologic diagnosis, although papillary thyroid carcinoma in children generally is not associated with hypothyroidism.

Complications

Loss in final height: may result due to late treatment, *ie*, treatment during the age appropriate for puberty will not provide sufficient time for "catch-up" growth.

Precocious puberty and galactorrhea: may complicate hypothyroidism.

Temporary loss of hair following treatment.

Excessive activity, similar to attention deficit disorder, after treatment: will ameliorate with time.

• Other autoimmune disorders, including Addison's disease, type I diabetes mellitus, vitiligo, may be associated with autoimmune hypothyroidism.

Differential diagnosis

Growth hormone deficiency and other causes of growth failure.

Depression.

Exogenous obesity.

Pregnancy.

Etiology

• Autoimmune thyroiditis accounts for 80%–90% of childhood acquired hypothyroidism.

• Brain tumors are the most common solid tumor in childhood. The location of the brain tumor (eg, craniopharyngioma) or brain tumor treatment, including surgery and cranial irradiation, are the major cause of secondary acquired hypothyroidism.

• Thyroid irradiation and thyroid surgery are relatively infrequent causes in childhood.

• Drugs, eg, amiodarone or lithium, used for various medical conditions can interfere with thyroid function.

Epidemiology

• Hypothyroidism is four times more frequent in females.

• Thyroid disorders, including hypothyroidism, are more common in children with Down syndrome and in girls with Turner's syndrome.

Treatment

Diet and lifestyle
• No changes are necessary.

Pharmacologic treatment

Standard dosage   L-thyroxine, 2–5 mug/kg/d (higher doses for younger children).

Special points   Titrate doses on basis of thyroid function tests.

General references

LaFranchi S: Thyroiditis and acquired hypothyroidism. *Pediatr Ann* 1992, **21**:29–39.

Ripkees SA, Bode HH, Crawford JD: Long term growth in juvenile acquired hypothyroidism: the failure to achieve normal adult stature. *N Engl J Med* 1988, **318**:599–602.

Diagnosis

Symptoms

Asymptomatic at birth.

If undiagnosed: will develop lethargy, poor feeding.

Signs

Open posterior fontanelle and/or large open anterior fontanelle.

Hypothermia.

Umbilical hernia.

Hypotonia.

Prolonged jaundice.

Investigations

Thyroid function tests: T4 will be low and thyroid-stimulating hormone (TSH) concentrations elevated in primary hypothyroidism. Low T4 and TSH suggest the possibility of thyroxine-binding globulin deficiency (or other decreased binding proteins), hypopituitarism or euthyroid sick syndrome.

Technetium or ^{123}I thyroid scan or ultrasound: is useful in demonstrating thyroid agenesis (dysgenesis) as opposed to an inborn error of thyroxine synthesis.

Thyroxine-binding globulin level and T3 resin uptake: useful in those cases of binding protein deficiency.

Complications

Untreated: severe mental retardation, neurologic complications, and growth failure.

Respiratory distress syndrome.

Differential diagnosis

Primary congenital hypothyroidism.
Hypopituitarism.
Thyroxine-binding globulin deficiency.
Euthyroid sick syndrome of neonates.
Transient hypothyroidism.
Prematurity.

Etiology

Thyroid agenesis or dysgenesis.
Inborn error of thyroxine synthesis.
Maternal drug ingestion (thiourea drugs).

Epidemiology

In North America, 1:3700 infants.
Two to three times more frequent in females.

Treatment

Lifestyle

• No changes necessary if treated within the first month of life.
• If treated at older age, educational needs must be assessed.

Pharmacologic treatment

Standard dosage   L-thyroxine, 10–15 µg/kg/d
Special points   Titrate dose to maintain T4 and TSH in normal range.

Treatment aims

To protect the child's brain development and overall growth.
To maintain T4 and TSH in normal range.
• During the first year of life, the TSH may be difficult to suppress without making the infant clinically and biochemically hyperthyroid.

Prognosis

Excellent if treated within the first month of life.
Significant decrease in intelligence quotient if treated after 3 months of life.

Follow-up and management

• The T4 and TSH should be monitored frequently (3-mo intervals) during first year of life and more frequently if needed to adjust thyroxine replacement.
T4 and TSH measurements less frequently after 2 y of age.
Growth, weight gain, head circumference at 3-mo intervals.
Developmental assessments at routine yearly visits.

General references

AAP Section on Endocrinology and Committee on Genetics, and American Thyroid Association Committee on Public Health: Newborn screening for congenital hypothyroidism: recommended guidelines. *Pediatrics* 1993, **91**:1201–1210.

Kooistra L, Lane C, Vulsma T, *et al.*: Motor and cognitive development in children with congenital hypothyroidism: a long-term evaluation of the effects of neonatal treatment. *J Pediatr* 1994, **124**:903–909.

Willi SM, Moshang T: Diagnostic dilemmas: results of screening tests for congenital hypothyroidism. *Pediatr Clin North Am* 1991, **38**:555–566.

Diagnosis

Symptoms

Reduced muscle tone: may be acute or chronic, congenital or acquired.

Lag in attainment (or loss) of motor milestones.

Other symptoms according to specific etiology.

• Acute hypotonia suggests infant botulism, Guillain-Barré syndrome, intoxication, systemic illness, acute central nervous system (CNS) insult, polio, tic paralysis.

• Chronic hypotonia suggests prior CNS insult or cerebral dysgenesis, spinal muscular atrophy, congenital myopathy.

Signs

Hypotonia of central origin

Weakness is absent or mild: assess withdrawal to noxious stimulus.

Normal muscle bulk.

Microcephaly.

Congenital malformations: note that club foot, torticollis, and other deformations are more common in central than in peripheral hypotonia.

Intrauterine growth retardation.

Cutaneous or ophthalmologic lesions.

Hypotonia of peripheral (neuromuscular) origin

Prominent weakness.

Muscle wasting.

Areflexia: suggests spinal muscular atrophy or Gullaine-Barré syndrome.

• Thorough general physical examination is essential to detect involvement outside the nervous system, including organ failure (renal, cardiac, pulmonary, hepatic), visceral abnormalities (*eg*, enlargement from storage disease), eye involvement (*eg*, congenital infection), skeletal abnormalities (*eg*, multiple congenital anomaly syndrome), skin lesions (*eg*, neurocutaneous syndrome).

Investigations

If central origin appears more likely

Neuroimaging (cranial CT or MRI without contrast).

Chromosome analysis.

Serum chemistries.

Blood pyruvate and lactate; plasma and urine amino/organic acids; lysosomal enzyme analysis.

If peripheral origin appears more likely

Electromyography/nerve conduction studies.

Muscle biopsy.

DNA testing for spinal muscular atrophy (Werdnig-Hoffmann disease).

Complications

Feeding difficulties.

Respiratory distress.

Aspiration pneumonia.

Joint contractures, scoliosis, functional limitation.

Other complications: according to specific etiology.

Differential diagnosis

Hypotonia of central origin:

Cerebral dysgenesis.

CNS insult (eg, stroke, hypoxic-ischemic or hypoglycemic encephalopathy).

Chromosomal disorder (especially trisomies, Prader-Willi syndrome).

Inborn error of metabolism.

"Benign congenital hypotonia" (diagnosis of exclusion if hypotonia gradually improves).

Idiopathic hypotonic cerebral palsy (a diagnosis of exclusion).

Peripheral hypotonia:

Congenital myopathy (show various specific histologic findings).

Metabolic myopathies, including acid maltase deficiency (Pompe's disease), cytochrome c oxidase deficiency, mitochondrial myopathies.

Congenital muscular dystrophy.

Congenital form of myotonic dystrophy.

Spinal muscular atrophy.

Polio.

Guillain-Barré syndrome (uncommon before 6–12 mo of age).

Congenital myasthenia gravis.

Infant botulism.

Hypomyelinating neuropathy.

Etiology

• Central hypotonia presumably results from imbalance between extrapyramidal and pyramidal influences on an intact motor unit.

• Peripheral hypotonia reflects impaired motor unit function.

Epidemiology

Varies according to specific disorder.

Treatment

Diet and lifestyle
• Optimize feeding and nutritional status; this may require high-calorie supplements or temporary or permanent gastrostomy placement, according to specific entity.
• Specific diets, supplements, or vitamin therapies are neccessary for some inborn errors of metabolism.

Pharmacologic treatment
• Specific therapies are not available in most cases.
• For congenital myasthenia gravis consider pyridostigmine.
• Agents producing neuromuscular blockade (*eg*, gentamicin) are contraindicated in infant botulism and myasthenia.

Nonpharmacologic treatment
• Diagnose and manage associated systemic disease.
• Optimize feeding and nutritional status.
• Encourage motor development in infant stimulation program.
• For infant botulism, most patients require mechanical ventilation for several weeks.
• For Guillain–Barré syndrome, plasma exchange (PE) appears to be effective in hastening recovery but it is not clear whether it will prove superior to intravenous immunoglobulin, which appears promising.

Treatment aims
To optimize motor development and correctly manage underlying condition. To prevent or minimize nutritional and respiratory complications.

Prognosis
• Outcome is determined by specific entity.
• Specific causes of peripheral hypotonia include the following:
Spinal muscular atrophy.
Early infantile form: (Werdnig-Hoffmann disease) nearly always fatal.
Intermediate type (symptoms usually appear after 6 months) is usually compatible with long-term survival with disability.
Infantile botulism and Guillain-Barré syndrome: complete recovery usually occurs with proper supportive care, including assisted ventilation if necessary.
Congenital muscular dystrophy, myotonia congenita: occasional early death; more commonly, survival with disability.
Congenital myasthenia gravis: autoimmune variety resolves within weeks as maternally derived antibodies wane; other forms may persist.
Congenital myopathy or hypomyelinating neuropathy: long-term survival with variable disability.

Follow-up and management
Periodic follow-up to monitor development and efficacy of early intervention. Genetic counseling where appropriate. Consider influenza vaccinations in family members.

General references
Fenichel GM: *Pediatric Neurology: A Signs and Symptoms Approach*, edn 3. Philadelphia: W.B. Saunders; 1997.

Parano E, Lovelace RE: Neonatal peripheral hypotonia: clinical and electromyographic characteristics. *Childs Nerv Syst* 1993, 9:166–171.

Diagnosis

Symptoms

• Onset of symptoms may be rapid or insidious. Insidious presentation more characteristic of chronic immune thrombocytopenic purpura (ITP).

Bruises.

Petechial rash.

Nose bleeds.

Blood in stool.

Hematuria (rare).

Signs

Bruising on trunk, extremities, head, neck.

Petechiae in any location.

Excessive bruising: after trauma.

Prolonged bleeding: after venipuncture.

Absence of hepatosplenomegaly.

Investigations

General investigations

Complete blood count: isolated thrombocytopenia; normal hemoglobin and leukocyte count; normal differential; may have mild anemia associated with blood loss.

Peripheral blood smear: erythrocytes and leukocytes appear normal. Platelets are decreased in number and may appear larger than normal.

Reticulocyte count: elevated with accompanying hemolysis (Evans syndrome is the combination of autoimmune hemolytic anemia with immune-mediated thrombocytopenia).

Special investigations

Bone marrow aspiration: megakaryocytes are present in normal or increased quantities. Erythrocyte and leukocyte cellularity and morphology should be normal. Routine performance of bone marrow aspirate to eliminate the possibility of acute leukemia is controversial. Some clinicians prefer to avoid the marrow and make the diagnosis on clinical history, physical findings, and laboratory data alone.

Direct antiglobulin test: to assess presence of antibody-mediated erythrocyte destruction.

Antinuclear antibodies: thrombocytopenia may be the presenting feature of lupus.

HIV antibody: thrombocytopenia may be an early manifestation of HIV infection.

Complications

Intracranial bleeding (rare, but leading cause of death).

Persistent epistaxis.

Gastrointestinal bleeding (unusual).

Development of chronic ITP, *ie*, persistence of thrombocytopenia 6 months after diagnosis.

Differential diagnosis

Acute lymphoblastic leukemia.

Viral suppression.

Drug-induced thrombocytopenia.

Evans syndrome.

Immune-mediated thrombocytopenia associated with systemic lupus erythematosus, antiphospholipid syndrome, HIV infection.

Etiotology

May occur 1–3 weeks after a viral infection or, rarely, after routine childhood immunization.

• Predicting patients at risk is not possible.

Epidemiology

Two peak ages in childhood, ages 2–5 and in adolescence.

For younger age group, male to female ratio 1:1; in adolescents, females more likely to develop ITP.

Treatment

Diet and lifestyle

• Active young children with low platelet counts (<15,000/μL) should wear protective gear. The home environment should be carpeted as much as possible and gates should block stairways. Activities that may incur head trauma (diving, bike riding, football) should be discouraged when platelet counts are low to minimize the risk of intracranial bleeding. Patients should not take aspirin, aspirin-containing products, or other medications known to adversely effect platelet function.

Pharmacologic treatment

Standard dosage Prednisone, 2 mg/kg/day with taper after 7–10 d. Repeat as necessary for excessive bruising or bleeding.

Intravenous immunoglobulin (IVIg), 600–1 000 mg/kg/d. Treat once, check platelet count, and if no improvement, consider retreatment. May repeat IVIg infusion when or if thrombocytopenia recurs.

Special points Some clinicians choose to carefully follow selected patients with ITP without prescribing medication(s).

Treatment aims

To minimize bleeding while waiting for spontaneous remission to occur. IVIg and corticosteroids temporarily raise the platelet count but do not cure ITP.

Other treatments

Splenectomy: reserved for patients >5 y of age with chronic ITP and severe thrombocytopenia. Results in "cure" approximately 50% of time.
Anti-D (Rh IgG): raises the platelet count in Rh (D)–positive patients.
Other medications for resistant, symptomatic ITP: Dexamethasone is useful for treatment in patients who have not responded to other therapies.

Prognosis

The prognosis is excellent for acute ITP, with 80% of patients having normal platelet counts 6 mo after diagnosis regardless of therapy received.

Follow-up and management

Patients with resolved ITP may have recrudescence of thrombocytopenia after a viral infection.

General references

Anderson JC: Response of resistant idiopathic thrombocytopenic purpura to pulsed high dose dexamethasone therapy. N Engl J Med 1994, **330:**1560–1564.

Bussel JB, Graziano JN, Kimberly RP, et al.: Intravenous anti-D treatment of immune thrombocytopenic purpura: analysis of efficacy, toxicity and mechanism of effect. Blood 1991, **77:**1884–1893.

Imbch P, Berchtold W, Hirt A, et al.: Intravenous immunoglobulin versus oral corticosteroids in acute for immune thrombocytopenia purpura in childhood. Lancet 1985, **2:**464–468.

Medeiros D, Buchanan GR: Current controversies in the management of idiopathic thrombocytopenic purpura. Pediatr Clin North Am 1996, **43:**757–772.

Diagnosis

Symptoms

Liquid stools: >3 movements and over 200 mL per day.

Blood (dysentery): implies active mucosal inflammation.

Abdominal pain: variable and often predefecatory.

Tenesmus: suggests proctitis.

Weight loss, malnutrition, dehydration, fever, secondary lactose intolerance, anorexia, flatulence, vomiting.

Oily stools with malabsorbed food: common in giardiasis.

Signs

Pyrexia: suggests active mucosal inflammation.

Clinical evidence of dehydration or malnutrition.

Mimics appendicitis: *Yersinia.*

Anal rash, excoriation: nonspecific irritation from alkaline stool; may also be due to infection by *Enterobius vermicularis* or *Strongyloides stercoralis.*

Arthropathy: occasionally seen with gram-negative infections.

Borborygmi.

Splenomegaly, rose spots: due to *Salmonella typhi* or *S. paratyphi* infection.

Rectal prolapse: *Shigella, Enterobius.*

Investigations

Hematology: severe bandemia (730%) suggests shigellosis; peripheral blood eosinophilia suggests invasive helminthic infection.

Fecal microscopy, parasitology, culture: fresh warm specimens yield highest positivity rate for *Entamoeba histolytica, Giardia lamblia* (three samples required); *Clostridium difficile* toxin A and B and culture (fresh, frozen specimen).

Upper GI endoscopy, including duodenal biopsy: for morphology and parasitology in chronic cases when symptoms persist >2 weeks and stool studies are negative.

Small-intestinal radiography: to check for ileocecal tuberculosis (TB) in patients at risk for TB or in those without diagnosis despite extensive evaluation.

HIV serology: in patients with risk factors or otherwise negative evaluation [1].

Colonoscopy with biopsy and culture: for morphology and microbiology in severe cases when diarrhea persists >2 weeks or in patients with increased bleeding and negative culture.

Complications

Dehydration, electrolyte disturbance, shock.

Gram-negative septicemia: rare.

"Hyperinfection syndrome": due to *Strongyloides stercoralis* infection.

Ileal perforation, hemorrhage, asymptomatic carrier: due to salmonellosis.

Mesenteric adenitis or ileitis, nonsuppurative arthritis, ankylosing spondylitis, erythema nodosum, Reiter's syndrome: due to *Yersinia enterocolitica* infection.

Acute necrotizing colitis, appendicitis, ameboma, hemorrhage, stricture: due to amebic colitis.

Colonic necrosis, toxic megacolon, bloody diarrhea in newborns: due to pseudomembranous colitis.

Seizures, intestinal perforation, Reiter's syndrome, arthritis, purulent keratitis: due to shigellosis [2].

Meningitis abscesses, pancreatitis, pneumonia, Guillan–Barré syndrome: due to *Campylobacter.*

Postviral enteritis, flat villous lesion: due to rotavirus.

Pseudomembranous colitis: *Clostridium difficile.*

Differential diagnosis

Inflammatory bowel disease (usually ulcerative colitis).

Drug-induced diarrhea: laxatives, magnesium compounds, quinidine, prostaglandins.

Lactose intolerance.

Endocrine-associated diarrhea (eg, diabetes, hyperthyroidism).

Other noninfective causes of bulky, fatty stools (malabsorption): severe malnutrition, intestinal resection, chronic pancreatitis, chronic hepatocellular dysfunction, sprue, Whipple's disease.

Idiopathic diarrhea.

Bacterial overgrowth syndrome.

NSAID enterpathy.

Celiac sprue.

Chronic nonspecific diarrhea of infancy.

Etiology

Travelers' diarrhea: clinical syndrome with many causes including viruses, bacteria, and protozoa.

Food poisoning (*Staphylococcus, Salmonella, Clostridium*).

Postinfective malabsorption.

Immunosuppression: CMV, *Cryptosporidium.*

Bacteria: Aeromonas spp., Campylobacter spp., *Clostridium difficile, Escherichia coli* (including 0157:H7), *Mycobacterium tuberculosis, Plesiomonas shigelloides,* Salmonella spp., Shigella spp., Vibrio spp., *Yersinia enterocolitica.*

Viruses: adenovirus, astrovirus, Norwalk virus, rotavirus, HIV [3].

Protozoa: *Entamoeba histolytica, Giardia lamblia,* Cryptosporidium spp., *Mycobacterium avium-intracellulare.*

Helminths: *Capillaria philippinensis, Enterobius vermicularis, Fasciolopsis buski, Schistosoma mansoni, S. japonicum, Strongyloides stercoralis,* Taenia spp., *Trichuris trichiuria,* Ascaris spp.

Epidemiology

• Intestinal infection occurs worldwide.

• Fecal-oral transmission.

• Travelers' diarrhea occurs more often in people who have travelled to an area where socioeconomic standards and hygiene are compromised (including most tropical and subtropical countries), although great geographical variations are found in prevalence rates.

Treatment

Diet and lifestyle

• Food hygiene must be strictly observed: most intestinal infections result from a contaminated environment, commonly food or drink (especially drinking water).

• Avoidance of milk and dairy products is advised due to secondary lactose intolerance complicating an intestinal infection of any cause.

• Aggressive intake of fluids while avoiding alcohol and caffeine is advised.

• Good handwashing must be stressed to avoid passage of the infection to others.

Pharmacologic treatment

• Most infectious diarrheas are self-limiting and require no pharmacological management.

Indications

Travelers' diarrhea: prophylaxis with bismuth subsalicylate; hydration only for loose stools; antimicrobial drugs not recommended in children. Traveler's should drink only boiled or carbonated water or other processed beverages; avoid ice, salads, and unpeeled fruit.

Clostridium difficile infection: vancomycin, 10 mg/kg every 6 h for 10 d, or metronidazole, 5 mg/kg 3 times daily for 10 d (maximum, 500 mg/kg 3 times daily).

Entamoeba histolytica infection: metronidazole, 15 mg/kg 3 times daily for 10 d (maximum, 500 mg/kg 3 times daily).

Giardia lamblia infection: metronidazole, 5–10 mg/kg 3 times daily for 7 d (maximum, 500 mg/kg 3 times daily).

Salmonella typhi or *paratyphi* infection: usually self-limiting. Antimicrobial treatment used for infants <3 mo old, immunosuppressed patients, and patients with severe colitis. Ampicillin, chloramphenicol, TMP, amoxacillin.

Schistosoma mansoni, japonicum, mekongi, intercalatum, or *matthei* infection: praziquantel.

Strongyloides stercoralis infection: albendazole or thiabendazole.

Cholera, watery (enterotoxigenic) diarrheas: oral rehydration (i.v. in extreme cases, *eg,* infection by *Vibrio cholerae*).

Selected regimens

Amoxicillin, 500 mg 3 times daily for 14 d (in *S. typhi* infection, reduced after defervescence).

Ampicillin, i.v. 100 mg/kg/d divided in 4 doses; orally 50 mg/kg/d divided in 4 doses (maximum, 500 mg/kg 4 times daily).

Chloramphenicol, 50 mg/kg daily in 4 divided doses for 14 d (maximum 1 g 4 times daily).

Mebendazole, 100 mg initially (for ascariasis second dose may be needed).

Thiabendazole, 25 mg/kg twice daily for 3 d (longer in "hyperinfection syndrome").

Praziquantel, 40–50 mg/kg initially; for *S. japonicum* infection, 60 mg/kg in three divided doses on a single day.

See manufacturer's current prescribing information for further details.

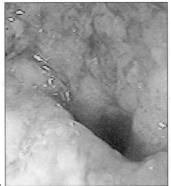

Colonoscopic view of infectious colitis.

Treatment aims

• Supportive treatment (clear fluids, Pedialyte).

To relieve diarrhea, abdominal colic, and other intestinal symptoms.

To rehydrate patient as rapidly as possible, preferably orally.

To ensure bacteriological or parasitic cure.

To return patient's nutritional status to normal, especially when clinically overt malabsorption has accompanied infection.

To prevent recurrences, especially of *Salmonella typhi* or *paratyphi* infections.

To relieve symptoms in untreatable immunosuppressed patients.

Prognosis

• In some severe infections (eg, shigellosis, *Entamoeba histolytica* colitis), specific chemotherapy results in complete recovery in almost all patients.

• If surgery is necessary for complications, the prognosis is less favorable.

Follow-up and management

• Most intestinal infections are acute; follow-up is unnecessary.

• *Salmonella typhi* or *paratyphi* infections should be followed up in order to establish that the carrier state has not ensued.

• Patients with overt malabsorption as a secondary manifestation of an intestinal infection should be followed up for maintenance therapy and ascertainment of ultimate cure.

Key references

1. Smith PD, Quinn TC, Strober W, *et al.*: Gastrointestinal infections in AIDS. *Ann Intern Med* 1992, **116**:63–77.

2. Kapala BS, Drummond KN: The hemolytic-uremic syndrome is a syndrome. *N Engl J Med* 1978, **290**:964–966.

3. Barnes GL: Viral infections. In *Pediatric Gastrointestinal Disease* Edited by Walker WA, Durie PR, Hamilton JR, *et al.*: BC Decker; Philadelphia; 1996:654–676.

4. Report of the Committee on Infectious Diseases: *The Red Book.* American Academy of Pediatrics: Chapel Hill, NC; 1991:207.

Diagnosis

Definitions

- Crohn's disease is a chronic inflammatory disease that affects the entire gastro-intestinal tract causing transmural disease and most commonly involving the terminal ileum [1].
- Ulcerative colitis is a chronic inflammatory disease of the colon.

Symptoms

Diarrhea, abdominal pain, tenesmus, weight loss: both Crohn's disease and ulcerative colitis.

Bloody diarrhea: ulcerative colitis or Crohn's.

Rectal or perianal abscess, growth failure, delayed puberty: Crohn's disease.

In ulcerative colitis

Mild attack: diarrhea up to 4 times daily or passage of small amounts of macroscopic blood *per rectum* without appreciable constitutional problems.

Moderate attack: diarrhea >4 times daily without severe bleeding or severe constitutional problems.

Severe attack: diarrhea ≥6 times daily; blood mixed with feces; and fever >37.5°C, abdominal pain, anorexia, or weight loss.

Signs

Pallor, fever, tachycardia, toxic megacolon, hypoalbuminemia: ulcerative colitis.

Extracolonic symptoms (all rare) include pyoderma gangrenosum of the skin, uveitis, erythema nodosum, episcleritis, arthritis, sclerosing cholangitis: both Crohn's and ulcerative colitis.

Aphthous ulcers in mouth, atrophic glossitis, right lower quadrant mass, perianal abscess and fistulas, arthritis, weight loss: in Crohn's disease.

Investigations

Stool studies: OVA and parasites × 3, culture, *Clostridia difficile* toxin.

Complete blood count: to check for normochromic anemia of chronic disease, microcytic anemia of iron deficiency, macrocytic anemia, (B_{12} and folate deficiency); increased platelets, and/or leukocytes may occur secondary to inflammation or infection.

ESR, CRP, ANCA measurement: inflammatory markers of disease activity.

Electrolytes, BUN, creatine: abnormal in patients with dehydration.

Serum albumin: decreased in patients with malnutrition.

Colonoscopy: allows assessment of colonic disease and usually visualization of the terminal ileum and appropriate biopsy; Crohn's is characterized by intermittent disease (*eg*, aphthous or serpiginous ulcers) separated by areas of normal mucosa. Ulcerative colitis is characterized by continuous mucosal inflammation from rectum to proximal colon (rectal sparing rarely occurs). Pseudopolyps and ulcers occur.

Upper gastrointestinal endoscopy with biopsy: if relevant symptoms; lesions must be biopsied to confirm that they are due to Crohn's disease. Histology reveals crypt abscess, granulomas, and inflammation.

Rose-thorn ulceration, string sign, skip lesions, cobblestone mucosa, stricture, fistulous tracts.

Contrast radiography: small-bowel follow-through (or enteroclysis) allows assessment of small-bowel mucosal disease; useful in assessing stricture formation and defining anatomy for surgery; barium enema may complement colonoscopy, particularly in checking for fistulas. Small bowel disease diagnostic of Crohn's disease.

Abdominal CT scan: useful when checking for extraintestinal inflammation (*eg*, abscesses).

Differential diagnosis [5]

Bacterial infections (*Salmonella, Shigella, Campylobacter spp., Escherichia coli, Yersinia, tuberculosis, Clostridium difficile*).

Viral gastroenteritis, cytomegalovirus.

Nonsteroidal anti-inflammatory drug enteropathy.

Amebic infection, *Giardia*.

Ischemia.

Colonic carcinoma (rare in children).

Lymphoma.

Hemolytic uremic syndrome (HUS).

Henoch–Schönlein purpura (HSP).

Etiology

- The cause is unknown, but the following may have a role:

Autoimmunity.

Defective mucosal barrier.

Altered neutrophil function.

Intestinal microflora.

- Crohn's disease is caused by multifocal granulomatous vasculitis.

Possible genetic influences: studies have shown familial clustering, suggesting a genetic predisposition.

Epidemiology

Crohn's disease: average age of onset, 7.5 y; incidence, 3.5:100,000 in 10–19 y of age; 25% of all patients present in childhood.

Ulcerative colitis: incidence 2–14:100,000; age of onset, 5.9 y.

Males and females equally affected.

Histology

Crohn's: cryptitis, granulomas, transmural inflammation.

Ulcerative colitis: crypt abscess formation, chronic inflammation, changes in lamina propria, eosinophils, and neutrophils.

Treatment

Diet and lifestyle

• Nutritional supplementation is needed in patients with severe illness, including total parenteral nutrition in advanced disease.

• Elemental diets by enteral feeding tube are effective for weight gain and have been shown to induce remission in children [3].

Pharmacological treatment [2–4]

Corticosteroids

Corticosteroids are the most efficacious medication in the treatment of patients with moderate to severe disease.

Standard dose	Prednisone, 1–2 mg/kg up to a daily maximum of 60 mg/kg wither tapering; 30–60 mg orally (consider i.v. administration in hospitalized patients with poor motility and absorptive function).
Contraindications	Overt sepsis; caution in hypertension and diabetes.
Special points	Steroid tapers should be instituted once the disease is in remission.
Main drug interactions	Significant immunosuppression with azathioprine: risk of opportunistic infections increased, immunization against varicella should be considered in patients without a history of chicken pox and negative antibody titer.
Main side effects	Fluid retention and hypertension, induction of glucose intolerance, osteoporosis, cushingoid features, mood lability, aseptic necrosis, hyperphagia, increased energy.

5-aminosalicylic acid preparations

Used as sole agents in patients with mild to moderate disease and as supplemental medications to regimens for patients with more severe disease [4].

Standard dosage	Sulfasalazine, 40–80 mg/kg daily in divided doses (contact pediatric gastroenterologist for details).
Contraindications	Salicylate hypersensitivity, sulfonamide sensitivity with sulfasalazine, renal impairment with mesalamine.
Special points	Sulfasalazine causes reversible oligospermia, may cause hemolysis; slow-release preparation of mesalamine of particular benefit in small-bowel Crohn's disease.
Main side effects	Nausea, rashes, occasional diarrhea, headache.

Other immunosuppressive drugs

Azathioprine is the best-studied but cyclosporine and methotrexate are also used in more refractory cases.

Special points	Risk of myelotoxicity maximal on starting treatment; whole blood count must be monitored closely, particularly in first few weeks, monthly thereafter.
Main drug interactions	Additive immunosuppressive effect with steroids.
Main side effects	Rashes, nausea, myelosuppression, increased risk of opportunistic infection, pancreatitis.

Antibiotics

Antibiotics are effective in some situations, particularly in perianal disease; they have recently been shown to have some benefit in small-bowel disease.

Standard dosage	Metronidazole, 15–30 mg/kg orally 3 times daily (maximum 500 mg 3 times daily).

Treatment aims

To suppress disease activity.

To restore quality of life.

To prevent complications.

To correct nutritional deficiencies.

Other treatments

• Conservative surgery (limited resection or stricturoplasty when possible to avoid short-bowel syndromes) is indicated for the following:

Acute: acute ileitis with signs of acute abdomen at presentation, fulminating colitis, uncontrolled or severe rectal hemorrhage (rare), intra-abdominal collections (abscesses), refractory to medical management, ruptured viscus with peritonism.

Chronic: subacute intestinal obstruction from fibrosis or scarring, fistulae, chronic debilitating disease unresponsive to medical treatment.

Prognosis

• Modern medical treatment, improved immunosuppressive regimens, and conservative surgery have greatly decreased the incidence of long-term complications.

• The risk of carcinoma is increased in Crohn's disease (lymphoma) and ulcerative colitis (adenocarcinoma).

Follow-up and management

• Close outpatient follow-up, every 6 mo.

Key references

1. Hyams JS: Crohn's disease. In *Pediatric Gastrointestinal Disease.* Edited by Wyllie R, Hyams JS. Philadelphia: WB Saunders; 1993:742–764.

2. McInerney GJ: Fulminating ulcerative colitis with marked colonic dilatation: a clinicopathologic study. *Gastroenterology* 1962, 42:2944–2957.

3. Sanderson IR, Udeen S, Davies PS, *et al.*: Remission induced by an elemental diet in small bowel Crohn's disease. *Arch Dis Child* 1987, 61:123–127.

4. Hanauer SB, Stathopoulos G: Risk benefit assessment of drugs used in the treatment of inflammatory bowel disease. *Drug Safety* 1991, 6:192–219.

Diagnosis

Symptoms

Gastrointestinal symptoms

Episodic abdominal pain: "drawing legs up."

Vomiting: may be bilious.

Diarrhea.

Currant jelly stool: late finding indicative of significant gut ischemia.

Nonspecific

Lethargy: from release of endogenous opioids secondary to intestinal ischemia.

Excessive crying, irritability.

Poor oral intake.

Signs

Vital signs: tachycardia due to pain, dehydration, hypotension.

Altered consciousness: lethargy, apathy, or unexpectedly cooperative with physical examination.

Abnormal bowel sounds: increased due to obstruction or decreased with ischemia.

Sausage-shaped mass or fullness palpated in the right middle portion of abdomen.

Digital rectal examination: gross or occult blood; may palpate tip of intussusceptum if it invaginates to the rectum.

Investigations

• Blood tests (CBC, serum electrolytes, BUN, blood type and crossmatch) are nondiagnostic; awaiting test results should not cause a delay in obtaining surgical evaluation and in alerting radiology personnel.

• Abdominal radiograph identifies intussusception in 50% of cases. Suggestive findings include small bowel obstruction (dilated loops of bowel, air fluid levels), paucity of bowel gas (especially right lower quadrant), soft tissue mass, meniscus sign (leading edge of the intussusceptum projecting into gas-filled colon), and presence of free air.

• Sonography is gaining popularity among radiologists due to the ease and accuracy in diagnosis or exclusion of intussusception. Other advantages include the ability to detect a lead point or other intra-abdominal pathology.

• Contrast enema is the gold standard for both the diagnosis and the treatment of intussusception. Contrast solutions include barium, water-based Gastrografin, saline, and air. The personal preference of the radiologist determines which modality is employed.

Complications

Delay in diagnosis or misdiagnosis.

Underlying malignancy or disease: can be missed if evaluation for lead point is not performed in older child.

Bowel ischemia and infarct requiring surgical resection.

Bowel perforation.

Recurrence.

Differential diagnosis

Incarcerated inguinal hernia.

Congenital anomalies (malrotation, duplication, atresia, Hirschsprung's).

Gastroenteritis.

Ileus.

Meckel's diverticulum.

Trauma (consider nonaccidental trauma).

Appendicitis.

Neoplasm.

Peptic ulcer disease.

Group A *Steptococcus pharyngitis*.

Diabetic ketoacidosis.

Urinary tract infection.

Lower lobe pneumonia.

Infant botulism.

Sepsis.

Etiology

• 90% of cases are idiopathic, probably secondary to lymphoid hyperplasia (Peyer's patches). Adenovirus and rotavirus have been implicated in preceding illnesses.

• Remaining 10% have an underlying cause—identifiable lead point such as in a Meckel's diverticulum, duplication, polyp, lymphoma, mesenteric adenitis. Patients with cystic fibrosis are predisposed due to abnormally viscid bowel contents, as are patients with Henoch–Schönlein Purpura in which intestinal wall hematomas serve as lead points.

Epidemiology

• Intussusception is the leading cause of acute intestinal obstruction in infants.

• 50% of cases are children aged <1 y.

• Peak incidence is between 5 and 9 months of age.

• 10% of cases are in children older than 5 years of age, underlying cause should be sought.

Treatment

Diet and lifestyle

Not applicable.

Pharmacologic treatment

• Initial therapy is supportive; establish intravascular access, volume resuscitation, and place nasogastric tube if there is evidence of obstruction.

• Most surgeons recommend that antibiotics be administered with the presumption that the reduction procedure might cause a translocation of bacteria through the ischemic intestinal wall, resulting in bacteremia. Ampicillin, gentamycin, and clindamycin, or ampicillin and cefoxitin are used commonly.

Standard dosage	Ampicillin, 25 mg/kg/dose.
	Gentamycin 2.5 mg/kg/dose.
	Clindamycin 10 mg/kg/dose.
	Cefoxitin 30 mg/kg/dose.
Contraindications	Known hypersensitivity.
Main drug interactions	*Gentamycin:* with concurrent diuretics can potentiate risk of ototoxicity and nephrotoxicity.
Main side effects	Diarrhea, rash, vomiting.

Nonpharmacologic treatment

• Contrast enema reduction is the main form of treatment for intussusception. The use of hydrostatic reduction (barium, Gastrografin, saline) or pneumatic reduction (air) depends on the expertise and experience of the radiologist responsible for the procedure. The surgeon should be in attendance while the enema is being performed in case of bowel perforation or unsuccessful reduction.

• Enema is contraindicated if free intraperitoneal air on abdominal plain film or if there is evidence of peritonitis.

• Surgical reduction.

Treatment aims

To correct dehydration.

To prevent bacteremia.

To relieve intestinal obstruction.

To relieve gut ischemia and prevent necrosis.

Prognosis

• Main determinant of outcome is the degree of intestinal ischemia. Mortality is less than 1% with early recognition, resuscitation, and prompt reduction. Success rates of hydrostatic and pneumatic reduction can be >90%. Decreased likelihood of success if 1) delay in presentation or diagnosis, 2) symptoms present >48 h, 3) patient has stooled gross blood, or 4) evidence of obstruction on abdominal plain film.

• Recurrence risk can be as high as 10% following radiological reduction; 4% following surgical reduction.

Follow-up management

• 24-hour admission following reduction to observe for recurrence, ileus.

• Evaluate for presence of a lead point in children over 2 y or with second recurrence.

General references

Daneman A, Alton DJ: Intussusception: issues and controversies related to diagnosis and reduction. *Radiol Clin North Am* 1996, **34**:743–756.

Ein SH, Stephens CA: Intussusception: 354 cases in 10 years. *J Pediatr Surg* 1971, **6**:16–27.

Marks RM, Sieber WK, et al.: Hydrostatic pressure in the treatment of ileocolic intussusception in infants and children. *J Pediatr Surg* 1966, **1**:566–570.

Pollack E.: Pediatric abdominal surgical emergencies. *Pediatr Ann* 1996, **25**:448–457.

Sargent MA, Babyn P, et al.: Plain abdominal radiography in suspected intussusception: a reassessment. *Pediatr Radiol* 1994, **24**:7–20.

Verscheldon P, Filiatrault D, et al.: Intussusception in children: reliability of US in diagnosis: a prospective study. *Pediatr Radiol* 1992, **184**:741–744.

West KW, Stephens B, et al.: Intussusception: current management in infants and children. *Surgery* 1987, **102**:704–710.

Diagnosis

• Jaundice in the newborn is common problem that the primary care physician must manage. With earlier discharges from the newborn nursery and more therapy taking place at home, many more jaundiced infants are being cared for by the non-neonatologist.

• Jaundice in the newborn continues to be a complex problem, with many elements in the differential diagnosis. The primary care physician must sort through the causes and know when to apply therapy. For the purposes of this section, only unconjugated hyperbilirubinemia will be considered. The long-term injury from jaundice comes in the complications of bilirubin encephalopathy and kernicterus.

Symptoms

• There are no specific symptoms associated with elevated bilirubin levels.

• Certain factors will influence neonatal jaundice and play a role in the development of symptoms and signs. These include race, method of nutrition (breast or bottle feeding), gestational age, and the presence of underlying disease states.

• If many symptoms are present, consider jaundice as secondary to some underlying condition (most often sepsis) of the newborn.

Signs

Yellow appearance of the skin, sclera, and mucus membranes.

Serum bilirubin levels of 5 mg/dL: indicative of jaundice.

Progression of jaundice: usually from the face to the feet proportionately to the serum levels.

Bilirubin increasing at a rate in excess of 0.5 mg/dL/h: usually indicative of an underlying nonphysiologic cause.

Pallor suggesting an anemia, plethora suggesting polycythemia, liver and spleen enlargement suggesting a congenital infection, lethargy, fever, and poor feeding suggesting sepsis or acute infection, or persistent vomiting suggesting upper gastrointestinal obstruction.

Time of the jaundice onset: jaundice that begins at the end of the first week is usually associated with breast milk and milder forms of hemolytic disease.

Investigations

• The initial investigation is the measurement of the bilirubin and determining the subelements of unconjugated and conjugated bilirubin. If the infant has elevated conjugated (direct) bilirubin, a different set of conditions and a different diagnostic evaluation must be considered.

• The following levels of hyperbilirubinemia in full-term newborns require further investigation and consideration of further action: those aged <24 hours with bilirubin level >10 mg/dL; those aged 49–72 hours with >13 mg/dL; those aged >72 hours with >17 mg/dL.

• Levels need to be adjusted for preterm infants and those with acidosis, hypoxemia, sepsis, birth asphyxia, or other conditions.

• Other investigations may include complete blood count, sepsis evaluation, mother and child's blood type, and Rh status, Coombs test.

• Other studies may be indicated based on clinical symptoms.

Complications

• The main short-term complication is the failure to consider sepsis or other infections in the differential diagnosis.

• Bilirubin encaphalopathy and kernicterus occur at high levels of bilirubin, but there is debate about exactly how high. Indications for exchange transfusion are currently set for levels above 30 mg/dL for full-term newborns on the second day of life.

Differential diagnosis

Physiologic jaundice of the newborn caused by increased bilirubin load. The following conditions are involved:

Polycythemia.

Hemolytic disease (ABO incompatibility).

Erythrocyte defects (G6PD, spherocytosis).

Infection: sepsis, urinary tract infection.

Hematoma breakdown.

Drugs.

Decreased bilirubin uptake and storage:

Hypothyroidism.

Hypopituitarism.

Acidosis.

Hypoxia.

Sepsis.

Congestive heart failure.

Congenital defects: Crigler–Najjar, Gilbert's disease.

Altered enterohepatic dirculation:

Breast milk jaundice.

Upper bowel obstruction.

Antibiotic administration.

Etiology

• In physiologic jaundice, the production of bilirubin is more rapid than what the newborn liver can conjugate.

• In nonphysiologic cases there is excessive production of bilirubin from hemolysis that may come from a variety of causes, including erythrocyte enzyme deficiency, blood group incompatibility, sepsis.

• Other mechanisms include binding-protein insufficiency in thyroid disease or breast milk jaundice or defective enterohepatic circulation, as in upper bowel obstruction.

Epidemiology

• Almost all newborns have some degree of physiologic jaundice and more than 50% become clinically jaundiced.

• Levels of bilirubin usually return to normal by 2 wk in full-term babies and slightly longer in premature babies.

Treatment

General treament

• The first step in therapy is to make sure the newborn is adequately hydrated and the bilirubin levels are not erroneously elevated by dehydration. This is especially true for newborns who are being breast-fed, in whom early jaundice may be "lack of breast milk jaundice" as differentiated from breast milk jaundice (discussed later). Nursing mothers should be encouraged to nurse more frequently to achieve good flow. Water and glucose water supplementation should not be used.

• There are no pharmacologic therapies for neonatal jaundice.

Nonpharmacologic treatment

For most cases of jaundice

• The primary treatment options are phototherapy and exchange transfusion.

Phototherapy: may be done in the hospital or at home. If this type of treatment is being offered there should be an evaluation as to the cause of the jaundice after a full examination of the newborn. Phototherapy should be considered in the following infant groups: those aged <24 hours with bilirubin level >10 mg/dL; those aged 49–72 hours with >13 mg/dL; those aged >72 hours with >17 mg/dL.

Exchange transfusion therapy: should be considered if total serum bilirubin levels reach levels of 20 mg/dL on the first day or 25 mg/dL on days 2 or 3, or if phototherapy fails to lower the serum bilirubin.

For breast milk jaundice

• For nursing babies whose jaundice increases at the end of the first week or is prolonged beyond the usual 2-week period, the cause may be breast milk jaundice. The treatment options are several: observe, continue nursing and initiate phototherapy, supplement breast feeding with or without phototherapy, or interrupt nursing temporarily. The last option may be the most advantageous. Nursing needs to be stopped for 12 hours and formula substituted. Bilirubin levels will fall sharply making this both a diagnostic and therapeutic strategy.

Treatment aims

To understand the cause of the jaundice.
To rule out acute infections such as sepsis.
To follow bilirubin levels as sequentially.
To initiate phototherapy when appropriate levels are reached.
To initiate exchange transfusion when appropriate levels are reached.
To support the family.
• Premature babies need close watching and modification of standards.

Prognosis

• The prognosis should be excellent if high levels of bilirubin are avoided.

Follow-up and management

• Once jaundice is resolved, no follow-up is needed. Although levels of bilirubin are rising, close and careful follow-up is needed. Once one abnormal bilirubin level is recorded, a second will need to be ordered to estimate the rate of rise or fall.

General references

Dodd KL: Neonatal jaundice: a lighted touch. *Arch Dis Child* 1993, **68:**529–533.

Gartner L: Neonatal jaundice. *Pediatr Rev* 1994, **15:**422–431.

Spivak W: Hyperbilirubinemia. In *Difficult Diagnosis in Pediatrics.* Edited by Stockman JA. Philadelphia: W.B. Saunders; 1990.

Newman TB, Maisels MJ: Evaluation and treatment of jaundice in the term infant: a kinder and gentler approach. *Pediatrics* 1992, **89:**809–818.

Diagnosis

Definition [1]

• Inflammatory condition comprised of a constellation of symptoms with serious cardiac involvement of myocardium and/or coronary arteries in 30%–50% of untreated patients.

Symptoms and signs [2]

Fever: of at least 5 days duration.

Presence of at least four of the following features:

Changes in the extremities: swelling of hands and feet and redness of palms and soles (desquamation occurs by 2–4 weeks).

Polymorphous exanthem.

Bilateral conjunctival injection.

Changes in lips and oral cavity: strawberry tongue, redness and fissuring of lips.

Cervical lymphadenopathy.

• Exclude other diseases with similar findings.

• In addition, patients are extremely irritable, may have severe joint pains and refuse to walk.

• **Tachycardia** is present from fever and is more pronounced in the presence of myocarditis.

• Associated clinical presentations include myocarditis, pericarditis, aseptic meningitis, diarrhea, gallbladder hydrops, obstructive jaundice, uveitis, urethritis.

Investigations

ECG: may show PR prolongation, QTc prolongation, low-voltage QRS, or ST-T wave abnormalities as signs of myocarditis; arrhythmias, including atrial and ventricular ectopy may be seen. Deep Q waves and marked ST segment elevation or depression along with abnormal R wave progression may indicate myocardial infarction.

Echocardiogram (ECHO): to determine whether coronary artery dilation or aneurysms have developed. To look for myocarditis evidenced by enlarged left ventricle or left atrium and/or decreased shortening fraction. Pericardial effusion may be present.

Blood laboratory studies: elevated erythrocyte sedimentation rate (ESR) and other acute phase reactants, C-reactive protein, $\alpha\text{-}_1$ antitrypsin; platelet count elevation >500,000 occurs after first week of illness. Sterile pyuria and proteinuria.

Exercise stress tests: to identify patients with myocardial ischemia, decreased myocardial performance associated with coronary lesions or myocardial dysfunction. Arrhythmias, especially ventricular may be noted.

Myocardial perfusion studies (^{201}Tl or ^{99m}Tc): may be combined with exercise to identify areas of regional myocardial ischemia.

Cardiac catheterization and angiography: recommended in children with large or multiple coronary aneurysms and evidence of myocardial ischemia or to follow possible stenosis or occlusion in patients with large or multiple aneurysms. Coronary angiography should be done after the acute phase has resolved and may be not be necessary unless the aneurysms fail to resolve within the expected 18–24 months.

Differential diagnosis

Viral or rickettsial exanthems (measles, Epstein–Barr viral infection, Rocky Mountain spotted fever), scarlet fever, toxic shock syndrome, juvenile rheumatoid arthritis, Stevens-Johnson syndrome, drug hypersensitivity reaction.

Etiology

Associated with immune response to toxin produced by virus or bacteria, possibly *Staphylococcus*.

Epidemiology

Attack rate in the US is 9.2:p100,000 children. Attack rate in Asian children is six times higher and black children is 1.5 times higher than in white children. Male:female ratio is 1.5:1. Occurs most frequently in winter and spring; 80% of cases occur in those under 5 y of age; 2% incidence of sudden death.

Complications

Coronary artery aneurysms [3]: occur most frequently in the left main coronary artery and proximal left anterior descending artery. Giant aneurysms (>8 mm) present a higher risk for infarction; 50% of all aneurysms regress within 2 y.

Axillary, iliofemoral, renal or other arterial aneurysms may occur.

Myocardial infarction (MI): may occur early due to thrombosis in aneurysm or later secondary to progressive stenosis. Mortality with first MI is 22%. Presentation is with shock, chest pain, vomiting, or abdominal pain.

Ventricular tachycardia/fibrillation.

Aneurysm rupture: most likely to occur in first 6–8 wk.

Pericarditis: occurs in 30% by ECHO.

Treatment

Diet and lifestyle

Limited activity or bed rest if myocarditis is present. Limited activity in the presence of coronary artery aneurysms in the first several weeks.

A heart-healthy lifestyle should be followed, with a low-fat diet, appropriate exercise levels, and no smoking (primary and secondary smoke should be avoided).

Pharmacologic treatment

Standard dosage   Aspirin, high dose (80–100 mg/kg) for first 3–10 d until signs of acute inflammation have subsided; reduce to low dose (2–5 mg/kg) once fever resolved for a few days to prevent platelet aggregation and thrombosis in coronary aneurysms; continue low-dose aspirin until ESR and platelet count normal (may take 8 weeks). Continue low-dose aspirin indefinitely, if aneurysms were ever present, or if they continue to be present.

Intravenous gamma globulin, 2 g/kg as a single dose over 12 h.

Coumadin, 0.05–0.34 mg/kg/d is recommended for anticoagulation in the presence of giant aneurysms.

Contraindications   *Intravenous gamma globulin*: patients with known hypersensitivity to immune globulin.

Special points   *Aspirin*: should be discontinued during an episode of influenza or chicken pox to prevent Reye's syndrome; the antiplatelet effect will be present for several weeks, but dipyridamole (2–3 mg/kg) may be substituted for anticoagulation.

Intravenous gamma-globulin: results in lower incidence of coronary artery aneurysms and more rapid resolution of symptomatology [4]; immunization with a live virus such as the MMR (measles, mumps, rubella) immunization should be delayed for 6 mo after receiving gamma globulin.

Coumadin: international normalized ratio (INR) in range of 2–3 is appropriate.

Main side effects   *Intravenous gamma-globulin*: hypersensitivity reaction, chills, fever.

Treatment aims

To induce resolution of symptoms.

To prevent development of myocardial and coronary involvement.

Other treatment options

Thrombotic therapy for MI with associated thrombosis.

Coronary artery bypass graft surgery.

Prognosis

Resolution of coronary aneurysms in 50%. Acute course responds well to gammaglobulin. Prognosis is unknown for those with giant or multiple persistent aneurysms.

Follow-up and management

For those with aneurysms, follow up every 6–12 mo with ECG and ECHO are indicated. Periodic exercise stress test, radionuclide testing and Holter monitoring are helpful. Coronary angiography may be indicated for positive tests or clinical symptoms suggestive of ischemia. For those with no prior aneurysms, periodic (3–5 y) follow-up is recommended through adolescence, with exercise stress testing prior to involvement in vigorous competitive sports.

Key references

1. Kawasaki T, Kosaki F, Okawa S, et al.: A new infantile acute febrile mucocutaneous lymph node syndrome (MLNS) prevailing in Japan. *Pediatrics* 1974, **54**:271–276.

2. Takahashi M: Kawasaki syndrome (mucocutaneous lymph node syndrome): Committee on Rheumatic Fever, Endocarditis, and Kawasaki Disease, Council on Cardiovascular Disease in the Young, American Heart Association. Diagnosis and therapy of Kawasaki disease in children. *Circulation* 1993, **87**:1776–1780.

3. Kato H, Ichinose E, Yoshioka F, et al.: Fate of coronary aneurysms in Kawasaki disease: serial coronary angiographic and long term follow-up study. *Am J Cardiol* 1982, **49**:1758–1766.

4. Newberger JW, Takahashi M, Burns JC, et al.: The treatment of Kawasaki syndrome with intravenous gammaglobulin. *N Engl J Med* 1986, **315**:341–347.

Diagnosis

Definitions
Lactose intolerance: inability to digest the disaccharidase lactose due to deficiency or interruption of the intestinal enzyme lactase.

Congenital lactase deficiency: rare, presents in newborns during first feeding with lactose.

Primary lactose intolerance: inherited disorder; late onset; symptoms almost always begin after 5 years of age but occur earlier in people of African descent.

Secondary lactose intolerance: acquired enzyme deficiency secondary to a disease process causing damage to the intestinal brush border with subsequent loss of function.

Symptoms [1]
Excessive flatus, abdominal distention, bloating: common; in varying degrees.

Recurrent abdominal pain: common; lower quadrants or periumbilical; crampy, occurring within 3 hours of lactose ingestion.

Diarrhea: watery, bulky, relieves cramps.

Weight loss, dehydration, vomiting: rare.

Signs
Borborygmi: loud, rumbling sounds secondary to intestinal gas.

Abdominal distention: tense, gaseous, tympanitic abdomen.

• Physical examination often not helpful.

Investigations
Dietary history: a detailed dietary history accompanied by abdominal symptoms may be helpful. This can be difficult to perform as many modern foods contain small amounts of lactose. The association between diet and symptoms is also hard to assess in children.

Lactose breath test: 2- to 3-hour test that involves collection of breath samples (every 30 minutes) after ingesting a lactose load. The breath is analyzed for hydrogen content. Normal individuals do produce a rise in hydrogen production, whereas those with lactose intolerance manifest a rise in breath hydrogen (>20 ppm). *Limitations:* some patients may have colonic non–hydrogen-producing bacteria. In these patients, the lactose breath test will be falsely normal; however, the patient will experience symptoms secondary to the breakdown of lactose into short-chain fatty acids. To perform test, patients must be off all antibiotics for 2 weeks and be NPO for 12 hours, off all lactose-containing foods for 24 hours and NPO 6 hours prior to the test [2].

Stool-reducing substances: an abnormal test indicates carbohydrate malabsorption; this test is not specific for lactose intolerance.

Fecal pH: low fecal pH (<6.0) indicates carbohydrate malabsorption but is not specific for lactose intolerance; fresh stool specimens must be collected and assayed immediately.

Measurement of intestinal lactase: lactase activity from intestinal biopsy specimens (third portion of duodenum to jejunum) obtained by upper endoscopy can be directly assayed; multiple biopsy specimens should be taken because patchy lactase activity may be present in secondary lactose intolerance[3].

Differential diagnosis
Children younger than 5 y of age with documented lactose intolerance should always be considered to have secondary lactose intolerance.

Infections: Bacterial and viral infections (causing mucosal damage and villous atrophy); parasites (*Giardia*) adhere to duodenal mucosa, disrupting lactase function.

Inflammatory: inflammatory bowel disease (Crohn's disease, ulcerative colitis), celiac disease, eosinophilic enteritis, immunodeficiency syndromes.

Pancreatic disorders: cystic fibrosis, Shwachman syndrome; can mimic lactose intolerance.

Congenital enzyme deficiencies: sucrase-isomaltase and glucose-galactose deficiency.

Epidemiology
Primary lactose intolerance develops in up to 80% of Africans and African-Americans, Eastern Asians, Native Americans, Jews, and Mediterranean whites.

Pathophysiology
Lactose passes into the colon and is fermented by intestinal flora producing hydrogen, carbon dioxide, and methane gas; short-chain fatty acids are produced, causing an osmotic diarrhea, low pH, and increased colonic peristalsis.

Treatment

Diet and lifestyle

• Symptoms can be prevented by the avoidance of all lactose-containing foods.

• Patients must be taught to read food labels to identify "unusual" nondairy sources of lactose.

• These include baked goods, candy, foods prepared with toppings, cereal, and luncheon meats.

Congenital lactose intolerance: avoidance of lactose.

Primary lactose intolerance: lactose-free diet or enzyme supplementation for remainder of life.

Secondary lactose intolerance: avoidance of lactose or lactase supplementation until resolution of primary intestinal disease.

Pharmacologic treatment

Lactaid milk: commercially available low-lactose milk (~70% reduced).

Lactase enzyme supplements: oral lactase supplements reduce symptoms and hydrogen production when taken with foods containing lactose; these substitutes are bacterial or yeast β-galactosidases and should be taken immediately before ingesting lactose; the effective dose ranges from one to four tablets per meal and depends on the degree of the individual's lactase deficiency and the amount of lactose ingested; liquid Lactaid enzyme can be added to 1 qt of milk 24 h before ingestion (five drops will reduce lactose by 70%; 10 drops will digest lactose completely).

Calcium supplementation: lactose-containing foods (milk, cheese, formula) comprise the major source of calories for children; calcium supplements should be administered if the dietary intake does not meet the recommended daily allowance for calcium (800 mg/d in children <10 y; 1200 mg/day in children >10 y) [4].

Treatment aims
To prevent further episodes of lactose intolerance.

Prognosis
• Symptoms can be prevented with avoidance of lactose-containing foods or with enzyme supplementation.

Follow-up and management
• No follow-up is necessary for primary lactose intolerance.
• Children with secondary lactose intolerance require follow-up for their underlying disease process.

Key references

1. Buller HA, *et al.*: Clinical aspects of lactose intolerance in children and adults. *Scand J Gastroenterol* 1991, **26 (suppl):**73–80.

2. Maffei HV, Metz G, Bampoe V, *et al.*: Lactose intolerance detected by the hydrogen breath test in infants and children with children with chronic diarrhea. *Arch Dis Child* 1977, **52:**766–771.

3. Montgomery RK, Jonas MM, Grand RJ: Carbohydrate intolerance in infancy. In *Intestinal Disaccharidases: Structure, Function and Deficiency.* Edited by Lifshitz R. New York: Marcel Dekker; 1982:75–94.

4. Stallings VA, Oddleifson NW, Negrini GY, *et al.*: Bone mineral content and dietary calcium intake in children prescribed a low-lactose diet. *J Pediatr Gastroenterol Nutr* 1994, **18:**440–445.

Diagnosis

Symptoms

• A constellation of symptoms is seen, many nonspecific and related to bone marrow failure.

Easy bruising, bone pain, fevers, pallor, lethargy, anorexia, malaise: due to bone marrow failure.

Abdominal distention: due to hepatosplenomegaly.

Shortness of breath, facial swelling: due to mediastinal mass (unusual).

Headache, vomiting: due to central nervous system (CNS) disease (unusual).

Signs

Fever, mucosal bleeding, purpura, pallor, congestive heart failure (rare): due to bone marrow failure.

Hepatosplenomegaly, lymphadenopathy, upper trunk and facial edema with distended superficial veins, skin infiltrates, testicular enlargement: due to leukemic "mass."

Cranial nerve palsies, papilledema, retinal hemorrhages, leukemic infiltrates: due to CNS disease (rare).

Investigations

Full blood count: shows pancytopenia, or isolated raised leukocyte count. (In 50% of patients, leukocyte count is >10,000/μL at diagnosis).

Peripheral blood smear: likely to show leukemic blasts.

Bone marrow morphology: confirms diagnosis in conjunction with cytochemistry and immunophenotyping (mature B cell varieties treated on lymphoma-type protocols).

Chest radiography: for mediastinal mass.

Lumbar puncture: for CNS disease.

Blood urea nitrogen, creatinine, electrolytes, calcium, phosphorous, and uric acid: to look for evidence of tumor lysis.

Complications

Early (in therapy)

• Early complications are usually related to drug side effects or further bone marrow suppression.

Tumor lysis syndrome, associated with hyperkalemia, hyperuricemia, hyperphosphatemia, renal dysfunction.

Infection of all types.

Bleeding.

Anemia.

Vomiting, hair loss, peripheral neuropathy and myopathy, mucositis.

Late (during or after therapy)

Learning difficulties: *eg*, problems with short-term memory or concentration due to cranial irradiation.

Cardiotoxicity: due to anthracycline treatment.

Cataracts, sterility, growth and hormone problems: due to cyclophosphamide treatment and total body irradiation bone marrow transplantation (BMT).

Secondary malignancies: due to epipodophyllotoxins, hair loss, peripheral neuropathy and myopathy, mucositis.

Differential diagnosis

Lymphadenopathy

Infections: eg, infectious mononucleosis.

Lymphomas or other tumors.

Hepatosplenomegaly

Macrophage, metabolic, hematologic, or infectious disorders.

Lymphomas.

Bone marrow failure

Aplastic anemia.

Myelodysplasia.

Hemophagocytic syndromes.

Autoimmune disorders.

Tumor metastatic to the bone marrow: eg, neuroblastoma.

Infections: eg, parvovirus, mononucleosis, tuberculosis, HIV, CMV.

Etiology [1]

• The cause is unknown.

• Increased risk for developing leukemia is associated with the following:

Down syndrome.

Faconi's anemia.

Bloom syndrome.

Ataxia telangiectasia and various immunodeficiency disorders.

Epidemiology [1]

• Acute lymphoblastic leukemia is the most common malignant disease of childhood and accounts for approximately 80% of childhood leukemias.

• Peak incidence is at 4 years of age.

• Slightly more boys than girls are affected.

Treatment

Diet and lifestyle

• Specialist support is needed for children and their families, including siblings, both in hospital during treatment and after discharge.

• Maintenance of nutrition is important.

Pharmacologic treatment [2]

• Treatment should be given under specialist supervision, in the context of a clinical trial if possible to allow evaluation of current treatment and the development of new therapies.

Treatment choice

• Treatment choice is stratified by risk group:

For standard risk group (age >1 and <10 with leukocyte count <50,000/μL): three-drug induction, one or two delayed intensification phases (see Principles of Treatment); total therapy approximately 2 y for girls and 3 y for boys.

For high-risk group (age ≥10 or leukocyte count ≥50,000 mm³): similar to standard treatment, with four-drug induction (daunorubicin is added; see Principles of Treatment); slow responders on day 7 receive augmented therapy and prophylactic cranial irradiation.

• Infants are treated with more intensive therapy.

• Transplantation in first remission for Philadelphia chromosome–positive and translocation (4;11).

• If bone marrow relapse occurs, HLA-identical sibling BMT is treatment of choice.

• CNS relapse curable without BMT if patient has not received prior CNS radiation therapy.

Principles of treatment

Induction: usually vincristine, asparaginase, steroids; remission in 97% of patients.

Consolidation: intensive treatment aimed at CNS.

Delayed intensification: recapitulation of induction and consolidation to eradicate residual leukemia.

Complications of specific drugs

Vincristine: extravasation injury, muscle and jaw pain, constipation, dysphagia, peripheral neuropathy.

Prednisone: Cushing syndrome and other steroidal side effects (including psychiatric).

L-Asparaginase: thrombotic episodes, pancreatitis, anaphylaxis.

Daunorubicin: extravasation injury, cardiomyopathy, bone marrow suppression, vomiting, gut toxicity.

Cytarabine: gut and bone marrow toxicity, rashes, cerebellar and pulmonary toxicity in high doses.

Thioguanine: hepatic and bone marrow toxicity.

VP16: allergic reactions and bone marrow toxicity.

Methotrexate: renal and hepatic dysfunction, bone marrow suppression, mucositis (depending on dose and mode of treatment); can affect intellect.

Mercaptopurine: bone marrow suppression, rashes, hepatic dysfunction.

Treatment aims

To cure patient at least risk (acute toxicity of specific drugs and late complications).

Other treatments

Transplantation.
Cranial irradiation.
See Pharmacologic treatment for indications.

Prognosis

• Adverse prognostic features include failure to achieve remission after 1 mo of treatment, Philadelphia chromosome–positive, near-haploid karyotype, age >10, male gender, high leukocyte count, infants <6 mo of age.

Follow-up and management

• Patients on treatment should be followed up every 1–4 wk, depending on the phase of treatment.

• After completion of treatment, all patients should be followed indefinitely; for the first 5 y, they must be checked carefully for signs of relapse (organomegaly, testicular swelling, low blood count, blasts on peripheral blood smear).

• Prophylactic cotrimoxazole should be given to prevent Pneumocystis carinii pneumonia while on chemotherapy.

• Childhood immunization can be restarted 6 mo to 1 y after completion of therapy.

Key references

1. Graves M: A natural history for pediatric acute leukemia. Blood 1993, **82:**1043–1051.
2. Pui C-H: Childhood leukemias. N Engl J Med 1995, **32:**1618–1630.

Diagnosis

Symptoms

Lethargy, irritability, fatigue, reduced exercise tolerance: symptoms of anemia.

Infection: due to neutropenia.

Spontaneous bleeding or bruising: due to thrombocytopenia.

Signs

Pallor, infections, bruising, petechiae.

Gum hypertrophy, skin infiltration: features of monocytic leukemia.

Hemorrhagic manifestations: feature of promyelocytic leukemia.

Lymphadenopathy or hepatosplenomegaly: occasionally.

Investigations

Full blood count: often shows reduced hemoglobin; thrombocytopenia frequent; leukocyte differential usually abnormal, with neutropenia and presence of "blast cells" (large cells, approximately 2–4 times diameter of erythrocytes); usually have significant amount of cytoplasm; nucleus of blast may contain at multiple nucleoli; Auer rods are pathognomonic.

Coagulation studies: prothrombin and partial thromboplastin time, fibrinogen, fibrin split products; all are intended to detect disseminated intravascular coagulation, especially in M3 and, less commonly, M5 FAB (French-American-British) subtypes.

Bone marrow analysis: increased proportion of blast cells; conventionally, >30% of bone marrow cellularity to distinguish from myelodysplasia.

Lumbar puncture: to detect blasts in cerebrospinal fluid (CSF), indicative of CNS disease.

Cytochemistry: useful to confirm myeloid or monocytic origin of blast cells: Sudan black, myeloperoxidase stains, or chloroacetate esterase can be positive.

Immunophenotying: expression of CD13, CD14, or CD33 indicates some myeloid maturation. Aberrant phenotypes have been identified that may be useful for monitoring remission status.

Cytogenetics: many structural chromosome abnormalities have been described; relationship between prognosis and cytogenic abnormality, *eg*, better prognosis with FAB M3 (15;17 translocation), some M2s (8;21 translocation), and inverted 16; worse prognosis with abnormalities or deletions of chromosomes 5 and 7.

Molecular genetics: molecular probes for the 15:17 and 8:21 translocations (among others) now available; polymerase chain reaction detection of minor cell populations therefore possible; such technology will be important in assessing quality of remission.

Complications

Early

Overwhelming infection.

Bleeding: especially intracranial in promyelocytic leukemia.

Hyperleukocytosis: with leukocyte count >200,000/μL, possibility of leukostasis and stroke.

Vomiting, hair loss, mucositis.

Late

Cardiotoxicity: due to anthracycline treatment.

Secondary malignancies: due to epipophyllotoxins.

Differential diagnosis

Aplastic anemia.

Acute lymphoblastic leukemia.

Etiology

• The risk is increased in the following:
Radiation exposure.
Chemotherapy for cancer, especially Hodgkin's disease.

Epidemiology

• Acute myeloid leukemia accounts for approximately 15% of acute leukemia in childhood.
• The frequency remains stable from birth to age 10 and then increases slightly in the teen years.
• The male to female ratio is equal.

Classification

• Based on morphological appearance, acute myeloid leukemia is divided into FAB types M0-7.
• The M3 type (promyelocytic) has a high of chance of remission and a lower risk of relapse.
• Although valuable in standardizing terminology, this classification has limited prognostic power except in the case of the M3 subtype.

Treatment

Diet and lifestyle

• Nutrition must be maintained, mucositis may lead to need for hyperalimentation, but this carries a higher risk of infections.

• Psychological support should be provided to patients and their families, especially siblings.

Pharmacologic treatment [1–3]

• Treatment should be given under specialist supervision in the context of a clinical trial if possible to allow evaluation and development of new treatments and supportive care.

• Drugs include anthracyclines, cytosine arabinoside, thioguanine, and etoposide; side effects include cardiotoxicity.

• Treatment for acute promyelocytic leukemia (APML) includes all-trans retinoic acid.

• Intensive supportive care is needed during remission induction; temperature >39.5°C or 38.0° three times in 24 h should be treated with broad-spectrum antibiotics, which should continue until bone marrow recovery. Amphotericin should be added empirically if fevers continue.

• Coagulation factor deficiency should be corrected by appropriate blood products or vitamin K supplements. Anticoagulation (*eg*, heparin) is not widely used for disseminated intravascular coagulation.

Complications of specific drugs

Idarubicin: extravasation injury, cardiomyopathy, bone marrow suppression, gut toxicity.

Cytarabine: gut and bone marrow toxicity, rashes, cerebellar and pulmonary toxicity in high doses.

Etoposide: allergic reactions and bone marrow toxicity.

Thioguanine: hepatic and bone marrow toxicity.

Treatment aims

To establish prolonged remission or cure.

Other treatments

Allogeneic bone marrow transplantation [1].
The risk of relapse is reduced.
Treatment-related mortality is now approximately 10% due to toxicity, infection, pneumonitis, and graft-versus-host disease.
Treatment is likely to result in infertility.
Allogeneic transplantation is available to only 10%–20% of patients.
Autologous transplantation is no longer standard therapy.

Prognosis [2,3]

• Current schedules achieve remission in 80% of patients.
• Survival is approximately 30%.
• Allogeneic bone marrow transplantation cures approximately 70% of all recipients.
• Most relapses occur while on therapy or in the first 2 years after completion of therapy.

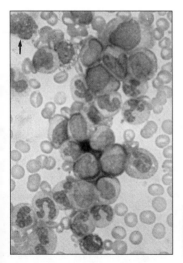

Bone marrow aspirate demonstrating acute myeloid leukemia (FAB subtype M3). *Arrows* indicate Auer rods.

Key references

1. Michel G, Socie G, Gebhard, *et al.*: Late effects of all allogeneic bone marrow transplantation for children with acute myeloblastic leukemia in first complete remission: the impact of conditioning regimen without total-body irradiation. A report from the Societé Francaise de Greffe de Moelle. *J Clin Oncol* 1997, **15:**2238–2246.

2. Tallman MS, Andersen JW, Schiffer CA, *et al.*: All-trans retinoic acid in acute promyelocytic leukemia. *N Engl J Med* 1997, **337:**1021–1028.

3. Woods WG, Kobrinsky N, Buckley JD, *et al.*: Timed-sequential induction therapy improves postremission in acute myeloid leukemia: a report from the Children's Cancer Group. *Blood* 1997, **87:**4979–4989.

Diagnosis

Symptoms

Adult (Philadelphia chromosome–positive) chronic myelogenous leukemia (CML): insidious and nonspecific complaints of fatigue, fever.

Juvenile myelomonocytic leukemia (JMML): ill-appearing child with rash or bleeding, respiratory complaints may be prominent.

• CML is largely an adult disease.

Signs

Adult CML: splenomegaly common; signs due to leukostasis such as papilledema or neurologic abnormalities, priapism, or tachypnea less common.

JMML: hepatosplenomegaly: cutaneous lesions (eczema, xanthomas, café-au-lait spots, other), lymphadenopathy, also tachypnea, cough, wheezing.

Investigations

Complete blood count:

In CML: marked leukocytosis with a "left shift," thrombocytosis, and a mild normochromic, normocytic anemia, also an increase in the number of basophils and eosinophils. Median leukocyte count at diagnosis is 250,000/mm^3.

In JMML: leukocytosis (but usually < 50,000/mm^3) with a relatively higher proportion of monocytes, anemia, thrombocytopenia; elevated hemoglobin F.

Leukocyte alkaline phosphatase: reduced in CML.

Bone marrow aspirate:

CML: hypercellular due to granulocytic hyperplasia. In the chronic phase, blasts are < 5% and in blast crisis they are > 30%. Accelerated phase has intermediate features.

JMML: immature cells of the monocytic series are prominent. Erythroid hyperplasia and a paucity of megakaryocytes can be seen. Hallmark is excessive production of granulocyte/macrophage colonies in the absence of exogenous growth factors.

Chromosomal analysis of bone marrow: reveals t(9;22) in CML; in JMML, most karyotypes are normal.

Complications

• Leukostasis: exchange transfusion rarely necessary as leukocyte count in CML often responds promptly to treatment with hydroxyurea.

Differential diagnosis

Leukemoid reaction.

Mononucleosis.

Acute leukemia: CML can be accompanied by either a myeloid or lymphoid crisis.

Etiology

• The cause is unknown.

Epidemiology

• Together, CML and JMML account for < 5% of all cases of pediatric leukemia.

• CML is more likely to occur in late childhood, whereas most patients with JMML are diagnosed before the age of 2.

• Neurofibromatosis type 1 is associated with JMML in 5%–10% of cases.

Treatment

Diet and lifestyle

• Specialist support is needed for children and their families (including siblings), both in the hospital during treatment and after discharge.

• Maintenance of nutrition is important.

General treatment

CML: hydroxyurea and alpha-interferon can help normalize blood counts but are not curative.

CML and JMML: are treated with allogenic bone marrow transplantation.

BMT and CML: is best done < year from diagnosis.

• CML in lymphoid blast crisis may respond to *all* therapy. CML is myeloid blast crisis may respond to AML therapy.

• Most investigators believe patients with JMML benefit from reduction of their tumor burden with chemotherapy prior to BMT because they are at high risk for relapse.

• Pre-BMT splenectomy is controversial.

Complications of specific drugs

Hydroxyurea: myelosuppression, nausea, elevations of liver function tests.

alpha-Interferon: flu-like symptoms, rashes.

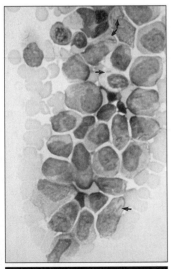

Chronic myelogenous leukemia.

Treatment aims

To establish prolonged remission or cure.

Prognosis

• Recent pediatric cure rates for CML after HLA-identical sibling transplants are 75% if done in chronic phase, 45% if done in accelerated phase, and 15% if done in blast crisis. However, HLA-identical sibling donors are available for a minority of patients. Unrelated donors are now more widely employed.

• Only a small series of patients transplanted for JMML have been published. Cure rates are estimated at 40%.

Follow-up and management

• Post-transplant patients should receive co-trimoxazole for pneumocystis prophylaxis for approx 1 y.

• Patients should be monitored for late effects of BMT, such as cataracts, growth failure, and hypothyroidism after total body irradiation (TBI) as well as primary ovarian failure following non-TBI regimens. Chronic graft-versus-host disease (GVHD) and second malignancies should be anticipated.

• Post-transplant patients with chronic GVHD are at risk for death from overwhelming infection, and all febrile episodes should be evaluated.

• Patients must be reimmunized for childhood illnesses, starting approx 1 y post-BMT if without GVHD.

General references

Gamis AS, Haake R, McGlare P, et al.: Unrelated donor bone marrow transplantation for Philadelphia chromosome-positive chronic myelogenous leukemia in children. *J Clin Oncol* 1993, 11:834–838.

Bunin NJ, Casper JT, Lawton C, et al.: Allogeneic marrow transplantation using T cell depletion for patients with juvenile chronic myelogenous leukemia without HLA-identical siblings. *Bone Marrow Transplant* 1992, 9:119–122.

Arico M, Biondi A, Pui C-H, et al.: Juvenile myelomonocytic leukemia. *Blood* 1997, 90:479–488.

Diagnosis

Definition

Inherited condition associated with prolonged corrected QT interval on the electrocardiogram, stress-related syncope, malignant ventricular arrhythmias, sudden death and/or family history of sudden death [1]. Also known as Romano–Ward syndrome or Jervell and Lange–Nielson syndrome.

Symptoms

• Symptoms are not always manifest.

Palpitations: episodes of rapid heartbeats, usually > 150 bpm, or of irregular or strong heartbeats.

Syncope or dizziness: sudden loss of consciousness (syncope) or near syncope (light-headedness or dizziness), associated with physical activity, emotional stress, anxiety, fear, or loud noises (doorbell, telephone, or alarm clock).

Cardiac arrest or sudden death: usually associated with torsades de pointes form of ventricular tachycardia (VT), which degenerates into ventricular fibrillation (*see* figure). Often there is a family history of sudden or accidental death (car accident, drowning) in young people.

Signs

• Signs are not always manifest.

Tachycardia: rapid (150–300 bpm), thready, often irregular pulse.

Hypotension: associated signs of pallor, clamminess, and diaphoresis.

Seizure: secondary to low cardiac output and poor cerebral perfusion from cardiac arrhythmia. Postictal state may occur if cerebral hypoxia was prolonged.

Hearing loss: congenital sensorineural hearing loss (severe) noted in Jervell and Lange–Nielson form of long QT syndrome.

Investigations [2]

12-Lead electrocardiograms (ECG): to calculate corrected QT interval using Bazett's formula: QTc = QT/(R-R interval; > 0.45 indicates abnormality. In some instances, resting 12-lead ECG may not show prolonged QTc. QT must be measured in regular rhythm, not sinus arrhythmia, and should be calculated because computerized ECG measurements may be incorrect. Analysis of T waves reveals flat T waves or broad, prolonged, notched bizarre-appearing T waves (*see* figure). T waves may be inappropriately inverted, especially in inferior and lateral leads, or may show T-wave alternans. ECG may show premature ventricular contractions or VT, especially polymorphic VT or torsades de pointes VT. Sinus bradycardia is common.

24-Hour ambulatory ECG monitoring: to determine presence or frequency of ventricular arrhythmias, including premature ventricular depolarizations, R-on-T premature ventricular contractions, ventricular couplets, sustained or nonsustained ventricular tachycardia, especially of the torsades de pointes or polymorphic variety. Other suggestive arrhythmias include marked sinus arrhythmia or sinus bradycardia and second- or third-degree AV block. T-wave abnormalities, T-wave inversion or alternans, and QT prolongation should be noted. QTc in the 0.45–0.49 range may be seen in normal patients on 24-hour ECGs.

Exercise stress test (EST): Under supervision of an arrhythmia specialist, as exercise may provoke serious ventricular arrhythmias including torsades de pointes type of VT or cardiac arrest. The EST is used to evaluate QTc at rest, during exercise, and exercise recovery. Often, the most prolonged QTc will occur at 1–2 minutes of recovery after exercise at heart rates of 110–130 bpm. T-wave abnormalities may be observed. After treatment with beta-blockade, EST may be used to evaluate effectiveness of treatment to suppress ventricular ectopy and blunt sinus tachycardia (<150–160 bpm), as evidence of adequate beta-blockade.

Audiogram: used to evaluate sensorineural hearing loss seen in the Jervell and Lange-Nielson form of long QT syndrome.

Differential diagnosis

• QT prolongation is associated with specific drugs, notably class I antiarrhythmics (quinidine, procainamide, flecainide, disopyramide), sotolol, tricyclic antidepressants, erythromycin, bactrim, cisipride, fluconazole, ketoconazole, antihistamines (eg, diphenhydramine, terfenadine, astemizole).

• Other causes of ventricular tachycardia: electrolyte abnormalities including hypocalcemia, hypokalemia, and hypomagnesemia; cardiomyopathy; myocarditis, tumors, pre- and postoperative congenital heart disease, hemosiderosis, and idiopathic VT.

Etiology [5,6]

• 90% of cases are familial, 15% sporadic. Genetic studies have identified abnormalities in genes that modulate potassium and sodium channels, altering repolarization and increasing the risk of ventricular arrhythmias. Currently identified abnormalities have been labeled LQT1 on chromosome 11 (KVLQT1:11p15.5) encoding a protein associated with a potassium channel, LQT2 (HERG-7q 35-36) encoding for a potassium channel, and LQT3 (SCN5A-3p21-24) encoding the cardiac sodium channel. A linkage to chromosome 4 has been reported. A homozygous mutation of KVLQT1 is felt to be responsible for Jervell and Lange-Nielson variety. Two to three additional genes are yet to be identified.

• Sympathetic nervous system imbalance plays a role, but precise mechanism unclear.

Complications

Cardiac arrest: from ventricular tachycardia/fibrillation or prolonged asystole. Cardiac arrest is initial presentation in 9% of children with long QT syndrome [4]. Sudden death: 10%–20% per year after initial presentation with syncope; 73% incidence untreated; 1%–5% incidence in patients treated with beta-blockers; sudden death is secondary to torsades de pointes VT, ventricular fibrillation, or asystole.

Treatment

Diet and lifestyle

• Avoid caffeine, chocolate, medications that stimulate heart (decongestants), medications that prolong the QT interval or those that stimulate the heart (sympathomimetic amines and epinephrine). Recreational activity allowed with moderation. No excessive or vigorous competitive sports. Less vigorous or modified competitive sports may be acceptable in specific cases.

Pharmacologic treatment

For acute treatment

For cardiac arrest: cardiopulmonary resuscitation with defibrillation, stabilization of airway and metabolic status; avoid epinephrine; may require intravenous β-blocker (*eg*, esmolol) and temporary transvenous pacing at rate approximately 20% greater than sinus rate.

For ventricular tachycardia: i.v. lidocaine (1 mg/kg) or phenytoin may control ventricular arrhythmias.

Chronic treatment

Standard dosage	*Beta-blockade:* Propranolol, 1–4 mg/kg/dose) every 6 h. Nadolol, 0.5–1 mg/kg every 12 h. Mexilitine, 5–15 mg/kg/d in 3 divided doses with blood level of 1–2 mg/L.
Contraindications	AV block, congestive heart failure, hypoglycemia, severe asthma. *Mexilitine:* cardiogenic shock; second- or third-degree AV block.
Special points	Beta-blockers may result in low heart rates, necessitating the implantation of a pacemaker; adolescents may require lower doses of beta-blockers than young children; long-acting or sustained-release β-blockers may not be effective. *Mexilitine:* effective to suppress ventricular ectopy not suppressed by β-blockers alone; may be most effective in patients with long QT 3 sydrome (sodium channel abnormality).
Main drug interactions	Avoid in combination with other drugs that suppress sinus rate or AV conduction.
Main side effects	Bradycardia, hypotension, AV block, ventricular dysfunction. *Mexilitine:* Central nervous system: dizziness, tremor, insomnia, coordination problems; cardiovascular: hypotension, bradycardia; gastrointestinal: nausea, vomiting.

Treatment aims

To suppress recurrence of ventricular arrhythmia and prevent sudden death. To treat episodes of ventricular tachycardia/ventricular fibrillation.

Other treatments

Potassium and magnesium supplements: potassium level should be above 4 mEq/L and magnesium above 1.8 mEq/L.
Pacemakers: can be effective by allowing the patient to tolerate sufficient beta-blockade. By raising the intrinsic heart rate, ventricular arrhythmias are suppressed. Atrial or dual-chamber pacing is preferred.
Automatic internal cardioverterdefibrillation (AICD): for patients who have sustained a cardiac arrest, AICD is recommended if technically possible. Medications (beta-blockade) must be continued.
Left-stellate sympathetic ganglionectomy: effective in controlling ventricular arrhythmia in some studies; efficacy is controversial.

Prognosis

Sudden death: 1%–5% in those on beta-blocker treatment; addition of other medications and AICD may lower mortality in refractory cases.

Follow-up and management

Patients should be referred to a center with pediatric arrhythmia specialists knowledgeable in this area. Long-term drug therapy is necessary and not be discontinued even if patient has no arrhythmia for years. Follow-up visits with periodic ECG, 24-h ECG monitoring, and exercise stress test should be scheduled every 6 mo.

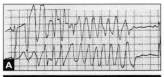
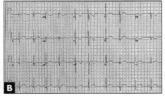

Electrocardiograms (ECGs). A, ECG of torsades de pointes ventricular tachycardia; B, ECG showing prolonged QTc interval and abnormal T waves.

Key references

1. Moss AJ, Robinson MS: Clinical features of the idiopathic long QT syndrome. *Circulation* 1992, **85:**140–144.

2. Schwartz PJ, Moss AJ, Vincent GM, Crampton RS: Diagnostic criteria for the long QT syndrome. *Circulation* 1993, **88:**782–784.

3. Garson A Jr., Dick M II, Fournier A, et al.: The long QT syndrome in children: an international study of 287 patients. *Circulation* 1993, **87:**1866–1872.

Diagnosis

Symptoms
• Patient may be asymptomatic early in course.

Fever.

Malaise.

Weight loss.

Cough: may or may not be productive for sputum.

Chest pain.

Dyspnea.

Shortness of breath.

Hemoptysis.

Signs
Examination may be normal.

Fever.

Tachypnea.

Dullness to percussion over the affected area.

Decreased breath sounds over the affected area.

Rhonchi and rales.

Respiratory distress.

Investigations
Chest radiograph: to visualize the lung abscess; may be opaque or have air-fluid level(s) present if communicates with the bronchial tree; the abscess is usually thick-walled.

Computed tomography scan of chest: to better delineate the abscess; helps to assess for underlying congenital lung malformations and evaluate the surrounding pulmonary parenchyma; useful to guide percutaneous drainage of the abscess.

Ultrasound: useful aid to guide in percutaneous drainage.

Sputum culture: does not always reflect the underlying infectious agent(s) causing the abscess.

Complications
Hypoxia.

Respiratory distress.

Ruptured abscess: soilage of the unaffected lung may occur with dissemination of the infection.

Reoccurrence of the abscess: if it does not entirely resorb with therapy.

Differential diagnosis
"Round" pneumonia.

Complicated pneumonia.

Pulmonary empyema (especially if loculations have developed).

Congenital malformation of the lung (especially cystic lesions: bronchogenic cyst, cystic adenomatoid malformation).

Postinfectious pneumatocele.

Tuberculosis with a cavitary lesion.

Neoplasm.

Etiology
Either primary (underlying healthy host) or secondary (child with a preexisting condition).

• Several bacteria are associated with abscess formation.

Staphylococcus aures: most common.

Oral anaerobes: common if abscess secondary to an aspiration event.

Streptococcus pneumoniae and *Haemophilus influenzae:* less common.

Gram-negative rods (ie, *Escherichia coli, Klebsiella pneumonia, Pseudomonas aeruginosa*) in neonates and chronically institutionalized patients.

Epidemiology
• Very uncommon.

• Risk factors depend on underlying disease processes that increase the risk for developing pulmonary abscess (ie, immunocompromised host, recurrent aspiration events secondary to altered swallowing reflex, bronchiectasis).

• Dependent lobes of the lung are more frequently affected (ie, in recumbent patient: right upper lobe, left upper lobe, and the apical segments of both lower lobes).

Treatment

Diet and lifestyle

• In general, no dietary or lifestyle modifications are required.

• If abscess is secondary to recurrent aspiration events (*ie*, swallowing dysfunction), avoiding oral feeding may be necessary.

Pharmacologic treatment

• Treat underlying disease process.

Antibiotic therapy: should be directed against the most common pathogens; therapy should initially be via the i.v. route.

In uncomplicated lung abscesses, therapy should be directed against *Staphylococcus aures*: oxacillin, cefuroxime, or clindamycin; if the *Staphylococcus aures is methicillin-resistant*, vancomycin should be used instead.

If aspiration is a concern, oral anaerobes should also be covered: clindamycin, penicillin G (if organisms are sensitive), ticarcillin/clavulanic acid.

If gram-negative rods are present or the patient is at higher risk for colonization, an aminogylcoside should be added: gentamicin, tobramycin.

• Total course of IV therapy should be until the patient is afebrile and improving (usually 2–3 weeks).

• Switch to oral antibiotics when improving and ready for discharge.

• Total duration of antibiotic therapy (i.v. and orally) is variable, but should be between 2–4 weeks (occasionally, longer courses are required).

Nonpharmacologic treatment

Drainage: controversial if needed; should be done if patient is failing to improve on i.v. antibiotics; may be via percutaneous route if the abscess is peripherally located or via bronchoscope if more centrally located.

Lobectomy: not done as frequently as in the past; should be reserved for stable patients who have failed conventional medical therapy and surgical drainage.

Treatment aims

To reverse any respiratory distress.

To treat underlying infection.

To address any underlying cause of abscess.

Prognosis

Excellent if simple, primary abscess. Dependent on the underlying disease process and the offending organism if more complicated secondary abscess.

Follow-up and management

• Chest radiographs can take 1–12 months to normalize.

• Treatment of underlying disease is key to preventing reoccurrence.

• Long-term pulmonary function is normal.

General references

Asher MI, Beaudry PH: *Kendig's Disorders of the Respiratory Tract in Children.* Philadelphia: WB Saunders; 1990:429•436.

Brook I: Lung abscesses and pleural empyema in children. *Adv Pediatr Infect Dis* 1993, **8**:159–176.

Campbell PW: *Pediatric Respiratory Disease: Diagnosis and Treatment.* Philadelphia: WB Saunders; 1990:257–262.

Klein JS, Schultz S, Heffner JE: Interventional radiology of the chest: image-guided percutaneous drainage of pleural effusions, lung abscess, and pneumothorax. *Am J Roentgenol* 1995, **164**:581–588.

Tan TQ, Seilheimer DK, Kaplan SL: Pediatric lung abscess: clinical management and outcome. *Pediatr Infect Dis J* 1995, **14**:51–55.

VanSonnenberg E, D'Agostino HB, Casola G, et al.: Lung abscess: CT-guided drainage. *Radiology* 1991, **178**:347–351.

Lyme disease

Diagnosis

Symptoms

• Patients may be asymptomatic.

Early, localized

• Symptoms occur 3–32 days after tick bite.

Influenza-like illness (malaise, pyrexia, myalgia, arthralgia, sore throat), **rash, stiff neck, photophobia.**

Early, disseminated

• Symptoms occur weeks or months later.

Rash (single or multiple); **headache, stiff neck, photophobia, confusion, concentration and memory impairment; chest pain, shortness of breath; joint pain and swelling; abdominal pain, tenderness, diarrhea.**

Late, chronic

Joint pain and swelling; memory impairment; fatigue, malaise.

Signs

Early, localized

Fever, tender muscles or joints, inflamed throat.

Erythema chronicum migrans: characteristic rash is an expanding lesion 5 cm or greater, red macule or papule at site of tick bite, enlarges peripherally with central clearing over several weeks; disseminated lesions may develop; lasts a few weeks.

Lymphadenopathy.

Meningismus.

Early, disseminated.

Meningitis, encephalitis, cranial neuritis (especially seventh-nerve palsy), radiculoneuritis, peripheral neuropathies; atrioventricular block, myoperi-carditis; arthritis; hepatomegaly, splenomegaly.

Late, chronic

Arthritis, arthralgra, myalgia; memory impairment, dementia; chronic encephylomyelitis, polyradiculopathy; acrodermatitis chronica atrophicans (vivid red lesions becoming sclerotic or atrophic [extremely rare]).

Investigations

Microscopy, histopathology, and culture: lack sensitivity and not widely available but may be diagnostic.

Serological tests: support clinical diagnosis; IgM tests positive 3–6 weeks after infection, may persist for many months, but may not be reproducible; IgG tests positive 6–8 weeks after infection, may remain positive for years.

• False-negative antibody results may occur early in illness, with antibiotic treatment; a negative antibody test does not exclude the diagnosis. False-positive results are due to other spirochete infections, other infections, or the test; Western blotting may distinguish true- from false-positive results.

Complications

CNS abnormalities.

Cardiac conduction disturbances.

Oligoarthitis.

Differential diagnosis

Erythema chronicum migrans
Erythema marginatum.
Erythema multiforme.
Granuloma annulare.
Tinia corporis.
Lymphadenopathy
Infectious mononucleosis.
Cytomegalovirus.
Toxoplasmosis.
Systemic lypus erythematosus.
Neurological symptoms
Infectious diseases.
Toxoplasmosis.
Guillain–Barré syndrome.
Multiple sclerosis.
Cardiac symptoms
Infectious diseases.
Chronic heart disease.
Rheumatic Fever.
Arthritis
Juvenile rheumatoid arthritis.
Reactive arthritis.
Other dermatological symptoms
Erythema nodosum.
Scleroderma (morphea variant)

Etiology

• Infection is transmitted by tick bites, usually *Ixodes scapularis* in the US.
• The causative organism is *Borrelia burgdorferi*, a spirochete.

Epidemiology

• Lyme disease is found in the USA, Europe, Russia, China, Japan, and Australia.
• Occurrence parallels distribution and infection in ticks.
• In forested areas, 5%–10% of the population have antibodies.
• Infection peaks in June and July, although may present clinically throughout the year.
• It is found in patients of all ages but especially in the most active and those exposed to ticks.
• Reinfection can occur.

Treatment

Diet and lifestyle

• No special precautions are necessary.

Pharmacologic treatment

Criteria for treatment

• The risk depends on infected tick attachment: <24 h, little risk; 48 h, 50% risk; 72 h, almost certain infection.

• Infection occurs in ~10% of people bitten by infected ticks, so empirical treatment is not justified in areas where infected ticks are rare.

• Erythema chronicum migrans must be treated; acute disease with positive serology and chronic disease when other causes are excluded warrant treatment.

• Treatment should be considered in anxious patients with possible infection but without high expectation of success.

• Asymptomatic individuals with positive serology probably should not be treated.

For acute disease

Standard dosage	Children >8 y Doxycycline, 100 mg/d orally divided in 2 doses for 2–4 wk. Children ≤8 y Amoxicillin, 50 mg/kg/d divided in 3 doses for 2–4 wk.
Contraindications	*Doxycycline*: pregnancy, lactation, children ≤8 y, SLE, porphyria. *Amoxicillin:* penicillin hypersensitivity.
Main drug interactions	*Doxycycline*: anticoagulants, antiepileptics, oral contraceptives. *Amoxicillin:* anticoagulants, oral contraceptives.
Main side effects	*Doxycycline*: nausea, vomiting, diarrhea, headache, photosensitivity. *Amoxicillin:* nausea, diarrhea, rashes.

• Erythromycin and clarithromycin are less effective but can be used in penicillin-sensitive children.

For chronic disease

• Chronic disease may be cardiac, neurologic, or rheumatologic.

Standard dosage	Ceftriaxone, 100 mg/kg/d for 2–4 weeks up to a maximum of 2 g/d. Penicillin G, 300,000 U/kg/d in divided doses to a maximum of 20,000,000 U in divided doses.
Contraindications	*Ceftriaxone:* hypersensitivity to cephalosporin. *Penicillin:* hypersensitivity.
Main drug interactions	*Ceftriaxone:* anticoagulants, probenecid. *Penicillin:* anticoagulants, oral contraceptives.
Main side effects	*Ceftriaxone:* gastrointestinal complaints, allergic reactions, rashes, hematological disturbance, liver dysfunction. *Penicillin:* sensitivity reactions, especially urticaria, angioedema, anaphylaxis.

Treatment aims

To kill organism.
To prevent disease progression.
To alleviate symptoms.

Prognosis

• Despite antibiotic treatment, symptoms recur in 10%–15% of patients, although severity and duration are greatly reduced; occasionally, recurrent symptoms may last several months, rarely years.

• Acute Lyme disease and carditis have good prognosis.

• Cranial nerve palsies and meningitis have good prognosis; radiculoneuritis, peripheral neuropathy, encephalitis, and encephalomyelitis usually have a favorable outcome, but a tendency toward chronic or recurrent disease is seen.

• Arthritis often resolves, but response may be slow, often needing further treatment.

• In chronic disease, recurrence is common.

Follow-up and management

• Patients may need careful monitoring for months or years, depending on the severity of the symptoms.

General references

Gerber MA, Shapiro ED, Burke GS, et al.: Lyme disease in children in Southeastern Connecticut. *N Engl J Med* 1996, **335**:1270–1274.

Guy EC: The laboratory diagnosis of Lyme borreliosis. *Review of Medical Microbiology* 1993, 4:89–96.

Sigal LM: Lyme disease: testing and treatment. *Rheum Dis Clin North Am* 1993, **19**:79–93.

Weber K, Pfister H: Clinical management of Lyme borreliosis. *Lancet* 1994, **343**:1017–1020.

Diagnosis

Symptoms

Classic Marfan syndrome

Chest pain: due to dissection/rupture of aorta (rare in childhood), pneumothorax, or cardiac arrhythmia.

Poor vision: subluxated lenses, high myopia.

Joint pain or delayed motor development: hyperextensible subluxable joints, scoliosis.

Headaches: frequent, severe.

Congenital Marfan syndrome

Congestive cardiac failure in neonatal period, occasionally early childhood.

Signs

Classic Marfan syndrome

Skeletal: tall (compared with unaffected family members or general population), disproportionately long limbs (dolichostenomelia) and hands and feet (arachnodactyly), dolichocephaly, deepset downslanting palpebral fissures of eyes, high nose bridge, pointed chin with horizontal chin crease, pectus excavatum/carinatum, scoliosis (often double curve); low muscle mass and adipose tissue; flexible joints, occasionally contractures.

Cardiovascular: mitral valve prolapse; later, aortic root dilatation, aneurysm, dissection; aortic valve incompetence.

Ocular: high myopia, flat corneas, subluxated lenses, detached retinas.

Other: frequent severe headaches, pneumothorax, dural ectasia, striae.

• Expression is variable: the extent and severity of each sign varies within and between families.

Congenital Marfan syndrome

Skeletal: long thin body, aged appearance (lack of subcutaneous tissue), wrinkled, sagging skin (cutis laxa). Characteristic facies include dolicocephaly, deepset eyes, large/small corneas, occasionally cataracts, high nose bridge, high palate, small pointed chin with horizontal skin crease, large simple/crumpled ears. Fingers and toes are long and thin (arachnodactyly).

Joints: hyperextensible or flexion contractures, causing equinovarus or -valgus, dislocated hips or adducted thumbs.

Hypotonia: with low muscle mass.

Cardiovascular: severe disease in most neonates; mitral and tricuspid valves prolapse and insufficiency, ascending aorta dilated and tortuous.

Hernias: occasional diaphragmatic or inguinal.

Ocular: retinal detachment; lenses are usually not subluxated at birth.

Complications

Classic Marfan syndrome

Aortic aneurysm rupture or aortic dissection: may occur during or after pregnancy. Early death if untreated; paralysis from descending aorta dissection.

Ocular lens subluxation and retinal detachment.

Cardiovascular compromise: if scoliosis is severe and untreated.

Dural ectasia.

Congenital Marfan syndrome

Congestive cardiac failure: most infants die in the first year; survivors have continuing hypotonia, contractures, inability to walk, and require repeated surgery.

Blood and skin: for gene mutation studies (not possible to detect mutation in each case); prenatal detection is possible in the second half of pregnancy.

• Most congenital cases are sporadic with one exception.

Differential diagnosis

Classic Marfan syndrome

Homocystinuria: similar body habitus, joint disease (including scoliosis), and dislocation of ocular lenses; some, but not all, have mental retardation; malar flush; vascular thromboses, causing stroke or early myocardial infarction or deep vein thromboses.
Autosomal recessive inheritance.
Measure homocysteine in plasma (amino acids).

Stickler syndrome: some have similar body and facial features, myopia, retinal detachment, and mitral valve prolapse. There is vitreoretinal degeneration, joint disease, cleft palate, deafness; no lens subluxation, aortic aneurysm, or dissection.

Shprintzen-Goldberg syndrome: similar body habitus, joint laxity, mild aortic dilatation. Sagittal craniosynostosis, causing dolichocephaly (increased anteroposterior diameter).

Beals congenital contractural arachnodactyly (CCA) syndrome: similar thin, wasted appearance, minimal muscle and fat mass, and contractures of large and small joints (which improve to some degree with time); cardiovascular involvement (mitral valve prolapse); normal lifespan; autosomal dominant inheritance, caused by mutations in fibrillin 2 (*FBN2*) gene, on chromosome 5 (5q23-31).

Congenital Marfan syndrome

Cutis laxa syndrome: the severe autosomal recessive form manifests at birth—loose, sagging skin, pulmonary emphysema, and gastrointestinal and urinary tract diverticula. No cardiovascular abnormality.

Beals syndrome.

Etiology

Autosomal dominant inheritance.
Mutations of a connective tissue, fibrillin, encoded by the fibrillin 1 (*FBN1*) gene on the long arm of chromosome 15 (15q21.1). Fibrillin and other proteins (microfibril-associated glycoproteins) are components of microfibrils in aorta, periosteum, perichondrium, cartilage, tendons, muscle, pleura, and meninges.

Epidemiology

• Classic disease occurs in 1:10,000.
• Congenital disease is rare.

Treatment

Lifestyle

• Avoid competitive sports, weight-lifting, and any exercise that puts excessive stress on heart and increases heart rate, to decrease the frequency of systole and stretching of the aorta. Avoid blows to head, as in contact sports to prevent dislocation of lenses and detachment of retina; use helmets with bicycling or skating.

Pharmacologic treatment

β-Adrenergic blockade drugs: atenolol or propanolol.

Other treatment options

Cardiac surgery: mitral valve repair or replacement.

Ascending aorta aneurysm and aortic valve: composite graft replacement; recommended electively if the aortic root (sinus) diameter is >55–60 mm, or if dissection or rupture occurs.

Descending aortic dissection: medical control of blood pressure and stress on aorta; surgical graft replacement if diameter >55–60 mm.

Bracing for scoliosis: if bracing is unable to control worsening of scoliosis, surgery is needed to prevent cardiopulmonary compromise.

Surgical lens extraction: usually contraindicated; may cause retinal detachment.

Support group

National Marfan Foundation, 382 Main Street, Port Washington, NY 11050; tel: 800-8-MARFAN; tel/fax: 516-883-8712; website: www.marfan.org.

General references

Dietz HC, Cutting GR, Pyeritz RE, et al.: Marfan syndrome caused by a recurrent de novo missense mutation in the fibrillin gene. *Nature* 1991, 352:337.

Godfrey M, Raghunath M, Cisler J, et al.: Abnormal morphology of fibrillin microfibrils in fibroblast cultures from patients with neonatal Marfan syndrome. *Am J Pathol* 1995, **146:**1414.

Morse RP, Rockenmacher S, Pyeritz RE, et al.: Diagnosis and management of infantile Marfan syndrome. *Pediatrics* 1990, **86:**888.

Pyeritz RE: Connective tissue and its heritable disorders. Edited by Royce PM, Steinmann B. In *The Marfan Syndrome.* New York: Wiley-Liss Inc.; 1995:437–468.

Shores J, Berger KR, Murphy EA, Pyeritz RE: Progression of aortic dilatation and the benefit of long term beta adrenergic blockade in Marfan's syndrome. *N Engl J Med* 1994, **330:**1384–1385.

Lopes LM, Cha SC, De Moraes EA, Zugaib M: Echocardiographic diagnosis of fetal Marfan syndrome at 34 weeks gestation. *Prenatal Diagnosis* 1995, **15:**183.

Diagnosis

Symptoms
• Symptoms depend on the underlying mass and its location.

May be asymptomatic.

Cough.

Wheeze.

Dyspnea.

Stridor.

Hoarseness.

Dysphagia.

Chest pain or fullness.

Signs
• Physical findings depend on the underlying mass and its location.

Examination may be normal.

Decreased breath sounds, rhonchi, rales, or dullness to percussion over the area of the mass.

Wheezing: usually unilateral.

Hoarseness.

Engorgement of head and neck veins.

Systemic symptoms such as fevers and night sweats if there is an underlying malignancy.

Investigations
Chest radiograph: useful for localizing the mass; frequently obtained for other reasons, with the mass being an incidental finding; both posteroanterior and lateral views are needed to localize the mass.

Computed tomography scan of the chest: also useful for further delineating the mass and for viewing its internal structures and its relationship to neighboring organs.

Barium swallow: useful for determining if the mass is compressing on nearby gastrointestinal structures.

Chest MRI: useful in posterior mediastinal masses for determining spinal cord and vertebral column involvement or in cases in which a vascular anomaly is suspected.

Angiography: useful in delineating any vascular lesion.

Bronchoscopy: if infection, foreign body, or bronchial obstruction is suspected.

Biopsy of the lesion: when indicated, can definitively establish the diagnosis.

Urine collection for catecholamines: if neuroblastoma is suspected.

Complications
Bronchial compression with secondary atelectasis or recurrent or chronic pneumonia.

Hemoptysis.

Esophageal compression with resultant dysphagia.

Vascular compression (*ie***, superior vena cava syndrome).**

Horner's syndrome.

Scoliosis.

Differential diagnosis

General

Round pneumonia

Foreign body with secondary atelectasis.

Anterior mediastinal masses

Thymic lesions (especially benign thymic hyperplasia)

Teratoma

Lymphomas (Hodgkin's and non-Hodgkin's)

Leukemic infiltrates

Lymphadenopathy

Vascular lesions (hemangiomas)

Middle mediastinal masses

Lymphomas (Hodgkin's and non-Hodgkin's)

Lymphadenopathy (tuberculosis, Histoplasmosis, sarcoidosis)

Metastases from other malignancies

Bronchogenic cysts

Cardiac tumors

Anomalies of the great vessels

Posterior mediastinal masses

Neurogenic tumors (especially neuroblastomas and ganglioneuorblastomas)

Esophageal cysts (duplication cysts)

Gastroenteric cysts

Etiology

Dependent on the underlying mass.

Epidemiology

Dependent on the underlying lesion.

• 40% of all lesions are located in the posterior mediastinum.

• Thymic lesions are the most common mediastinal masses in children.

• Teratomas are the most common anterior mediastinal tumors in children.

• Lymphomas are the most common middle mediastinal tumors in children.

• Neurogenic tumors are the most common posterior mediastinal tumors in children.

Treatment

Diet and lifestyle
• No specific dietary or lifestyle changes are required.

Pharmacologic treatment
Dependent on the underlying mass.

• Antibiotics if infection is present (*ie*, pneumonia, tuberculosis, lung abscess).

• Hemotherapy and/or radiation therapy for certain malignancies.

• Surgery to correct any vascular anomaly or to remove a benign lesion (*ie*, bronchogenic cyst, pulmonary sequestration, or isolated tumor such as a teratoma).

• Observation is sometimes an option if the mass is benign and delay in treatment will not adversely effect the outcome (*ie*, benign thymic enlargement, Histoplasmosis).

Treatment aims
To alleviate symptoms.
To treat underlying pathology.
To prevent reoccurrence of lesion or recurrent infections secondary to bronchial obstruction.

Prognosis
Dependent on the underlying mass.
• Excellent if congenital lung malformation or gastrointestinal anomaly.
• Good if vascular anomaly or benign tumor.
• Variable if malignant tumor.

Follow-up and management
• If benign mass, follow-up is short term. Follow-up chest radiographs and pulmonary function tests can prove useful for following pulmonary involvement.
• If malignant mass, follow-up is as per the oncologic protocol.
Posterior: esophagus, sympathetic ganglions, paraspinal lymph nodes, descending aorta.

General references

Brooks JW: *Kendig's Disorders of the Respiratory Tract in Children.* Philadelphia: WB Saunders; 1990:614–648.

Meza MP, Benson M, Slovis TL: Imaging of mediastinal masses in children. *Radiol Clin N Am* 1993, **31**:583–604.

Watterson J, Kubic P, Dehner LP, Priest JR: *Pediatric Respiratory Disease: Diagnosis and Treatment.* Philadelphia: WB Saunders; 1993:590–620.

Diagnosis

Symptoms
Fever: anorexia, vomiting.

Irritability: headache.

Lethargy: altered mental status.

Seizures: additional symptoms attributable to primary source of infection (*eg*, ear pain, cough)

Signs
High-pitched, irritable cry.

Nuchal rigidity.

Kernig's sign: pain and hamstring spasm on passive knee extension with hip flexed.

Brudzinski's sign: spontaneous knee and hip flexion on attempted neck flexion.

Cranial nerve palsies: especially affecting the abducens (VIth) nerve.

Other focal neurological signs: *eg*, hemiparesis in complicated cases.

Bulging fontanel.

papilledema.

Fever, tachycardia, shock, and evidence of primary source of infection: *eg*, pneumonia, otitis media, sinusitis, endocarditis.

Investigations
Lumbar puncture for cerebrospinal fluid (CSF) examination: manometry (opening pressure often elevated), inspection (turbid cerebrospinal fluid), Gram's stain, determination of cell count and differential and of protein and glucose levels, culture and antigen immunoassay for specific organism. Relative contraindications include papilledema, deteriorating level of consciousness, and focal neurologic signs; prepuncture cranial CT or MRI is needed in such patients to exclude mass lesion.

Complete blood count: to detect neutrophilic leukocytosis.

Serum electrolyte analysis.

Neuroimaging (cranial CT, MRI): generally indicated if focal findings are present to exclude abscess, subdural empyema, encephalitis, infarction, septic thrombosis of dural sinuses.

Electroencephalography: for seizures.

CSF findings in meningitis

Type	Typical cellular profile	Protein	Glucose
Bacterial	Markedly elevated with polymorphonuclear predominance	Markedly elevated (often >1 mg/dL)	Low
Partially treated bacterial	Variable	Elevated	Low
Tuberculous	Lymphocytic predominance (but may have polymorphonumclear predominance in the first day or so)	Elevated	Low
Viral	Moderately elevated with mononuclear predominance (but may have polymorphonuclear predominance in the first few hours)	Normal or mildly elevated	Normal or mildly depressed

Complications
Cerebral infarction (stroke), epilepsy, hearing loss, mental retardation, focal neurologic deficits.

Differential diagnosis
• The presentation of acute bacterial meningitis is generally distinctive in older children but may be mimicked by intracranial abscess, subarachnoid hemorrhage, and chemical meningitis.

• Symptoms and signs may be subtle and nonspecific in young infants or immuno-compromised patients.

Etiology
• After the neonatal period, 70%–90% of bacterial meningitis is attributable to one of three organisms: *Neisseria mengitidis*, *Haemophilus influenzae* type b (declining incidence since introduction of vaccine), and *Streptococcus pneumoniae*.

• Other bacterial organisms are found in specific settings, especially:

Enterobacteriaceae, group B streptococci in neonates.

Listeria monocytogenes in neonates and immunocompromised patients.

Mycobacterium tuberculosis in patients from developing countries or in high-risk areas.

Staphylococci and other unusual organisms in patients with ventriculoperitoneal shunts or with unusual portals of entry (eg, occult nasal encephalocele or sacral dermal sinus tract).

The most common cause of aseptic meningitis is enterovirus infection [2].

• Less common causes of treatable meningitis should also be considered, especially in immunosuppressed patients: fungal or parasitic infection, autoimmune disorders, chemical irritation (eg, due to ruptured dermoid cyst or intrathecal chemotherapy), or neoplasm with meningeal involvement.

Epidemiology
• The incidence of bacterial meningitis is 5–10:100,000 annually in developed countries and is higher during the winter months

• The incidence of aseptic (presumed viral) meningitis is higher in the summer months.

Treatment

Diet and lifestyle
• No special precautions are necessary.

General measures
• Support respiratory and cardiovascular function as indicated.
• Avoid excessive administration of hypotonic fluids, which may produce or exacerbate brain edema.

Pharmacologic treatment

Bacterial meningitis
• Bacterial meningitis may prove fatal within hours; successful treatment depends on early diagnosis and i.v. administration of appropriate antibiotics in antimeningitic doses (intrathecal antibiotics are not recommended).
• If lumbar puncture is delayed by the need for prepuncture CT, antibiotic treatment should be started before the scan, but after blood cultures.
• Recommendations for initial therapy are given below; subsequent therapy should always be guided by *in vitro* sensitivity testing [3]. Duration is based on clinical response, and is at least 21 days in neonates and generally 10 to 14 days in older children.

For infection with *N. meningitidis* or *S. pneumoniae* beyond the newborn period: high-dose penicillin G intravenously, 250,000–400,000 units/kg/d divided in 4–6 doses.

For infection with *H. influenzae* type b: ceftriaxone (80–100 mg/kg/d divided in 1–2 doses beyond the newborn period); cefotaxime, or ampicillin in combination with chloramphenicol are acceptable alternatives, but ampicillin alone may be ineffective.

For infection with *Listeria monocytogenes* in neonates: ampicillin in combination with an aminoglycoside.

For infection with gram-negative bacilli in neonates: initial empiric therapy consists of ampicillin and an aminoglycoside; an alternative consists of ampicillin and a cephalosporin such as cefotaxime or ceftazidime, but rapid emergence of cephalosporin-resistant strains may occur as a result of frequent use in a nursery.

• Dexamethasone is recommended for children with *H. influenzae* type b infections to decrease the incidence of deafness and possibly of other neurologic complications. Some experts do not recommend dexamethasone in meningo-coccal or pneumococcal meningitis because of unproven efficacy and concerns about possible adverse effects [3,4].

Tuberculous meningitis
• A combination of four drugs (isoniazid, rifampin, pyrazinamide, and streptomycin) is given initially to protect against drug-resistance and the severe consequences of treatment failure.

Viral meningitis
• No specific antimicrobial therapy is recommended.

Prevention
• In bacterial meningitis in certain settings, chemoprevention of household contacts and index patients before hospital discharge is indicated [3].
• Immunization against *H. influenzae* infection (using *H. influenzae* type b vaccine) is recommended routinely for children at 2, 4, and 6 months of age (or at 2 and 4 months, depending on the specific vaccine product), with an additional booster dose at 12–15 months of age [3].

Treatment aims
To secure survival and prevent persistent neurologic complications.
To reduce the risk of recurrence by treating any predisposing cause.
To prevent spread to close contacts.

Prognosis
• Mortality of bacterial meningitis is 5%–10%, but up to 20% of survivors have long-term sequelae, the most common of which is hearing impairment.
• Patients with viral meningitis typically recover fully.

Follow-up and management
• Brainstem auditory evoked potentials or audiogram should be performed to detect hearing loss.
• Repeat lumbar puncture to monitor treatment is not necessary if the patient is improving.
• Bacteriological relapse needs immediate reinstitution of treatment.
• Older children should generally be reevaluated at 3 months and neonates periodically for several years to detect any long-term sequelae.

Key references
1. Brown LW, Feigin RD: Bacterial meningitis: fluid balance and therapy. *Pediatr Ann* 1994, 23:93–98.
2. Rotbart HA: Enteroviral infections of the central nervous system. *Clin Inf Dis* 1995, 20:971–981.
3. Peter G (ed.): *1997 Red Book: Report of the Committee on Infectious Diseases*, edn 24. Elk Grove Village, IL: American Academy of Pediatrics; 1997.
4. Schaad UB, Kaplan SL, McCracken GH Jr: Steroid therapy for bacterial meningitis. *Clin Inf Dis* 1995, 20:685–690.

Diagnosis

Definition

Detection of microscopic amounts of blood in urine of well child.

Blood found by dipstick method during routine examination should alarm patient, parents, and physician.

Symptoms

Usually asymptomatic.

• Take more seriously if there are urinary symptoms, other symptoms, butterfly rash, Henoch–Schönlein purpura rash, hypertension, proteinura, erythrocyte casts, oliguria, episodes of macroscopic hematuria, flank pain.

• Take careful history for recent trauma, strenuous exercise, menstruation, bladder catheterization.

• Take careful family history for hematuria, hearing loss, nephrolithiasis, renal diseases, renal cystic diseases, bleeding disorders, sickle cell trait.

Signs

Usually no signs.

• Take more seriously if there is fever, costovertebral angle tenderness, abdominal mass, tumor, hydronephrosis, multicystic kidney, polycystic kidney, rash, arthritis, edema.

Investigations

• Aim to detect major or treatable problems while limiting anxiety, cost, energy entailed by unnecessary testing.

Positive dipstick result: erythrocytes, hemoglobin, myoglobin.

False-positive: oxidizing contaminants, *eg*, bacterial peroxidases; dipstick may deteriorate with age.

Renal ultrasonography: costly and time-consuming but the value provided by a normal renal ultrasound examination in terms of reassurance may justify its cost and time.

Complications

Acute renal failure: uncommon.
Chronic renal failure: uncommon.

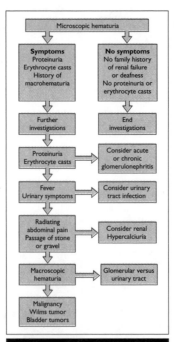

Investigation of microscopic hematuria.

Differential diagnosis

Microscopic hematuria and significant proteinuria: evaluate for nephrotic syndrome.

Recent sore throat or skin infection or viral infection: evaluate for postinfectious glomerulonephritis.

Microscopic hematuria and significant proteinuria and erythrocyte casts: evaluate for glomerulonephritis.

History of dysuria, frequency, abdominal pain: evaluate for urinary tract infection or urolithiasis.

Etiology

Usually idiopathic.
IgA nephropathy.
Hypercalciuria.
Thin basement membrane disease.

Epidemiology

School-aged children: 4%–6% had detectable blood on a single urine sample.

Fewer than half had blood when urinalysis repeated in 7 d.

Annual incidence of new cases with five or more erythrocytes per high-powered field on two of three consecutive specimens estimated at 0.4% in children 6–12 y of age.

Course

May persist for years.
End-stage renal failure is rare.

Treatment

Diet and lifestyle

No changes needed.

Serious conditions must not be overlooked.

Unnecessary and expensive laboratory studies must be avoided.

Physician must be able to reassure family.

Physician must provide guidelines for additional studies in case there is a change in course.

Pharmacologic treatment

None.

Nonpharmacologic treatment

Reassurance: parents must be reassured that there are no life-threatening conditions, that there is time to plan a stepwise evaluation, and that most causes of isolated microscopic hematuria in children do not warrant treatment.

Education: of patient/family regarding causes for concern, which may include symptoms, macroscopic hematuria, hypertension, or proteinuria.

Treatment aims

To reassure.

To avoid psychologic stress.

To support child and family.

Precautions

Rule out infection if febrile.

Rule out serious glomerulopathies if proteinuric, erythrocyte casts, family history of chronic renal failure and/or deafness.

Rule out calculi if abdominal pain.

Rule out bladder tumor if there are urinary symptoms.

Rule out Wilms' tumor if there is an abdominal mass.

Prognosis

Excellent.

Follow-up and management

Regular urine dipstick examinations.

Reevaluate if patient becomes hypertensive, or develops macroscopic hematuria, or erythrocyte casts, or significant proteinuria.

General references

Lieu TA, Grasmeder HM, Kaplan BS: An approach to the evaluation and treatment of microscopic hematuria. *Pediatr Clin North Am* 1991, **38**:579–592.

Yadin O: Hematuria in children. *Pediatr Ann* 1994, **23**:474–478, 481–485.

Diagnosis

Definition

Migraine without aura (common migraine): episodic headache, typically lasting several hours to 1–2 days, in which several of the following features are prominent: 1) unilaterality, 2) throbbing cephalalgia, 3) photophobia or phonophobia, 4) nausea or vomiting, 5) intense desire for and relief by sleep. Family history is usually positive.

Migraine without aura (classic migraine): as above, but the attacks are heralded by an aura (*see* below) that typically lasts 10–20 minutes but can persist up to 1 hour.

Ophthalmoplegic migraine: recurrent attacks of III or VI cranial nerve palsies associated with headache; resolution of deficit may be delayed by several days.

Confusional migraine: an uncommon disorder resembling a toxic-metabolic psychosis, with recurrent bouts of delirium in which the child is agitated and appears uncomfortable, but may not complain of head pain. Gradual evolution to recognizable migraine typically occurs over several months.

Hemiplegic migraine: recurrent attacks of hemiparesis of rapid onset followed by headache: weakness may last hours. This syndrome is in some cases inherited as an autosomal dominant trait due to a mutation involving one type of calcium channel.

• The relationship of so-called "migraine variants" (*eg*, "abdominal migraine," paroxysmal vertigo, cyclic vomiting syndrome) to common and classic migraine is unclear. Other more serious causes of the clinical picture (*eg*, stroke, aneurysmal leak, transient ischemic attack, hemorrhage into tumor) must be excluded, especially if the pain is severe, before the diagnosis is accepted.

Symptoms

• The aura of classic migraine is most commonly visual, and may include visual field defects (hemianopia or scotoma), often associated with sparkling lights (scintillating scotoma), or bright, multicolored jagged lines (fortification spectra). Less commonly, hemisensory symptoms (numbness, paresthesias, more often in an upper than a lower limb), transient hemiparesis, or even aphasia occur. The laterality of the neurological disturbance is not necessarily related to that of the headache and may not be consistent from one attack to the next.

• Diagnosis is facilitated when the attacks are stereotyped, disabling, and discrete (*ie*, separated by periods of complete wellness).

Signs

• Common migraine may have no signs.

• The scotomas, hemianopia, and sensorimotor phenomena of classic migraine may be detected if the aura is still present at the time of examination.

• Prolonged neurologic deficit requires exclusion of other causes.

Investigations

• Investigation is often not needed, but the following studies should be considered with the aim of excluding alternative diagnoses in selected cases.

Neuroimaging (cranial CT, MRI, or MRA): for tumor, vascular malformation, hydrocephalus, vasculitis

Electroencephalography: for seizures.

CSF analysis: for subarachnoid hemorrhage, meningoencephalitis.

Complications

Complicated migraine: rarely, focal neurologic signs occurring in association with migraine continue as permanent deficits or stroke.

Dehydration.

Differential diagnosis

Chronic daily headache: dull, usually generalized cephalgia that may last for weeks or months. This syndrome is often accompanied by depression, and is extremely common in adolescents (especially females) but infrequent in younger children. This headache pattern is often triggered by difficulties in peer relations, domestic discord, or poor academic achievement, and is commonly associated with school avoidance. When migraine coexists—as is often the case—the result is a pattern of prolonged or constant headaches with episodic exacerbations.

Tumor, pseudotumor cerebri, and hydrocephalus: raised intracranial pressure, when subacute or chronic, usually causes headache with early morning occurrence or accentuation that may be associated with vomiting and is accompanied by papilledema. Persistent, focal neurologic deficits (especially VI cranial nerve palsy) may be present.

Local disease: nasopharyngeal lesions, dental problems, sinusitis, and glaucoma.

Systemic disease: fever is the most common cause of acute headache in childhood. Rarely, disorders such as pheochromocytoma cause recurrent headaches mimicking migraine.

Hemorrhage: abrupt onset of severe headache, usually occipital and associated with neck stiffness and photophobia.

Etiology

• Migraine is probably due to a combination of genetic predisposition and environmental triggers (eg, stress, certain foods) causing changes in neurotransmitter release (5-hydroxytryptamine), with alteration in cerebral blood flow and pain in the distribution of the trigeminal nerve.

Epidemiology

• The prevalence is between 2%–10% in children aged 5–15 y. Migraine is more common in males before puberty and in females after puberty.

Migraines may occur in infants as young as 24 mo, but are difficult to diagnose at this age.

Treatment

Diet and lifestyle

• Dietary precipitants, *eg*, cheese, chocolate, cured meats, nuts, and certain other foods may precipitate migraine in susceptible individuals. Acute withdrawal headaches may occur in children consuming large amounts of caffeine and related stimulants.

• Stress may precipitate migraines in some individuals, and appropriate measures may reduce the frequency of attacks.

• Oral contraceptives are best avoided, and are contraindicated in migraine with focal neurological deficits.

Pharmacologic treatment

• Many patients respond satisfactorily to rest, darkness, and simple analgesics such as nonsteroidal anti-inflammatory agents or acetaminophen. Combination agents, which include mild sedatives such as Midrin (isometheptane mucate, a vasoconstrictor; dichloralphenazone, a sedative; and acetaminophen) or Fioricet (butalbital, caffeine, and acetaminophen) may also be effective, but formulations of these agents for younger children are not available.

For migraine with and without aura: acute

• Patients with gastrointestinal disturbance and more severe headache may benefit from a combination of an analgesic and an antiemetic/sedative, which may need to be administered parenterally (*eg*, promethazine suppositories [Phenergan]).

• More severe attacks unresponsive to this treatment may, in older children, be treated with ergotamine or sumatriptan.

Standard dosage   Ergotamine, in varying doses according to route. Sumatriptan, 25–100 mg orally at onset or 6 mg s.c. by auto-injector.

Contraindications   *Ergotamine*: vascular disease (*eg*, vasculitis or Raynaud's syndrome), hemiplegic migraine.

     Sumatriptan: uncontrolled hypertension, hemiplegic migraine.

Main drug interactions: *Ergotamine, sumatriptan*: the concomitant use of these two agents should probably be avoided because of a theoretically increased risk of precipitating vasospasm.

Main side effects: *Ergotamine*: nausea, vomiting, dizziness, headache, chest tightness (particularly with overuse).

     Sumatriptan: chest, jaw, or neck pain or tightness, light-headedness, transient pain at site of injection.

For migraine with and without aura: prophylactic

• β-Blockers (*eg*, propranolol) or tricyclic antidepressants (*eg*, amitryptiline) should be considered for two attacks monthly; 6–12 months effective treatment may allow withdrawal. Tricyclic antidepressants are useful in mixed headache syndromes (ie, migraine plus tension headache) because of the frequent coexistence of depression, which may be exacerbated by propranolol.

Standard dosage   Short-acting propranolol, 10–20 mg 3 times daily in children ≤35 kg, and 20–40 mg 3 times daily in children >35 kg. If this is tolerated, consider change to a long-acting formulation.

Contraindications: Insulin-dependent diabetes, asthma (depending on severity), cardiac failure or heart block, allergies undergoing desensitization, history of anaphylactic reaction (*eg*, bee sting allergy).

Main drug interactions   *See* manufacturer's current prescribing information.

Main side effects   Bradycardia, orthostasis, fatigue, depression.

Treatment aims

To provide adequate relief from symptoms.

To adjust treatment appropriately to the severity and frequency of attacks.

To minimize effect of migraine on school performance and leisure activities.

Prognosis

• A majority of children with migraine experience a substantial reduction in headache frequency and severity within 6 months of evaluation, regardless of therapy. Relapses may occur in adolescence and adulthood, but if a syndrome of very frequent, recurrent headaches persists for years, tension or psychosomatic headache should be suspected.

Follow-up and management

• Prophylactic agents should generally be continued for 6 mo, assuming reasonable efficacy, before withdrawal.

• Outpatient follow-up within a few weeks of initiation of prophylaxis is usually indicated.

• For mixed headache syndromes with migrainous and tension components, consider psychotherapy and/or behavioral management techniques, such as biofeedback. In children with school avoidance, steady and gradual resumption of full academic activities is essential.

General references

Rothner AD: The migraine syndrome in children and adolescents. *Pediatr Neurol* 1986, **2**:121–126.

Singer HS: Migraine headaches in children. *Pediatr Rev* 1994, **15**:94–101.

Minimal-change nephrotic syndrome

Diagnosis

Definition
Nephrotic syndrome: edema, proteinuria, hypolalbuminemia, hyperlipidemia.
Minimal change nephrotic syndrome (MCNS): biopsies rarely needed; the terms *steroid-sensitive* or *steroid-responsive* nephrotic syndrome are used to denote MCNS.

Symptoms
Fatigue, general malaise.
Edema: severity and extent fluctuates in the early stages.
Reduced appetite, diarrhea, and/or bulky stools.

Signs
Edema: periorbital, pedal, scrotal.
Ascites and/or pleural effusions.
Hypertension: absent or mild.
Urine: decreased output, frothy, gross hematuria unusual.

Investigations
Serum albumin: usually <2.4 g/dL.
Hyperlipidemia: occurs during relapses; persists during remission.
Serum electrolyte: sodium level is often decreased.
Serum potassium: thrombocytosis can spuriously elevate potassium levels by *in vitro* release of potassium.
Serum calcium: decreased as a result of hypoalbuminemia.
Serum creatinine and BUN: transiently increased in 33% of children.
Hemoglobin: often increased as a result of intravascular depletion.
Platelets: increased to as high as 1,000,000/mL.
Erythrocyte sedimentation rate: markedly elevated.
Proteinuria: >2 plus by dipstick test; protein excretion > 4 mg/m^2/h; U prot/creat >1.0 mg/mg.
Hematuria: microscopic hematuria in 23% with MCNS.

Complications
Psychological: anxiety in patients and parents because of uncertain cause; likelihood of recurrence, fear of end-stage renal failure, and loathing of corticosteroids.
Infections: increased risk for primary peritonitis.
Thrombosis: venous, arterial thromboses.
Acute renal failure: uncommon complication of MCNS.
Growth failure: caused by corticosteroids.
Focal glomerulosclerosis: in a small percentage of patients.
Chronic renal failure: never in patients with MCNS unless they develop focal segmental glomerulosclerosis.

Differential diagnosis
Frequently misdiagnosed as "an allergy."
Focal glomerulosclerosis (FSGS): histopathological lesion; usually begins in juxtamedullary region, is often progressive, is usually steroid-resistant, may recur after renal transplantation.
Occurs with or without features of nephrotic syndrome.
Protein-losing enteropathy: normal urine and cholesterol.

Etiology
No definite cause.
Associations: nonsteroidal anti-inflammatory agents, lithium, Hodgkin's disease.

Epidemiology
1.5:100,000 children.
Occurs predominantly in those 2–8 years of age.
Male to female ratio, 2:1.

Progression
Usually responds to steroid treatment.
Course: relapsing and remitting.
End-stage renal failure: rare.

Treatment

Diet and lifestyle

Sodium restriction: 1–2 g/d reduces edema formation, minimizes risk of hypertension while on steroids.

Protein intake: recommended daily allowance.

Calorie intake: control to reduce obesity while on steroids.

Hyperlipidemia: dietary manipulation to reduce risk of cardiovascular complications.

Normal lifestyle.

Pharmacologic treatment

Diuretics: only for gross edema.

Prednisone: initial high daily dose of steroids is required to achieve remission: 60 mg/m^2 for 4 wk followed by 40 mg/m^2 every second morning for another 4 wk.

Relapses: first three relapses are managed the same way as the first episode. Once the dose of steroids required to maintain a remission is established, the patient with frequent relapses is given prednisone every second morning for 6 months in a dose of 0.1 to 0.5 mg/kg and the dose is gradually tapered.

Alkylating agents: alkylating agents can induce prolonged remissions but are used judiciously because of potential side-effects.

Cyclosporin A: used to treat steroid-dependent nephrotic syndrome if there are serious side-effects of steroids and failure to respond to cyclophosphamide.

Nonpharmacologic treatment

Tuberculosis: rule out before starting steroids.

General management: provide psychosocial support; admit at first presentation for treatment, counseling, and education; parents and patients taught how to monitor the condition; potential side effects of steroids (mood, behavior, appetite changes, weight gain, acne, growth delay, hypertension, hair changes) are explained in detail.

Hypovolemia: corrected with infusions of saline, plasma, or 5% albumin.

Inoculations: while in remission off steroids; especially pneumococcal and hemophilus vaccines.

Treatment aims

To induce remissions.
To maintain remissions.
To support child and family.

Precautions

Rule out infection if febrile.
Avoid/treat varicella if on alkylating agents, prednisone.
Avoid volume depletion while on diuretics.
Monitor side-effects of steroids.

Prognosis

Antibiotics have reduced mortality rate.
Tendency to relapse declines with age.
Incidence of relapses over 18 y is 5.5% if onset was under 6 y.

Follow-up and management

Most patients can be treated over the telephone.
Regular serum chemistries are not needed.

General references

Consensus Statement on Management and Audit Potential for Steroid Responsive Nephrotic Syndrome. *Arch Dis Child* 1994, **70:**151–157.

Meyers KW, Kujubu D, Kaplan BS: Minimal change nephrotic syndrome. In *Immunologic Renal Diseases*. Edited by Neilsen EG, Couser WG. New York: Lippincott-Raven Press; 1997:975–992.

Schnaper HW: Primary nephrotic syndrome of childhood. *Curr Opin Pediatr* 1996, **8(2):**141–147.

Diagnosis

Definitions

• The mucopolysaccharidoses (MPS) are a group of lysosomal storage diseases in which the degradation of the glycosaminoglycans (GAGs), a class of mucopolysaccharides, keratan sulfate, dermatan sulfate, and/or chondroitin sulfate is perturbed. (*See* table.)

Symptoms and signs

• There are many common signs and symptoms, but each type of MPS has a somewhat different clinical presentation. In the "classic" presentation of the types with mental retardation (types I-H, II, III), development is normal in the first 6 months to 2 years of life, and then acquisition of milestones slows or ceases. This is followed, over a variable time (months to years), by loss of abilities. Growth retardation occurs in the more severe forms, although growth may be above average for the first few years in Hunter and Sanfilippo syndromes. Coarse facial features are obvious in MPS I-H, II-A, and VI by late infancy and may be more subtle in MPS II and III. When skeletal signs are present, they often affect multiple bones and are referred to radiologically as dysostosis multiplex. Umbilical or inguinal hernias may occur.

Investigations

• Each type of MPS has a characteristic pattern of urinary glycosaminoglycans (GAGs). Screening consists of analysis of urine for excretion of the GAGs. However, false-negative results can occur, especially in MPS II, III, and IV. A more reliable method uses quantitative electrophoretic assay of GAGs in a urine specimen collected for 8–24 hours. Determination of enzyme activity in lymphocytes or fibroblasts must be performed to confirm the diagnosis.

Complications

• Limitation of joint movement may occur in MPS I-H, I-S, II-A, III, and VI. The severe forms may have macroglossia and hypertrophied alveolar ridges and gums due to accumulation of GAGs. Macrocephaly and scaphocephaly (increased anteroposterior diameter) can occur. Heart disease (affecting myocardium and/or valves), obstructive airway disease, hydrocephalus, and hearing loss may also occur.

Differential diagnosis

• A similar presentation may be seen with oligosaccharidoses, GM_1 gangliosidosis, mucolipidoses, and multiple sulfatase deficiency. The skeletal anomalies in MPS type IV are similar to those in spondyloepiphyseal dysplasia. Coarse facial features, macroglossia, developmental delay, obstructive airway disease, and umbilical hernia can also occur in congenital hypothyroidism, but affected individuals generally have signs and symptoms in the first few months of life and may have neonatal feeding problems and prolonged hyperbilirubinemia. Coarse facies, joint stiffness, and a deep voice may also be present in Williams syndrome (due to a deletion of chromosome 7q11.23).

Etiology

• Deficiency in the activity of enzymes catabolizing the GAGs results in the accumulation of metabolic intermediates and resultant clinical and neurologic manifestations. MPS II is X-linked. All other MPS types are inherited as autosomal recessive conditions.

Classification, enzyme defects, and major clinical features of the mucopolysaccharidoses.

Eponym (number)	Enzyme Defect	Organ System Involvement			
		Corneal Clouding	Organomegaly	Skeletal Abnormalities	Neurologic Impairment
Hurler (I-H)	α-L-iduronidase	+	+	+	Severe
Scheie (I-S)	α-L-iduronidase	+	–	–	None
Hurler-Scheie (I-H/S)	α-L-iduronidase	+	+	+	Mild or none
Hunter (II-A)	Iduronate-2-sulfatase	–	+	+	Severe
Hunter (II-B)	Iduronate-2-sulfatase	–	–	–	None
Sanfilippo A (IIIA)	Heparan N-sulfatase	–	–	Mild	Severe
Sanfilippo B (IIIB)	α-N-acetylglucosaminidase	–	–	Mild	Severe
Sanfilippo C (IIIC)	Acetyl CoA: α-glucosaminide-N-acetyl-transferase	–	–	Mild	Severe
Sanfilippo D (IIID)	N-acetyl-glucosamine-6-sulfatase	–	–	Mild	Severe
Morquio A (IVA)	Galactose-6-sulfatase	+	–	Severe, extensive	None
Morquio B (IVB)	β-Galactosidase	+	–	Variable	None
V (no longer used)					
Maroteaux-Lamy (VI)	N-acetylgalactosamine-4-sulfatase	+	–	+	None
Sly (VII)	β-Glucuronidase	–	+	+	Variable

Plus sign indicates present; minus sign indicates absent.

Treatment

General information

• Treatment is supportive. However, the quality of life can be substantially improved with early diagnosis and treatment of the associated complications. Bone marrow transplantation (BMT) has been used in the last decade and seems to improve some of the somatic abnormalities in types I, II, and VI. The outcome varies with the type of MPS, the degree of involvement, and the age of the patient. The effect on neurologic outcome is not consistent. BMT may be beneficial in type I but does not prevent neuroregression in type III. In type I, BMT under 1 year of age and in type II BMT before 2 years of age seem to have better outcomes. However, long-term outcome is not yet known. Prenatal diagnosis is possible with all of the MPS types.

Prognosis/natural history

• Although survival is shortened in the severe forms, a normal life span may be achieved with MPS I-S, I-H/S, II-B, and the mild forms of VI and VII. MPS III has profound mental retardation but relatively few somatic findings. Conversely, MPS IV has severe somatic and skeletal abnormalities with secondary cardiorespiratory involvement. Intelligence is normal in this type. MPS VII is extremely variable and in the most severe case may present as neonatal hydrops.

General references

Hopwood JJ, Morris CP: The mucopolysaccharidoses: diagnosis, molecular genetics, and treatment. *Mol Biol Med* 1990, **7:**381–404.

Kaplan P, Kirschner M, Watters G, et al.: Contractures in Williams syndrome. *Pediatrics* 1989, **84:**895–899.

Neufeld EF, Meuzer J: The mucopolysaccharidoses. In *The Metabolic and Molecular Bases of Inherited Disease.* Edited by Scriver CR, Beaudet AL, Sly WS, Valle D. New York: McGraw-Hill; 1995:2465–2494.

Shapiro EG, Lockman LA, Balthazar M, et al.: Neuropsychological outcomes of several storage diseases with and without bone marrow transplantation. *J Inherit Metab Dis* 1995, **18:**413–429.

Wraith JE: The mucopolysaccharidoses: a clinical review and guide to management. *Arch Dis Child* 1995, **72:**263–267.

Diagnosis

Symptoms

Functional ("innocent") murmurs

• Patients are generally asymptomatic.

• Most common between the ages of 2 and 6 years, but also common in adolescence.

• Louder during times or illness, with anemia.

• No demonstrable structural heart disease or cardiac dysfunction.

Organic heart murmurs

• Due to structural or functional cardiac abnormalities, congenital or acquired.

• Although many have cardiac symptoms, some minor forms of heart disease are asymptomatic.

• Symptoms relate to patient age and location and severity of the cardiac defect.

• Younger patients may have feeding problems, slow growth, tachypnea, pallor, or cyanosis.

• Older patients may have changing exercise tolerance, dyspnea, chest pain, palpitations, dizziness, or syncope.

Signs

Functional ("innocent") murmurs

• Murmur is vibratory, generally localized to left lower sternal border in younger patients.

• Infants < 6 months of age may have murmur transmission to posterior lung fields

• Murmur takes on an ejection quality at the base (in older children and adolescents) but not in back.

• Second heart sound splits variably with respiration. No clicks or gallops heard

• Overall heart rate, blood pressure, and four-extremity pulses are normal for age

Organic murmurs

• May first present in infancy, especially if associated with outflow tract obstruction, ductal dependent pulmonary or systemic circulation, or with cyanosis; however, age at first diagnosis is quite variable, ranging from first year of life to teens and young adults, depending on the lesion.

• Most commonly due to a ventricular septal defect (VSD), although other common cardiac problems include bicuspid aortic valve, pulmonary valve stenosis, atrial septal defect, coarctation of the aorta, and patent ductus arteriosus.

• Systolic murmur takes on an ejection ("crescendo–decrescendo") quality with outflow tract lesions and atrial septal defects or a holosystolic quality with VSD or atrioventricular valve leakage.

• Diastolic murmurs should always be considered pathologic

• Murmurs that are audible in the back should always be of concern

• In general, organic murmurs are harsher than vibratory innocent murmurs

• Listen for valve clicks and especially for the presence of splitting and quality of the second heart sound! A widely split S2 suggests an atrial septal defect (ASD), whereas a narrowly split or loud, accentuated S2 suggests associated pulmonary artery hypertension.

• Always feel all four extremity pulses; femoral pulses need not be absent in coarctation of the aorta, just diminished.

Differential diagnosis

Systolic murmurs

Lower sternal border: innocent murmur, ventricular septal defect, atrioventricular canal defect, tricuspid regurgitation, mitral regurgitation.

Upper sternal border: innocent murmur, pulmonary stenosis, atrial septal defect, aortic stenosis, coarctation.

Posterior chest: pulmonary stenosis, ASD, coarctation, PDA, mitral regurgitation, large VSD, TOF.

Diastolic murmurs

Should be considered pathologic.

Early diastole (at the base): aortic insufficiency is best heard when erect; pulmonary insufficiency is best heard when supine.

Mid-diastole: "rumble" from an ASD, a VSD, or mitral stenosis.

Continuous murmurs

Should be considered pathologic.

Patent ductus arteriosus: best heard under left clavicle and in left posterior chest

Collaterals: heard in the back in a number of conditions, including coarctation and TOF.

Etiology

Functional murmurs: cause unclear, likely audible "flow" of blood through a normal heart; may be accentuated by anemia, fever, increased cardiac output, left ventricular "false tendons."

Organic murmurs: multifactorial causes: 1) genetic predisposition to congenital heart disease with trisomies, gene deletion syndromes; and 2) environmental predisposition to heart disease with certain drug exposures, infectious diseases.

Epidemiology

Functional murmurs: occurs in approximately 1:3 normal children.

Organic murmurs: congenital heart disease occurs in approx. 8:1000 live births.

Treatment

Investigations

Electrocardiography: should be "normal" for age in innocent murmurs, and may also be normal in some minor congenital heart defects. *Remember*: in infancy through approximately 6 months, the cardiac axis is rightward (90°–150°) with right ventricular dominance, after which the axis "normalizes" (0°–90°) with left heart dominance.

• A rightward axis (RAD) with right ventricular hypertrophy (RVH) indicates right ventricular (RV) and/or pulmonary artery hypertension; large VSD, ASD, atrioventricular canal defects; RV outflow obstruction (valvar, subvalvar or supravalvar pulmonary stenosis, tetralogy of Fallot [TOF]), severe obstruction to systemic circulation (critical coarctation, aortic stenosis or hypoplastic left heart syndrome).

• A leftward axis (LAD) for age (<90° in a neonate or <0° in any child) may be seen in some normal patients or patients with small VSDs. If voltage criteria for LVH are present, there is left ventricular dominance/hypertrophy (*Note*: in the neonate, this is highly suggestive of tricuspid valve atresia). If criteria for RVH are present, a primum ASD (incomplete AV canal) is likely.

Chest radiography: check for heart size and contour, pulmonary vascular markings and symmetry, aortic arch sidedness, and abdominal situs in relationship to cardiac situs. Cardiomegaly may be seen with large left-to-right shunt lesions, dilated cardiomyopathy, severe mitral or tricuspid regurgitation, aortic valve regurgitation, pericardial effusion, or chronic cardiac arrhythmias; pulmonary edema is due to limited left ventricular output due to either cardiomyopathy or severe left heart outflow obstruction.

• A right aortic arch may occur with TOF, truncus arteriosus, VSD, vascular ring, or complex single ventricle, and may have an association with Di George syndrome. If cardiac situs is discordant with abdominal situs, there should be high suspicion for congenital heart disease.

Two-dimensional and Doppler echocardiography: This test is safe and generally available in most hospitals but is expensive and may require sedation of young patients in order to obtain accurate results. A thoroughly performed two-dimensional, color, and Doppler examination can accurately evaluate the anatomy and physiology of most forms of congenital and acquired cardiac disease in children.

Cardiac catheterization: this invasive cardiac test is reserved for patients with significant structural heart disease for confirming diagnosis (pre- and postoperatively) and therapy (balloon valvuloplasty and angioplasty, coil and stent insertion, etc).

Diet and lifestyle

• With the exception of congestive heart failure due to dilated cardiomyopathy, no specific salt restrictions are necessary in childhood. After 2 years of age, a "prudent diet" that avoids excessive intake of fat calories is advisable for all children with and without heart disease and especially in those with a family history of hyperlipidemia.

Pharmacologic treatment

Functional murmurs

• No special precautions are needed.

Organic murmurs

• Except with isolated ASD, antibiotic prophylaxis against SBE is recommended.

• CHF symptoms may require digoxin, diuretics, afterload reduction

• Associated cardiac arrhythmias may require anti-arrhythmic medications

• Anticoagulants (aspirin, dipyridamole, warfarin) may be needed for prosthetic heart valves or in situations where cardiac blood flow is sluggish (cardiomyopathies, Fontan physiology, arrhythmias).

Treatment aims

• The goal of evaluation is either 1) to confirm that a child has a normal heart or 2) to identify children with cardiac abnormalities and provide appropriate management guidelines for their particular condition, thus avoiding worsening function of the cardiopulmonary system.

• In particular, try to normalize cardiac size and function and pulmonary artery pressure as much as possible.

Prognosis

Functional murmurs: excellent; may be "outgrown" over time.

Organic murmurs: prognosis dependent on type and severity of cardiac involvement.

Follow-up and management

Functional murmurs: none required.

Organic murmurs: timing of checkups and management (medical and/or surgical) depend on the type and severity of heart involvement.

Nonpharmacologic treatment

Interventional cardiac catheterization

• Certain heart lesions are successfully treated with catheter intervention (balloon dilation of pulmonary valve stenosis and aortic valve stenosis, balloon angioplasty of recurrent coarctation of the aorta [some centers also dilate native coarctation], balloon angioplasty, and stenting of branch pulmonary stenosis.

General references

Lehrer S. *Understanding pediatric heart sounds.* Philadelphia: WB Saunders; 1992.

Rosenthal A. How to distinguish between innocent and pathologic murmurs in childhood. *Pediatr Clin North Am* 1984, **31**:1229–1240.

Veasey G: Innocent heart murmurs in children. In *Moss and Adams' Heart Disease in Infants, Children and Adolescents*, ed 5. Edited by Emmanouilides G, Allen H, Riemenschneider T, Gutgesell H. Williams and Wilkins: Baltimore; 1995:650–653.

Diagnosis

Symptoms

Slowly progressive weakness, in most cases involving proximal muscles more than distal. The distribution and rate of progression of weakness depends on the subtype.

Duchenne: proximal weakness apparent by age 5–6, typically nonambulatory by age 12 and with respiratory failure by mid- to late adolescence; learning disability or reduced intelligence sometimes present; limited to males with rare exceptions.

Becker: proximal weakness apparent late in first decade, but progression slower and disability less than in Duchenne; limited to males with rare exceptions.

Limb-girdle: variable onset, severity, and progression of proximal weakness; typically much milder than Duchenne muscular dystrophy.

Congenital: weakness at birth, often with joint contractures; depending on subtype, central nervous system abnormalities may also be present.

Myotonic (adults): variable, slowly progressive weakness, distal greater than proximal.

Myotonic (children): severe, generalized weakness and hypotonia in infancy, often associated with mental retardation; occurs when the disease is inherited from the mother rather than the father.

Other syndromes: variable severity and progression; distribution as indicated by designation (fascioscapulohumeral, scapuloperoneal, oculopharyngeal).

Signs

• Findings vary according to subtype.

In syndromes of proximal weakness (especially Duchenne and Becker): findings include characteristic gait (excessive lumbar lordosis, wide base, "waddle") and Gower sign (child "climbs up his legs" when rising from seated position on floor).

Gradual muscle wasting.

Pseudohypertrophy of calves in Duchenne and Becker dystrophies.

Joint contractures: early in congenital muscular dystrophy and late in Duchenne and other types.

Myotonia (delayed relaxation, eg, of grip): in older individuals with myotonic dystrophy, but typically not in infants.

Hypotonia: in congenital muscular dystrophy and congenital myotonic dystrophy.

Evidence of muscular dystrophy in relatives.

Investigations

Serum creatine kinase (of skeletal muscle origin): is massively elevated in Duchenne and Becker muscular dystrophy. Lesser elevations are seen in other types.

Electromyography: shows myopathic changes. In myotonic dystrophy, myotonic discharges are present in older individuals, but may be absent in infants.

Muscle biopsy: shows myopathic changes, muscle degeneration (usually accompanied by some regeneration), and variable fibrosis and fatty infiltration.

Western blot analysis of muscle biopsy: in Duchenne and Becker dystrophies shows absent, reduced, or truncated dystrophin protein.

DNA analysis: currently has roughly 75% sensitivity to detect deletions in the dystrophin gene in Duchenne and Becker dystrophy, may obviate need for muscle biopsy, and may help identify carrier status. In myotonic dystrophy, DNA analysis shows expansion of unstable trinucleotide repeat sequence.

Differential diagnosis

Spinal muscular atrophy (spinal motor neuronopathies).

Other spinal cord syndromes, including syringomyelia, diastematomyelia.

Polymyositis.

Central hypotonia.

Etiology

• Duchenne and Becker muscular dystrophies are due to mutations (usually deletions) affecting the dystrophin gene on chromosome Xp.

• Myotonic dystrophy is dominantly inherited and results from excessive expansion of an unstable trinucleotide repeat sequence on chromosome 19p.

• Fascioscapulohumeral dystrophy is dominantly inherited and caused by a mutation affecting an as yet uncloned gene on chromosome 4q. Other muscular dystrophies are genetic in origin, and often show autosomal dominant inheritance with high penetrance.

• Merosin, a basal lamina protein, is deficient in some cases of congenital muscular dystrophy.

Epidemiology

• Duchenne dystrophy is the most prevalent variety, affecting roughly 1:4000 live-born males; one third of cases represent new mutations; Becker muscular dystrophy is roughly one eighth as common.

Complications

Scoliosis and other deformities: tend to occur in sedentary patients with muscular dystrophy.

Respiratory infections and failure: nearly always occur in Duchenne dystrophy and may complicate other types (especially congenital myotonic dystrophy); is attributable to weakness and restrictive disease (from scoliosis).

Gut and cardiac myopathy: may occur in Duchenne and Becker dystrophies.

Treatment

Diet and lifestyle

• Moderate exercise does not appear to hasten progression and may help to preserve function.

• Attention to diet is indicated to minimize the obesity which often develops in sedentary patients.

Pharmacologic treatment

• Prednisone (daily dose of 0.5 mg/kg; alternate-day regimens are significantly less effective) has been shown to slow the progression of weakness in Duchenne muscular dystrophy, and this option should be offered to families. However, it is often declined because side effects may be unacceptable given the relatively mild and temporary functional impact. A variety of other medications have been studied in controlled trials and afford no clear benefit.

• Mexilitene and other antiarrhythmic drugs can improve myotonia, but do not halt progression of weakness in myotonic dystrophy. Because mytonia is rarely disabling in children, these agents are seldom indicated.

Nonpharmacologic treatment

Physical therapy to limit contractures.

Bracing: including ankle–foot or knee–ankle–foot orthoses to improve ambulation and thoracolumbosacral orthoses (not always well tolerated) to slow progression of scoliosis.

Orthopedic surgery: including tendon releases and spine stabilization, to improve function and prevent progression of scoliosis.

Respiratory support: the degree of which should generally be determined by the desires of the patient or family.

Treatment aims
To preserve and maximize function.
To prevent or delay complications.

Prognosis
• Duchenne muscular dystrophy typically results in death late in the second decade in the absence of mechanical ventilation.
• Other types of muscular dystrophy are generally compatible with a long lifespan but varying degrees of disability. Patients with severe forms of congenital myotonic dystrophy, fascioscapulohumeral dystrophy, or congenital muscular dystrophy are also at risk for early death.

Follow-up and management
• Genetic evaluation is indicated to identify and advise carriers and reassure noncarriers.
• Regular follow-up in a multidisciplinary clinic is advised.

General references
Dubowitz V: *Muscle Disorders in Childhood*, edn 2. Philadelphia: W.B. Saunders; 1995.
Hilton T, Orr RD, Perkin RM, Ashwal S: End of life care in Duchenne muscular dystrophy. *Pediatr Neurol* 1993, **9:**165–177.

Diagnosis

Definition
• Inflammation of myocardium in association with myocellular necrosis.

Presentation
Mild to moderate congestive heart failure (CHF).

Severe CHF or shock.

Non-CHF: arrhythmia [1], sudden death.

History of prior gastrointestinal or flu-like illness.

Symptoms
Poor feeding or decreased appetite, shortness of breath or dyspnea, easy fatigability or general malaise: indicate CHF.

Palpitations with sensation of increased, irregular heart rate or skipped or hard beats; chest pain; dizziness, presyncope, or syncope; cardiac arrest/sudden death: indicate arrhythmia.

Signs
Tachycardia, irregular pulse.

Soft, indistinct heart sounds.

Mitral or tricuspid regurgitation.

Systolic murmur of atrioventricular (AV) valve regurgitation.

Tachypnea.

Rales: associated with pulmonary edema.

Hepatomegaly.

Hypotension: associated with shock.

Weak peripheral pulses.

Poor perfusion.

Jugular venous distention.

Pallor or cyanosis.

Investigations
ECG: low-voltage QRS complexes frequently present; nonspecific ST-T wave elevation or depression or T-wave flattening or inversion may be seen.

Chest radiography: cardiac size may be normal or enlarged; in severe CHF, pulmonary venous congestion and pulmonary edema are present.

Echocardiography (ECHO): used to evaluate left ventricular function. Left ventricular (LV) end-diastolic and end-systolic dimensions may be increased. Shortening fraction is diminished <28%. Global hypokinesis is common. Mitral insufficiency may be seen by color and pulsed-wave Doppler interrogation. Pericardial effusion may be present and indicates associated pericarditis. ECHO can be used to exclude other causes of LV dysfunction.

Radionuclide studies: ^{67}Ga scintigraphy identifies chronic inflammation and may show positive findings in myocarditis. This test has a high sensitivity but low specificity. ^{111}In-antibody cardiac imaging has a high sensitivity for myocardial necrosis but low specificity.

Laboratory studies: Erythrocyte sedimentation rate and CPK-MB (creatine phosphokinase of muscle band) fraction may be elevated. Rising sequential titers of viral neutralizing antibodies may suggest a viral cause. Positive viral nasopharyngeal or rectal cultures are circumstantial support.

Endomyocardial biopsy: these findings may be focal, necessitating submission of 4–6 specimens for histologic evaluation. Viral infection may be identified by new molecular techniques of *in situ* hybridization assays and polymerase chain reaction gene amplification to look for evidence of enteroviral infection.

Differential diagnosis
Cardiomyopathy.

Anomalous origin of left coronary artery from the pulmonary artery.

Left heart obstructive lesions: coarctation of the aorta, aortic stenosis, hypoplastic left heart syndrome.

Etiology
Bacterial, viral (enterovirus, coxsackie, echovirus, adenovirus), fungal, parasitic, autoimmune disease: systemic lupus erythematosus, rheumatoid arthritis, rheumatic fever, Kawasaki disease, and sarcoidosis.

Pathogenesis: in early stages, direct viral cytopathic effect results in myocardial necrosis. Later, an immune-mediated cellular injury occurs manifested by interstitial lymphocytic infiltrates.

Epidemiology
Autopsy information: myocarditis present in 16%–20% of children dying with sudden death [2]; 4%–5% of young men dying with trauma. Overall incidence of myocarditis in population in Myocarditis Treatment Trial is 9%. Myocarditis occurs in 1% of all enteroviral infections and 4% of coxsackie B infections. Ten percent of patients presenting with acute onset congenital heart failure after infancy have myocarditis.

Complications
Congestive heart failure secondary to LV dysfunction.

Ventricular tachycardia.

Sudden death secondary to ventricular fibrillation or complete heart block.

Cardiac arrest.

Treatment

Diet and lifestyle

• Limit vigorous and competitive sports activity until significant arrhythmias resolved for 6 months and LV function normalized for 6 months.

Pharmacologic treatment

Digoxin

Standard dosage	Digoxin, 30 μg/kg IV or 40 mg/kg oral total digitalizing dose (TDD) maximum dose, 1 mg. Initial dose, one-half TDD; second dose, one-quarter TDD; third dose, one-quarter TDD; maintenance, 10–15 μg/kg in 2 divided doses daily.
Contraindications	Relative: hypokalemia, hypocalcemia, renal failure.
Special points	Second and third doses may be given every 6–8 h and maintenance initiated in 8–12 h.

Diuretics

Standard dosage	Furosemide, 1–2 mg/kg every 6–12 h to 6 mg/kg/d.
	Aldactone, *infants and children*: 1.5–3.5 mg/kg/d in 2 divided doses; *older children and adolescents*: 25–200 mg/d in 2 divided doses.
Contraindications	*Furosemide*: hypersensitivity.
	Relative: renal failure, hypokalemia.
	Aldactone: renal failure; hypokalemia (both relative contraindications).
Special points	Aldactone: may result in hyperkalemia; should not be used in presence of hyperkalemia.

Afterload-reducing agents

• Used in patients with significant LV dysfunction.

Standard dosage	Enalapril, *infants and children*: 0.1–0.5 mg/kg/d in 2 divided doses; *adolescents*: 2–5 mg/d increased to 10–40 mg/d as tolerated in 1–2 divided doses.
	Captopril, *infants*: 0.05–0.3 mg/kg/dose every 6–8 h initially titrated to maximum of 6 mg/kg/d; *children and adolescents*: 6.25–12.5 mg/dose every 8 h; increase to 25 mg/kg/dose and by 25 mg/dose to maximum of 450 mg/d.
Contraindications:	Worsening renal failure, hypersensitivity.
Special points:	Lower dosage in patients with renal impairment, severe congestive heart failure. Administration in volume-depleted patients may cause severe hypotension.

Phosphodiesterase inhibitors, afterload-reducing agents (for severe CHF)

Standard dosage	Milrinone i.v.: Load, 25–75 μg/kg over 20–30 min; infusion, 0.5–1.2 μg/kg/min.
	Amrinone i.v.: load, 0.75 mg/kg over 2–3 min; infusion: 3–10 μg/kg/min.
	Nitroprusside, 0.3–10 μg/kg/min.
Main side effects	Hypotension, nausea, vomiting, abdominal pain, ventricular arrhythmias.
	Amrinone thrombocytopenia, hepatic toxicity.

Sympathomimetics and immunosuppressive agents

Standard dosage	Dopamine, 1–20 μg/kg/min; dobutamine, 2–20 μg/kg/min.
	Intravenous gamma-globulin [3], 2 g/kg over 12–24 h.
	Prednisone [4], 2 mg/kg/d in 2 divided doses.
Special points	Digoxin is usually not used in combination with sympathomimetics due to arrhythmogenic potential

---

Treatment aims

To treat symptoms of CHF.

To suppress arrhythmias, treat arrhythmia symptoms, prevent sudden death.

Other treatments

Antiarrhythmics: for ventricular arrhythmias or AV block.

O_2 or ventilator support: may be used when alveolar edema is present.

Pacemaker for complete heart block: temporary; used initially as AV conduction may return.

Heart transplantation, or extracorporeal membrane oxygenator or LV assist device while awaiting transplant.

Prognosis

• 70%–80% of patients have mild-to-moderate myocarditis with either no symptoms or moderate signs and symptoms of congestive heart failure; 70% of these recover completely, 10%–20% develop a dilated cardiomyopathy, and 10% progress to more severe disease, requiring transplant or dying. Of the 20%–30% presenting with severe CHF or shock, 60%–70% will recover, 10%–20% develop a cardiomyopathy, and 10% die or require cardiac transplant; 10% of patients present only with arrhythmias. Most of these recover, but some may progress to more severe arrhythmias or a dilated cardiomyopathy.

Follow-up and management

Regular office visits with ECG, periodic ECHO, chest radiography, Holter monitoring, and exercise stress test.

Key references

1. Wiles HB, Gillette PC, Harley RA, Upshur JK: Cardiomyopathy and myocarditis in children with ventricular ectopic rhythm. *J Am Coll Cardiol* 1992, **20:**359–362.

2. Drucker NA, Colan SD, Lewis AB, *et al.*: gamma-globulin treatment of acute myocarditis in the pediatric population. *Circulation* 1994, **89:**252–257.

3. Balaji S, Wiles HB, Sens MA, Gillette PC: Immunosuppressive treatment for myocarditis and borderline myocarditis in children with ventricular ectopic rhythm. *Br Heart J* 1994, **72:**354–359.

Neuroblastoma

Diagnosis

Symptoms

• Signs and symptoms depend on location and stage of disease at presentation.

Mass symptoms

Abdominal/pelvic: constipation, abdominal pain, fullness.

Thoracic/cervical (20%): respiratory compromise, Horner's syndrome.

Spinal cord compression: pain, paraplegia, bowel/bladder dysfunction.

Disseminated disease (common)

Fevers, bone pain, pancytopenia, skin nodules.

Paraneoplastic syndromes (infrequent)

Opsoclonus-myoclonus: "dancing eyes/dancing feet," cerebellar ataxia.

Vasoactive intestinal peptide secretion: profuse watery diarrhea.

Signs

Localized masses: palpable abdominal mass, adenopathy, thoracic mass on chest radiography.

Disseminated: "raccoon eyes"/proptosis from orbital tumor infiltration, organomegaly, skin nodules, bone lesions.

Miscellaneous: hypertension, failure to thrive.

Investigations

Imaging of the primary tumor site: plain radiography, CT scan, and/or MRI.

Diagnosis: must be confirmed by tissue histology from the primary mass (preferred) or from metastatic sites, including bone marrow (a compatible radiographic picture with elevated urine catecholamines is not sufficient for diagnosis).

Complete blood count: decreased hemoglobin, platelets, or leukocytes may suggest bone marrow infiltration.

Serum ferritin, lactic dehydrogenase, neuron-specific enolase: elevated levels are associated with poor outcome.

Urine catecholamines (homovanillic acid [HVA] and vanillymandelic acid [VMA]): spot urine analysis or 24-hour quantitation; elevated in neuroblastoma; can be used to follow disease progression/therapeutic response.

Liver function tests: may indicate liver involvement.

Staging tests: chest radiography (pulmonary metastases rare), bone marrow aspirate and biopsy, bone scan or skeletal survey, MIBG (radioiodinated metaiodobenzyl guanidine) nuclear scan (if available).

MIBG nuclear scan: very specific for neuroblastoma.

Complications

• Complications are related to the site of the primary tumor and the presence or absence of metastatic disease.

• Biologically aggressive advanced stage neuroblastoma has a 5-year survival rate of approximately 25%.

• The majority of children (approximately 60%) present with disseminated disease at the time of diagnosis.

Differential diagnosis

Depends on the site of primary tumor and disease stage.

Differential diagnosis of abdominal masses in children includes Wilms' tumor, other renal masses (non-neoplastic), germ cell tumor, constipation, enteric duplication cysts, and others.

Histology: the differential diagnosis for small, round, blue cell tumors includes neuroblastoma, lymphoma/leukemia, Ewing's sarcoma, primitive neuroectodermal tumor, and rhabdomyosarcoma.

Staging

• Staging is done using the International Neuroblastoma Staging System (INSS) and has stage 1 (localized and grossly excised) through 4 (disseminated/metastatic).

• Stage 4S is a special metastatic stage with favorable prognosis for infants — months of age with dissemination limited to the skin, bone marrow (minimal involvement), and/or liver.

Etiology

• Neuroblastoma is a malignancy of the peripheral nervous system, arising in neural crest–derived cells, which are primarily located along the sympathetic ganglia (paraspinal) and within the adrenal gland.

Epidemiology

8%–10% of childhood cancers, 15% of childhood cancer deaths.

Incidence: 1:10,000 children.

• Majority of children are diagnosed before 4 years of age.

• Localized tumors in younger children tend to be biologically benign, whereas advanced tumors occurring in children >2 years of age are likely to be biologically aggressive.

Neuroblastoma

Treatment

Pharmacologic treatment

• Patient evaluation and therapy should occur at a pediatric cancer center to optimize outcome.

• Treatment protocols (designed by collaborative groups) are based on risk stratification.

• Almost all patients will require surgery for resection and/or biopsy, whereas decisions regarding the use of chemotherapy or radiotherapy depend on the prognostic grouping.

• Low risk group: low stage disease (nonmetastatic) with favorable prognostic markers and 4S patients can achieve a >90% cure rate with surgery alone or surgery combined with a short course of cytotoxic chemotherapy.

• High-risk group: all non–4S metastatic disease patients, and those patients with localized tumors with unfavorable biologic markers and incomplete resections require intensive therapy. This includes dose-intensified multiagent chemoradiotherapy, followed by autologous bone marrow transplantation in many instances.

• Children <1 year of age with metastatic disease and favorable markers may not require as fully intensive a therapy.

Other treatments

• Many novel treatment options are being investigated in hopes of improving the outcome in children with high-risk disease.

• These options include monoclonal antibodies reactive against neuroblastoma-specific surface antigens, buthionine sulfoximine (BSO), desferrioxamine, retinoic acid, and newer chemotherapeutic agents.

• Refractory and multiply recurrent disease may necessitate palliative or supportive care alone.

Follow-up and management

• Posttherapy management is designed for two purposes: to evaluate for disease recurrence and to assess for toxicities incurred by the therapy.

• Patients are routinely assessed for recurrence by radiographic studies of the primary disease site, and by the evaluation of serum and urine markers, such as catecholamine excretion levels (VMA and HVA).

• Recurrences beyond 2 y off therapy are rare.

• Children receiving chemoradiotherapy will require long-term oncologic follow-up for side effects such as poor growth and endocrine disturbances, and assessment for organ dysfunction and other toxicities, which depend on the specific therapies used.

• Immunizations to prevent childhood diseases may be resumed after immuno-competence is restored following therapy.

Treatment aims

• The goal of treatment in children with low-risk neuroblastoma is to maintain the excellent overall survival while minimizing the potential side effects of therapy.

• By utilizing known risk markers, both biological and clinical, many children in the best prognostic groups may be spared chemotherapy.

• In high-risk patients, newer modalities are necessary as the survival rate with current therapy remains dismal.

Prognosis

• Age at diagnosis and stage of disease remain the most important.

• Obtaining the proper specimens for biological studies is critical to the appropriate risk stratification of these children.

Tumor histology: using the Shimada classification for "favorable" and "unfavorable."

MYCN gene copy number: amplification of the MYCN proto-oncogene (>10 copies) is strongly correlated with aggressive disease.

Ferritin, neuron-specific enolase and lactic dehydrogenase: elevated in poor-prognosis neuroblastoma.

General references

Evans AE, et al.: Successful management of low stage neuroblastoma without adjuvant therapies. J Clin Oncol 1996, 14:2405–2410.

Stram DO, et al.: Consolidation chemoradiotherapy and autologous bone marrow transplantation versus continued chemotherapy for metastatic neuroblastoma: a report of two concurrent Children's Cancer Group studies. J Clin Oncol 1996, 14:2417–2426.

Diagnosis

Symptoms and signs

- Diagnosis of neurofibromatosis 1 (NF1) requires two of the following seven criteria:

At least six cafe-au-lait spots greater than 5 mm in diameter (prepubertal) or greater than 15 mm (postpubertal).

At least two neurofibromas or one plexiform neurofibroma: generally do not present until after the first decade.

Axillary or inguinal freckling.

Optic nerve glioma: develops in 15%.

At least two Lisch nodules (iris hamartomas): may not be present until age 5 years, resent in almost all adults.

Distinctive bony lesion: such as sphenoid wing dysplasia or thinning of the long bone cortex, with or without pseudoarthrosis.

A first-degree relative with NF1.

- Other associated features include macrocephaly (even in the absence of hydrocephalus), mild short stature, delayed gross motor milestones, and mild mental retardation. The skin lesions may not be present at birth but are generally present by age 6 years. Neurofibromas and Lisch nodules usually are not present until adolescence.

- A few individuals have been reported with features seen in Noonan's syndrome who had large deletions in the NF1 gene.

Investigations

- Although brain MRI is not needed in the absence of symptoms, unidentified bright objects (UBOs) can be seen in some patients and may be confused with leukodystrophy. This finding is most likely caused by a glioma or hamartoma.

Complications

Tumors, including optic nerve gliomas (15%), meningiomas, schwannoma, neurofibrosarcoma (5%), and pheochromocytoma.

Scoliosis.

Segmental hypertrophy.

Seizures/abnormal electroencephalogram (20%).

Hydrocephalus.

Differential diagnosis

- A less common type of neurofibromatosis, NF2, is characterized by acoustic neuromas. It shows autosomal dominant inheritance and the gene is located on chromosome 22. Cafe au lait spots are not as prevalent as in NF1. Affected individuals are at risk for tumors such as neurofibromas, schwannomas, and intracranial tumors.

Multiple areas of hyperpigmentation can be seen in a variety of conditions, including Russell-Silver, multiple lentigenes, McCune-Albright, and Bannayan-Riley-Ruvalcaba syndromes.

Etiology

- Autosomal dominant inheritance with very high penetrance (clinical manifestation of the abnormal gene) but great variability of expression (specific signs or symptoms present in an individual). The gene, neurofibromin, is located on chromosome 17 and may act as a tumor suppressor. NF1 can be caused by point mutations, deletions, or insertions. DNA analysis is needed to detect mutations or deletions but cannot detect all abnormalities.

Epidemiology

- Frequency is 1:3500; ~50% of cases are due to new mutations.

Treatment

General information

• Treatment is focused on the complications of NF1.

• Regular monitoring is important for early detection of treatable problems. For example, spinal cord impingement and optic gliomas can be detected through annual neurologic and ophthalmologic examinations. Blood pressure should be monitored carefully because of the risk of pheochromocytoma. Assessment for learning disabilities should be performed if indicated. Psychologic and genetic counseling are important. Orthopedic intreatment for kyphoscoliosis and tibial bowing may be needed. The parents should be carefully assessed to determine if they show any manifestations of NF1 so that a recurrence risk may be estimated for future pregnancies.

Prognosis/natural history

• Most individuals have a normal lifespan and do not suffer significant morbidity. Some patients are diagnosed incidentally. There is great clinical variability between affected persons, even within a family. The degree of involvement in one family member is not predictive of the severity of another affected family member. Although the frequency of mild mental retardation and learning disabilities seems to be higher in affected individuals compared with the general population, the precise incidence has not been determined.

General references

Korf BR: Diagnostic outcome in children with multiple cafe au lait spots. *Pediatrics* 1992, 90:924–927.

Mouridsen SE, Sorensen SA: Psychological aspects of von Recklinghausen neurofibromatosis (NF1). *J Med Genet* 1995, 32:921–924.

Shen MH, Harper PS, Upadhyaya M: Molecular genetics of neurofibromatosis type 1 (NF1). *J Med Genet* 1996, 33:2–7.

Leppig KA, Kaplan P, Viskochil D, et al.: Familial NF1 contiguous gene deletions: cosegregation with distinctive facial features and early onset of cutaneous neurofibromas. *Am J Med Genet*, in press.

Stumpf DA, Alksne JF, Annegers JF, et al.: Neurofibromatosis Conference Statement. *Arch Neurol* 1988, 45:575–578.

Diagnosis

Diagnosis

- Childhood neutropenias are either congenital (cyclic, Kostmann, Schwachman-Diamond syndrome, chronic benign neutropenia of childhood) or acquired (autoimmune, drug-induced, viral suppression, systemic lupus erythematosus, HIV).

Signs

- Many patients have no obvious symptoms. Neutropenia is detected on complete blood count (CBC) performed as part of the laboratory evaluation for infection or for unrelated complaint.

Red, swollen gums.

Skin infection.

Fever.

Pneumonia.

Symptoms

Skin infections (pustules, furuncles, carbuncles).

Swollen red gums.

Oral ulcerations.

Cellulitis.

Perirectal abscess.

Vaginal abscess.

- Kostmann syndrome, cyclic neutropenia, and Schwachman syndrome are associated with a propensity for severe infection. Despite absolute neutropenia, chronic benign neutropenia, and autoimmune neutropenia are usually associated with minimal risk for serious infections.

Investigations

General investigations

Complete blood count: the hemoglobin and platelet count are normal. The total leukocyte count may be normal or decreased. The absolute neutrophil count (ANC is calculated as follows: total leukocyte count x% neutrophils + bands = ANC) is <1000/μL. All cell lines may be decreased in Schwachman syndrome.

The CBC should be repeated to document persistent or cyclic nature of neutropenia.

Antinuclear antibody (ANA): neutropenia may be presenting feature of systemic lupus erythematosus (SLE).

Anti-HIV antibody: neutropenia is common with HIV infection.

Antineutrophil antibodies: to diagnose immune-mediated neutropenia (autoimmune neutropenia, SLE).

Special investigations

Bone marrow aspirate: assessment of morphology demonstrates no leukemic blasts and no megaloblastic changes. Neutrophil precursors do not mature beyond myelocyte stage in Kostmann syndrome.

Complications

Susceptibility to infection: severely neutropenic (ANC < 500)

- Schwachman and Kostman syndromes are rare autosomal recessive disorders of uncertain cause.

Differential diagnosis

Neutropenia may be a prominent feature in the following:

Aplastic anemia.

Megaloblastic anemia.

Leukemia.

Systemic lupus erythematosus.

HIV infection.

Hypersplenism.

Etiology

Congenital neutropenias

- Kostmann syndrome and Schwachman syndrome are autosomal-recessive disorders without known cause.
- Kostmann's syndrome is characterized by ANC <200/μL.
- Schwachman syndrome patients have ANC 200–400/μL and pancreatic insufficiency; may develop aplastic anemia.
- Cyclic neutropenia is an autosomal dominant disorder due to regulatory abnormalities of hematopoietic precursor cells. Neutrophil counts fall every 21 days.
- All three syndromes are associated with high risk of infection.
- Chronic benign neutropenia is poorly understood; the risk of infection is proportional to the degree of neutropenia.

Acquired neutropenias

Autoimmune acquired neutropenias: a common cause of neutropenia in infants and toddlers; the neutrophilic equivalent of ITP, splenomegaly may be present. Neutrophil antibodies are present on cell surface or in patient's serum.

Drug-induced acquired neutropenias: due to 1) suppression from indomethacin, phenylbutazone, penicillin, sulfonamides, phenothiaxines, cimetidine, and ranitidine; and 2) immune destruction in association with the use of ibuprofen, indomethacin, penicillin, phenytoin, propylthiouracil, quinidine, and others.

Viral suppression: the most common cause of transient neutropenia.

Systemic lupus erythematosus.

HIV infection.

Epidemiology

- Kostmann and Schwachman syndromes are rare autosomal recessive disorders of uncertain cause.

Treatment

Diet and lifestyle

• For serious neutropenia syndromes, when neutrophil count if < 1000/μL, all febrile episodes deserve evaluation by a physician with a physical examination, CBC, and blood culture. When < 500/μL, patient is admitted to hospital although prophylactic antibiotics are not recommended.

Pharmacologic treatment

For chronic benign neutropenia or autoimmune neutropenia

• No definitive treatment required.

• Patients with serious infections need reevaluation for another cause of neutropenia.

• Rare patients with chronic benign neutropenia or autoimmune neutropenia will require corticosteroids.

• Granulocyte colony-stimulating factor (G-CSF) has proven useful in autoimmune neutropenia patients with chronic infections.

For Kostmann syndrome, Schwachman syndrome, cyclic neutropenia

• Granulocyte-colony stimulating factors have been documented to increase neutrophil counts into the normal range in cyclic and Kostmann neutropenia. May work in Schwachman syndrome. G-CSF is started at 5 μg/kg, given parenterally. Patients require yearly bone marrow aspirations. Potential for transformation into myelofibrosis or leukemia.

• Granulocyte transfusions are reserved for treatment of culture-proven sepsis episodes.

Treatment aims

To aggressively treat infections associated with neutropenia.

To restore neutrophil count to normal range.

Other treatments

Bone marrow transplantation.

Prognosis

• The outlook for patients with Kostmann syndrome and cyclic neutropenia has improved with the successful use of cytokines to improve neutrophil counts.

Follow-up and management

• Patients with serious chronic neutropenia syndromes should be followed by a pediatric hematologist familiar with such rare syndromes. Those patients on cytokines require careful follow-up. Others require aggressive evaluation of febrile episodes and treatment of infections.

General references

Bernini JC: Diagnosis and management of chronic neutropenia during childhood. *Pediatr Clin North Am* 1996, **43**:773–792.

Curnette JT: Disorders of granulocyte function and granulopoiesis. In *Hematology of Infancy and Childhood*, edn 4. Edited by Nathan DG, Oski FA. Philadelphia: W.B. Saunders Co.; 1993.

Jonsson OG, Buchanan GR: Chronic neutropenia during childhood. *American Journal of Diseases of Childhood* 1991, **145**:232–235.

Osteomyelitis

Diagnosis

Symptoms [1,2]
• Signs and symptoms are related to age, location, and duration of infection.
Fever.
Bone pain.
• Neonatal symptoms vary (irritability, poor feeding, sepsis).

Signs [1,2]
Toddlers and young children
General appearance varies from nontoxic to highly toxic.
Point tenderness: in 50% of patients.
Limp/refusal to walk: lower extremity involvement in 50% of patients.
Limited joint motion: sympathetic joint effusion, joint extension, muscle spasm.
Erythema/edema: infection in periosteal region.

Infants
Multiple infection sites: not uncommon; pseudoparalysis limb.
Erythema, edema, and discoloration of limb: due to rapid invasion.

Investigations [1–3]
Laboratory studies
Complete blood count with differential: may be normal or show leukocytosis with mild left shift, thrombocytosis.
Erythrocyte sedimentation rate: elevated within 24 hours; slowly declines to normal within 3–4 weeks.
C-reactive protein: elevated within 6 hours; begins decline with appropriate treatment in 6 hours.
Blood culture: positive in 60%.
Bone aspirate: positive in 80%; invasive; risk of injury to epiphyseal plate; may be reserved for patients with radiographic findings suggestive of increased pressure within bone (*ie*, sequestrum); consider in patients with puncture wound to foot (higher incidence of *Pseudomonas* spp.).
Hemoglobin electrophoresis: patients with gram-negative osteomyelitis.

Imaging studies
Plain films: help to rule out malignancy and fracture.
Bony changes: take 7–10 days (*ie*, metaphyseal rarefaction, periosteal elevation, or new bone formation).
Soft tissue changes: present within 3–7 days (*ie*, muscle plane displacement, obliteration of intermuscular fat planes).
Bone scan: sensitive but not specific positive within 24–48 hours
MRI: expensive, requires sedation.
Helpful in spinal, pelvic, and chronic osteomyelitis.
Ultrasound: distinguishes between superficial cellulitis, soft-tissue abscess, and subperiosteal abscess.

Complications [1,2]
Complications increase with delayed diagnosis, inadequate treatment.
Growth disturbances: overgrowth, shortening, and angulation due to growth plate damage.
Septic arthritis: when metaphysis is intracapsular (*eg*, hip, ankle).
Dissection of infection to nonosseous sites; pathologic fractures.
Chronic osteomyelitis.

Differential diagnosis [1,2]
Septic arthritis.
Toxic synovitis.
Cellulitis.
Bone infarction (hemoglobinopathies).
Rheumatic fever.
Fracture.
Malignancy (leukemia, Ewing's sarcoma, metastatic neuroblastoma).

Etiology [1,2]
Hematogenous seeding (most common)
Bacteremia results in deposition of bacterium in metaphysis with migration through cortex to subperiosteal space.
Vascular compromise results in formation of sequestrum (dead bone).
Trauma may be precipitating factor.
Local invasion: contiguous infected structures.
Direct inoculation of bone: surgical or traumatic.
Most common organisms
Staphylococcus aureus, streptococci, group B streptococci (in neonates), salmonellae and other gram-negative organisms (hemoglobinopathies), *Pseudomonas* spp. (from foot puncture wounds), and *H. influenza* (decreasing in frequency).

Epidemiology [1,2]
Occurs in 1 in 5000 children <13 y of age per year.
Male:female ratio, 2.5:1.
Most common in infants and young children.
Predilection for metaphyseal area of long bones, especially lower extremities.

Treatment

Diet and lifestyle
• Not applicable.

Pharmacologic treatment [1,2,4]
• Key to definitive therapy is identification of organism.
• Empiric therapy consists of parenteral antibiotics to cover *Staphylococcus aureus*.

In infants and children
Standard dosage	Oxacillin, 100–200 mg/kg/d in divided doses every 6 h.
	Nafcillin, 100–200 mg/kg/d in divided doses every 4–6 h.
	Ampicillin, 100–200 mg/kg/d in divided doses every 6 h; based on ampicillin component.
	Cephalosporin, 50–100 mg/kg/d in divided doses every 8 h.
Contraindications	*Oxacillin:* allergy.
	Nafcillin: allergy; caution in patients with combined renal and hepatic impairment.
	Ampicillin: allergy; adjust dose in renal failure.
	Cephalosporin: allergy (cross-reactivity with penicillin allergy); caution in renal insufficiency.
Main drug interactions	*Oxacillin:* Ampicillin, Cephalosporin: none
	Nafcillin: may increase elimination of warfarin.
Main side effects	*Oxacillin:* allergy, GI symptoms, leukopenia, hepatotoxicity.
	Nafcillin: phlebitis, rash, bone marrow suppression.
	Ampicillin: rash in 5–10 d, interstitial nephritis, anaphylaxis, urticaria, hemolytic anemia.
	Cephalosporin: phlebitis, leukopenia, thrombocytopenia, elevated liver enzymes.

In neonates
Standard dosage	*Oxacillin, nafcillin:* age ≤7 d, weight <2 kg: 50 mg/kg/d in divided doses every 12 h.
	Age ≤7 d, weight >2 kg: 75 mg/kg/d in divided doses every 8 h.
	Age >7 d, weight <1.2 kg: 50 mg/kg/d in divided doses every 12 h.
	Age >7 d, weight 1.2–2 kg: 75 mg/kg/d in divided doses every 8 h.
	Age >7 d, weight ≥2 kg: 100 mg/kg/d in divided doses every 6 h.
	Cephalosporins: age ≤7 d: 40 mg/kg/d in divided doses every 12 h.
	Age >7 d, weight ≤2 kg: 40 mg/kg/d in divided doses every 12 h.
	Age >7 d, weight> 2 kg: 60 mg/kg/d in divided doses every 8 h.
Contraindications	Same as for infants and children.
Main drug interactions	Same as for infants and children.
Major side effects	Same as for infants and children.

• Therapy should last a minimum of 4 wk—i.v. therapy for 5–7 d followed by home i.v. or p.o. therapy.

Treatment aims [1,2]
To eradicate infection and prevent further tissue destruction.

Other treatments [1,2]
Surgical debridement is required in conjunction with antibiotics when pus is obtained on aspiration, presence of a local abscess or intramedullary debris/sequestra, or failure to improve in 48 h. The use of oral antibiotics is controversial and they are not recommended to initiate treatment; requires identification of organism, parent–patient compliance, adequate absorption from the gut, and close outpatient follow-up.

Prognosis [1,2]
Early identification and treatment generally result in good prognosis.
Neonates incur more epiphyseal plate damage, growth disturbances, and joint abnormalities.
Higher treatment failure rates have been related to shortened treatment duration.

Follow-up and management [1,2]
Bony changes lag behind pathophysiologic changes, so radiologic changes may progress despite adequate therapy.
Physical examination and laboratory parameters used to confirm therapy adequacy.
Erythrocyte sedimentation rate and C-reactive protein should be monitored as an index of successful treatment.
Peak and trough serum bactericidal titers, renal function, and hearing function may require monitoring with the use of certain antibiotics.
Neonates should be followed for a period of 1 y for growth disturbances.

Key references
1. Sonnen GM, Henry NK: Pediatric bone and joint infections. *Pediatr Clin North Am* 1996, 43:933–947.
2. Roy DR: Osteomyelitis. *Pediatr Rev* 1995, 16:380–384.
3. Unkila-Kallio L: Serum C-reactive protein, erythrocyte sedimentation rate, and white blood cell count in acute hematogenous osteomyelitis of children. *Pediatrics* 1994, 93:59–62.
4. Barone MA (ed): Formulary: drug doses. In *The Harriet Lane Handbook*, ed 14. St. Louis: Mosby-Year Book, Inc.; 1996:486–592.

Pericarditis and tamponade

Diagnosis

Symptoms and signs

Pericarditis

Mild to severe precordial pain on inspiration or worse on inspiration: may radiate to neck and shoulders; worse on coughing, swallowing, or sneezing; improved by leaning forward.

Fever.

Pericardial, often pleuropericardial, coarse rub: best heard at left sternal edge with patient leaning forward; may come and go over minutes to hours, may decrease with development of effusion.

Pericardial effusion: varies from small to large.

Tamponade

Symptoms similar to pericarditis: pain, cough, hoarseness, tachypnea, dysphagia; malaise, cyanosis, dyspnea, sweating, anxiety.

Tachycardias.

Low blood and pulse pressures.

Pulsus paradoxus: exaggerated reduction (>10 mm Hg) of the normal inspiratory decrease in systolic blood pressure; pulse may disappear on inspiration.

Hypotension: accompanied by signs of low cardiac output (pallor, diaphoresis, poor perfusion with cool extremities).

Jugular venous distention: may increase on inspiration.

Hepatomegaly.

Muffled heart sounds.

Tachypnea.

Friction rub: heard with small to moderate effusions (may not be present with large effusions or tamponade).

Investigations

• For any pericardial disease, the underlying cause must always be sought.

Pericarditis

Complete blood count, erythrocyte sedimentation rate.

Antistreptolysin O titer, antineutrophil factor, rheumatoid factor analysis.

Cardiac enzyme tests: enzymes may be normal or increased, but creatinine phosphokinase of muscle band probably not significantly increased unless there is accompanying myocarditis.

Paired viral antibody screening: increase in neutralizing antibodies (up to 4 times) within 3–4 weeks of onset.

Mantoux test.

ECG: changes throughout all leads: raised ST segment, inverted T waves only in some patients, pericardial effusion (low-voltage QRS and T wave in large effusions), electrical alternans.

Chest radiography: normal unless pericardial fluid ≥250 mL; cardiac contour may be globular, with no congestion in lungs.

Tamponade

Echocardiography: essential in any patient in whom pericardial fluid is suspected (eg, cardiomegaly on chest radiography with hypotension); right ventricular or right atrial collapse characteristic of tamponade [1] (see figure).

Complications

Relapsing or constrictive pericarditis, pericardial effusion, and tamponade: complications of pericarditis.

Hypotension, renal failure: complications of tamponade.

Differential diagnosis

Pericarditis: consider in children with chest pain and/or cardiomegaly on chest radiography, especially in the presence of fever; pneumothorax; pulmonary embolus.

Tamponade: cardiomyopathy or constrictive pericarditis.

Etiology

Causes of pericarditis

Infection: viral [2] (coxsackie, echovirus, adenovirus, influenza, mumps, varicella, Epstein–Barr virus, AIDS virus); bacterial (known as purulent pericarditis; [3] *Staphylococcus aureus, Haemophilus influenzae* type B, *Neisseria meningitides* are the three most common bacterial causes) tuberculous pericarditis; fungi, rickettsiae, protozoa.

Postpericardiotomy syndrome: more frequent after atrial septal defect surgery and Fontan repairs. May be seen after any surgical procedure. Associated with fever, malaise, anorexia and signs and symptoms of pericarditis or pericardial effusion.

Chyloperidium: may occur with congenital thoracic cystic hygroma or after congenital heart surgery.

Collagen vascular disease: juvenile rheumatoid arthritis, systemic lupus erythematosus.

Rheumatic fever.

Kawasaki disease.

Chronic renal failure: uremic pericarditis.

Hypothyroidism.

Malignancy: leukemia, lymphoma; intrapericardial tumors; radiation pericarditis (occur with >4000 cGy delivered to the heart).

Causes of tamponade

Any of the above, but particularly the following: cardiac surgery; viral infection.

Epidemiology

Viral pericarditis is associated with an antecedent viral infection in 40%–75%. Purulent pericarditis may be primary or secondary to pneumonia, septic arthritis meningitis, or osteomyelitis.

226

Treatment

Diet and lifestyle
• Bed rest or limited activity is recommended during acute inflammation and until symptoms have resolved.

Pharmacologic treatment
• Drugs are indicated for pericarditis with significant symptoms or effusion.
• Aspirin usually improves both pain and fever; a short course of steroids may be needed for large effusions.
• Specific treatment is needed for any related condition.

Standard dosage
Aspirin, 60–90 mg/kg/d every 3–4 h.

Indomethacin, 25–200 mg in 3 divided doses in older children and adolescents; increase by 25–50 mg weekly.

Ibuprofen, 30–50 mg/kg/d in 3–4 divided doses maximum, 2–3 g.

Prednisone, 1–2 mg/kg/d in 1–4 divided doses for 2–3 wk, then reduced depending on symptoms.

Contraindications
Aspirin: peptic ulceration, hypersensitivity.

Ibuprofen: hypersensitivity.

Indomethacin: peptic ulceration.

Prednisone: osteoporosis, history of gastrointestinal symptoms, active infection, tuberculosis, pregnancy; caution in renal or hepatic impairment.

Special points
Indomethacin: not generally recommended for children <14 y of age. If used, dose is 2–4 mg/kg/d in 3 divided doses. Maximal dose, 150–200 mg/d.

Main drug interactions
All: warfarin.

Ibuprofen: digoxin levels may increase.

Indomethacin: aspirin, steroids.

Prednisone: aspirin.

Main side effects
Aspirin: dyspepsia, nausea, vomiting, epigastric pain.

Ibuprofen: dizziness, dyspepsia, abdominal pain, hepatitis.

Indomethacin: gastrointestinal problems, including bleeding, headache, dizziness.

Prednisone: edema, hypertension, weight gain, seizures, psychosis, acne, glucose intolerance, hypokalemia, alkalosis.

Treatment aims
To prevent tamponade and cardiac arrest.
To alleviate symptoms.
To diagnose and treat underlying condition.

Other treatments
Purulent pericarditis: drain pericardium [4]. Treat with i.v. antibiotics for 4 wk. May require pericardial window or stripping or pericardiectomy [5].
Viral pericarditis: bed rest and anti-inflammatory agents.

Prognosis
Depends on underlying condition. Excellent for viral pericarditis with recovery in 2–4 wk. Constriction is rare.
• Mortality of purulent pericarditis is 25%–75%. Constriction common if window or pericardiectomy not performed at initial treatment.
• Surgical postpericardiotomy syndrome is self-limited, but may be acutely life-threatening if not diagnosed quickly.
• For tamponade, pericardial aspiration may be life-saving.
• As much fluid as possible should be drained.
• Recurrent effusions may need pericardiectomy.

Follow-up and management
• Regular clinical echocardiographic follow-up is necessary for patients with pericardial effusions until medication discontinued and process resolved.

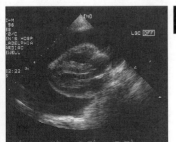

Large pericardial effusion surrounding heart.

Key references
1. Fowler NO: Cardiac tamponade: a clinical or an echocardiographic diagnosis. *Circulation* 1993, **87:**1738–1741.
2. Friman G, Hohlman J: The epidemiology of viral heart disease. *Scand J Infect Dis* 1993, **88:**7–10.
3. Feldman WE: Bacterial etiology and mortality of purulent pericarditis in pediatric patients. *Am J Dis Child* 1979, **133:**641–644.
4. Zahn EM, Honde C, Benson L, Freedom RM: Percutaneous pericardial catheter drainage in childhood. *Am J Cardiol* 1985, **55:**476–479.

Diagnosis

Symptoms

• Basic disease determines most of systemic symptoms. Patients may be asymptomatic until amount of fluid is large enough to cause cardiorespiratory distress.

Dyspnea, cough, fever, and pleuritic pain.

Signs

• Dependent on the size of the effusion; may be normal in small effusions.

Pleural rub: during early phase; resolves as fluid accumulates the in pleural space.

Decreased thoracic wall excursion, dull or flat percussion, decreased tactile and vocal fremitus, decreased whispering pectoriloquy, fullness of intercostal spaces, decreased breath sounds on affected side, trachea and cardiac apex displaced toward the contralateral side, tachycardia, tachypnea, shortness of breath, and respiratory distress.

Investigations

Chest radiograph: to determine the size of the effusion.

Upright films: anteroposterior projection can see >400 cm^3; lateral projection can see >200 cm^3.

Lateral decubitus films: can check for free-flowing pleural fluid; can see as little as 50 cm^3 of fluid.

Ultrasound: can diagnose small (>10 cm^3) loculated collections of pleural fluid; useful as a guide for thoracentesis; can distinguish between pleural thickening and pleural effusion.

Computed tomography scan: useful for defining extent of loculated effusions; visualizes the underlying lung parenchyma.

Thoracentesis: indicated whenever etiology is unclear or the patient is symptomatic.

Pleural fluid analysis: *see* table.

Sedimentation rate (ESR): to follow degree of inflammation and response to therapy.

Pleural biopsy: if thoracentesis is non-diagnostic; most useful for diseases that cause extensive involvement of the pleura (*ie*, tuberculosis, malignancies) confirms neoplastic involvement in 40%−70% of cases.

Complications

Hypoxia.

Respiratory distress.

Trapped lung (secondary to a constrictive fibrosis) with restrictive lung diseases.

Decreased cardiac function.

Shock: secondary to blood loss in cases of hemothorax.

Malnutrition: seen in chylothorax.

Pleural fluid analysis

Test	Transudate	Exudate
pH	7.4	<7.3
Protein, g/100 cm^3	<3.0	>3.0
Pleural/serum protein	<0.5	>0.5
Pleural/serum LDH	<0.6	>0.6
LDH, *IU*	<200	>200
Pleural/serum amylase	<1	>1
Glucose, *mg/dL*	>40	<40
Red blood cell count, mm^3	<5000	>5000
White blood cell count, mm^3	<1000	>1000
	(mostly monos)	(mostly polyps)

LDH—lactate dehydrogenase.

Differential diagnosis

Transudate

Cardiovascular: congestive heart failure, constrictive pericarditis.

Nephrotic syndrome with hypoalbuminemia.

Cirrhosis.

Atelectasis.

Exudate

Infections: parapneumonic effusions (*Staphylococcus aureus* is most common organism), tuberculous effusion, viral effusions (adenovirus, influenza), fungal effusions (most not associated with effusions; *Nocardia* and *Actinomyces* are most common), and parasitic effusions.

Neoplasms: uncommon in children; seen mostly in leukemia and lymphoma.

Connective tissue disease.

Pulmonary embolus: intraabdominal disease, subdiaphragmatic abscess, pancreatitis.

Others: sarcoidosis, esophageal rupture, hemothorax, chylothorax, drugs, chemical injury, postirradiation effusion.

Etiology

• There is normally 1−15 cm^3 of fluid in the pleural space.

• Alterations in the flow and/or absorption of this fluid leads to accumulation.

• Six mechanisms influence fluid flow:

1) increased capillary hydrostatic pressure.

2) decreased pleural space hydrostatic pressure.

3) decreased plasma oncotic pressure.

4) increased capillary permeability.

5) impaired lymphatic drainage from the pleural space.

6) passage of fluid from the peritoneal cavity through the diaphragm to the pleural space.

• Etiology is dependent on the underlying disease.

• There are two types of pleural effusion are described.

1) Transudate: mechanical forces of hydrostatic and oncotic pressures are altered favoring liquid filtration.

2) Exudate: damage to the pleural surface occurs that alters its ability to filter pleural fluid lymphatic drainage is diminished.

Epidemiology

• For empyema, major organisms include:

Staphylococcus aureus, 28%.

Streptococcus pneumoniae, 20%.

Haemophilus influenzae, 13%.

Treatment

Diet and lifestyle

• In general, no special precautions are necessary.

• If a chylothorax is present, patient's diet should include medium chain triglycerides as the primary source of fat for 4–5 weeks.

Pharmacologic treatment

• Treatment is dependent on the etiology; the underlying disease process must be adequately treated.

Antibiotics

• Antibiotics are administered depending on the organism identified and degree of illness

• Clinical improvement usually occurs in 48–72 h.

Staphylococcus aureus: 3–4 wk minimum.

Streptococcus pneumoniae: 2 wk minimum.

Haemophilus influenzae: 2 wk minimum.

• Patients should remain on i.v. antibiotics until afebrile. Complete remainder of therapy on oral antibiotics (usually between 2–4 wk total of i.v. and oral treatment).

Pharmacologic treatment

Drainage

Thoracentesis: for diagnosis and relief of dyspnea or cardiorespiratory distress.

Chest tube drainage: for large effusions; reduces reaccumulation; drainage of empyema.

fiberoptic thoracoscopy: to remove the pleural rind to aid with chest tube drainage; helpful if loculated effusions are present.

Open thoracotomy with rib resection: performed less now that fiberoptic thoracoscopy is available.

Decortication: symptomatic chronic empyema; relief of thick fibrous peal.

Pleurectomy: chylothorax, malignant effusions.

– Drainage should be stopped when patient is asymptomatic. Thick, loculated empyema requires prolonged drainage.

Treatment aims

To remove pleural fluid.

To decrease respiratory distress.

• Earlier intervention is associated with a better prognosis.

• Prevent long term complications, such as trapped lung.

Prognosis

• Prognosis is dependent on underlying disease process.

If properly treated for infectious etiology: excellent.

If malignancy: poor.

Follow-up management

• Clinical improvement usually occurs within 1–2 wk.

• Fever spikes may last up to 2–3 wk.

• It may take up to 6 mo for the chest radiograph to normalize, dependent on the extent and etiology of the effusion (serial films are helpful at following the patient's course).

• Pulmonary function tests will start to normalize as the underlying cause resolves; dependent on the extent and etiology of the effusion.

General references

Chin TW, Nussbaum E, Marks M: *Pediatric Respiratory Disease: Diagnosis and Treatment.* Philadelphia: WB Saunders Co.; 1993:271–281.

Mathur PN, Loddenkemper R: Medical Thoracoscopy: Role in pleural and lung diseases. *Clin Chest Med* 1995, **16**:487–496.

Pagtakhan RD, Chernick V: *Kendig's Disorders of the Respiratory Tract in Children.* Philadelphia: WB Saunders Co.; 1990:545–556.

Pagtakhan RD, Montgomery MD: *Kendig's Disorders of the Respiratory Tract in Children.* Philadelphia: WB Saunders Co.; 1990:436–445.

5. Rosa U: Pleural effusion. *Postgrad Med* 1984, **75**:252–275.

6. Rubin SA, Winer-Muram HT, Ellis JV: Diagnostic imaging of pneumonia and its complications in the critically ill patient. *Clin Chest Med* 1995, **16**:45–59.

7. Sahn SA: The pleura. *Am Rev Resp Dis* 1988, **138**:184–234.

8. Zeitlin PL: *Respiratory Diseases in Children.* Baltimore: Williams and Wilkins; 1994:453–464.

Pneumonia, bacterial

Diagnosis

Symptoms
Cough, fever, chest pain, dyspnea.
Abdominal pain, nausea, vomiting: less common.

Signs
Increased respiratory rate, grunting, retractions.
Dullness on percussion.
Crackles, abdominal pain, distention, dehydration.

Investigations
Chest radiography: anteroposterior and lateral.
Decubitus: if suspect effusion.
• *Note*: Chest radiograph resolution can lag behind physical findings.

To assess severity
Arterial blood gas: low PO_2, inversed PCO_2, decreased pH.
Pulse oximetry : helpful for O_2 saturation.
Complete blood count: white blood cell count >15,000 often found (<5000 can be associated with severe infection).

To assess cause
Blood culture: will be positive in less than 15% of cases.
Serology: cold agglutinins (mycoplasma).
Acute: convalescent titers for specific antibodies.
Serum stain and culture of sputum: usually difficult to obtain.

Complications
Respiratory failure.
Pleural effusion.
Lung abscess.
Pneumothorax.
Empyema.
Pneumatocele.
Bacteremia.
Sepsis.

Differential diagnosis
Viral pneumonia (adenovirus, influenza, para-influenza, respiratory syncytial virus, echovirus, coxsackie).
Fungal pneumonia.
Rickettsia and *Chlamydia.*
Tuberculosis.
Pulmonary sequestration.
Congenital heart disease/failure.
Atelectasis.
Sarcoidosis.
Cystic fibrosis.
Drug reaction.
Aspiration/inhalation of toxin or foreign body.
Collagen vascular disease.
Reactive airway disease.

Etiology
• Etiology is age-dependent.
Neonates
Group B *Streptococcus*, mechanically ventilated and gram-negative.
Ages 2 mo to 2 y
S. pneumonia.
Type B *Haemophilus influenza.*
Bordetella pertussis (unimmunized).
Ages 2–5 y
S. pneumonia.
Type B *Haemophilus influenza.*
Staphylococcus.
Age >5 y
Mycoplasma pneumonia.
Nosocomial in institutionalized children.
Anaerobic bacteria.
S. aureus.

Epidemiology
• Conditions that can predispose include:
Congenital anomalies (cleft palate, tracheoesophageal fistula, sequestration).
Congenital defects of immune system, sickle cell disease.
Cystic fibrosis.
Otherwise normal, healthy children, with younger children 2 y of age more susceptible.
• May follow epidemic of viral infections.
• Human transmission via droplet spread more common in winter.

Treatment

Pharmacologic treatment

Oxygen to maintain PO$_2$ >60 mmHg.

Oral or parenteral fluids to correct dehydration.

• Initial treatment with antibiotics is empirical.

• Oral antibiotics are appropriate in mild infection, parenteral if severe infection or if vomiting.

• Bronchodilator may be of benefit.

• Treatment is for at least 7 days.

Neonates (sepsis: infants >2000 g)

Standard dosage   Ampicillin, 25–50 mg/kg i.v. every 6 h.

Gentamicin, 2.5 mg/kg i.v. every 12 (0–7 d of age) to 8 (>7 d of age) h.

• After sepsis or meningitis is ruled out, the antibiotic regimen may be adjusted to the specific organism isolated and/or site involved.

Older children

Standard dosage   Empiric therapy until etiology established (especially in children <5 y old).

Cefuroxine, 100–150 mg/kg/d i.v. or i.v. divided into every 8-hour doses, *or*

Ampicillin, 150 mg/kg/d i.v. or i.v. divided into every 6-hour doses plus chloramphenicose, 50–75 mg/kg/d i.v. divided into every 6-h doses, *or*

Ceftriaxone, 50 mg/kg/d i.v. or i.v. once daily.

• The antibiotic regimen is adjusted according to organism isolated, resistance pattern, and types/sites of infection finally identified.

Outpatient

Standard dosage   Penicillin V, 25–50 mg/kg divided every 8 h.

Erythromycin, 20–40 mg/kg divided doses every 8 h.

Second generation cephalosporin or semisynthetic macrolides.

Clarithromycin, 15 mg/kg divided in doses every 12 h, or

Azithromycin, 10 mg/kg first day, then 5 mg/kg/d for 4 d.

Specific treatment

Mycoplasma: erythromycin.

Gram-negative pneumonia: must consider aminoglycoside.

Anaerobic: penicillin or clindamycin.

Prevention

• Prophylactic antibiotics and vaccinations for children at elevated risk (*H. influenza* type B for all children; pneumococcal vaccine for immunocompromised and sickle cell patients).

Treatment aims

To improve oxygenation.

To achieve rapid resolution.

To maintain nutritional support.

Prognosis

• Pyrexia usually resolves within 48 h of beginning antibiotics.

• Radiographic findings are slow to clear and lag behind clinical recovery.

• Prognosis is excellent in uncomplicated cases of Pneumococcal pneumonia, but longer recovery with other pathogens.

• Bacterial resistance and poor response to choice of antimicrobial requires reassessment.

Follow-up and management

• Patients should be seen routinely following treatment completion.

• Follow-up chest radiography indicated for child with recurrent pneumonias, persistent symptoms, severe atelectasis, unusually located infiltrates, pneumothorax, or effusion.

• Admit to hospital if 1) patient presents dehydration, hypoxia, or significant respiratory distress; 2) outpatient management fails (24–72 hours), or if 3) less than 6 mo of age.

General references:

Nelson JD: *1996–1997 Pocket Book of Pediatric Antimicrobial Therapy*, ed 12. Baltimore: Williams and Wilkins; 1996.

Peter G: The child with pneumonia: diagnostic and therapeutic considerations. *Pediatric Infect Dis J* 1988, 7:453–462.

Prober CG: Pneumonia. In *Nelson Textbook of Pediatrics*, ed 15. Edited by Behrman PE, Kliegman RM, Arvin AM. Philadelphia: WB Saunders; 1996:716–721.

Schutze GE, Jacobs RF: Management of community-acquired pneumonia in hospitalized children. *Pediatr Infect Dis J* 1992, 11:160–167.

Diagnosis

Symptoms

Coryza, cough.

Hoarseness.

Myalgias, malaise.

Fever: can be afebrile.

Signs.

Increased respiratory rate, retractions.

Wheezing or rales.

Decreased breath sounds.

• Signs and symptoms of viral pneumonia may be indistinguishable from that of bacterial pneumonia.

Investigations

Chest radiograph: anteroposterior and lateral.

To assess severity

Arterial blood gas.

Complete blood count: white blood cell count may be normal to elevated.

Viral diagnostic tests

Fluorescent antibody test for respiratory syncytial virus (RSV).

On nasopharyngeal secretions can perform antibody test for specific virus.

Tracheal aspirate culture.

Complications

Severe chronic respiratory failure.

Bronchiolitis obliterans.

Bronchiectasis.

Persistent interstitial lung disease.

Differential diagnoses

Bacterial pneumonia.

Chlamydia: 50% will have inclusion conjunctivitis.

Parasitic pneumonia.

Tuberculosis.

Drug reactions.

Aspiration or inhalation of toxin.

Reactive airway disease.

Etiology

RSV (very young).

Adenovirus.

Influenza A and B.

Parainfluenza 1, 2, and 3.

Cytomegalovirus.

Epidemiology

RSV common in infants.

More common in winter months.

Majority of pediatric pulmonary infections.

Congenital anomalies can predispose.

Treatment

Pharmacologic treatment

Oxygenation: to maintain $PO_2 > 60$.

Oral or parenteral fluids: to correct dehydration.

Bronchodilator: may be of benefit.

Antibiotics: may be used empirically as bacterial pneumonia can complicate viral pneumonias.

For RSV infection

Standard dosage   *In high-risk infant*: ribavirin, 6 g vial diluted in 300 mL preservative-free sterile water administered via small particle aerosol generator 12–18 h/d for 3–7 d.

For influenza infection

Standard dosage   Amantadine, 5–8 mg/kg in divided doses every 12 h.

Prevention

• RSV can be prevented with RSV immunoglobulin monthly beginning in Fall through Winter.

• Influenza can be prevented with an annual vaccination.

• Amantadine in above dosage can also be used as prophylaxis.

Treatment aims

To improve oxygenation.
Achieve rapid resolution of symptoms.

Prognosis

• Almost all children recover uneventfully.

• Worsening reactive airways, abnormal pulmonary function, or persistent respiratory insufficiency can occur in high risk patients such as newborns or those with underlying lung, cardiac, or immunodeficiency disease.

• Patients with adenovirus or concomitantly infected with RSV and second pathogen have a less favorable prognosis.

Follow-up and management

• Patients should be seen routinely following treatment completion.

• Patient admitted to hospital if dehydration, hypoxia or significant respiratory distress or very young.

• Children with suspected viral pneumonia should be placed in respiratory isolation.

General references

Brasfield, D: Infant pneumonitis associated with CMV, Chlamydia, Pneumocystitis, and Ureaplasma. *Pediatrics* 1987, **79**:76–83.

Steele, R: A clinical manual of pediatric infectious disease: approach to pneumonia in infants, children and adolescents. *Imm Allergy Clin North Am* 1993,

Diagnosis

Symptoms

- Patients may be asymptomatic.

Shortness of breath.

Dyspnea.

Cough.

Pleuritic chest pain: usually sudden in onset; localized to the apices (referred pain to shoulders).

Respiratory distress.

Signs

- Patient may be normal.

Decreased breath sounds on the affected side.

Hyperresonance to percussion on the affected side.

Decreased vocal fremitus.

Tachypnea.

Shortness of breath.

Shifting of the trachea away from the affected side.

Subcutaneous emphysema.

Respiratory distress.

Tachycardia.

Shifting of the cardiac point of maximal impulse away from the affected side.

Scratch sign: when listening through the stethoscope, a loud scratching sound is heard when a finger is gently stroked over the area of the pneumothorax.

Cyanosis.

Investigations

Chest radiography: to assess the extent of the pneumothorax; findings include radiolucency of the affected lung, lack of lung markings in the periphery of the affected lung, collapsed lung on the affected side, possible pneumomediastinum with subcutaneous emphysema.

Computed tomography scan: useful for finding small pneumothoraces; can also help distinguish a pneumothorax from a bleb or cyst.

Arterial blood gas: PO_2 can frequently be decreased (though pulse oximetry can obtain this information in a noninvasive manner); PCO_2 can be elevated with respiratory compromise or decreased from hyperventilation.

Electrocardiogram: may show diminished amplitude of the QRS voltage; in a left-sided pneumothorax, the QRS complex will be shifted to the right.

Complications

Pain.

Hypoxia.

Respiratory distress.

Tension pneumothorax: can develop rapidly and lead to hypercarbia with acidosis and eventual cardiopulmonary failure.

Pneumomediastinum with subcutaneous emphysema.

Bronchopulmonary fistula: either as a result of the pneumothorax or of the treatment.

Differential diagnosis

Pulmonary: congenital lung malformations (ie, bronchogenic cysts, cystic adenomatoid malformations, congenital lobar emphysema), acquired emphysema, hyperinflation of the lung, bullae formation, pleurisy.

Gastrointestinal: diaphragmatic hernia.

Infection: pulmonary abscess, post-infectious pneumatocele.

Miscellaneous: muscle strain, rib fracture.

Etiology

Spontaneous: usually secondary to the rupture of congenital apical blebs.

Trauma: from a penetrating injury (ie, knife or bullet wound) or blunt trauma (ie, auto accident).

Barotrauma: from mechanical ventilation, foreign body, mucus plugging (seen in asthmatics) or meconium aspiration.

Iatrogenic: ie, central venous catheter placement or bronchoscopy (especially with transbronchial biopsy).

Infection: most common organisms are Staphylococcus aureus, Streptococcus pneumoniae, Mycobacterium tuberculosis, Bordetella pertussis, and Pneumocystis carnii.

Bleb formation: complication of cystic fibrosis, malignancy.

Epidemiology

- Epidemiology is dependent on the underlying lung disease.

Spontaneous pneumothorax

Incidence: 5–10:100,000.

Male:female ratio: 6:1.

Peak incidence: 16–24 years of age.

Cystic fibrosis

Incidence: 20% of patients > 18 years of age.

Treatment

Diet and lifestyle
• No special precautions needed.

Pharmacologic treatment
Initial treatment: stabilization of the patient, evacuation of the pleural air (should be done urgently if tension pneumothorax is suspected) and treating the underlying condition predisposing for the pneumothorax (*ie*, antibiotics for infection; bronchodilator and anti-inflammatory agents for asthma attacks).

Nonpharmacologic treatment
For small, asymptomatic pneumothoraces: observation of the patient is indicated (many will self-resorb).

Oxygen therapy: should be used to keep $SaO_2 > 95\%$; breathing 100% O_2 can speed the intrapleural air's reabsorption into the bloodstream (especially useful for treating smaller pneumothoraces and in neonates).

Surgical management
Needle thoracentesis: useful for evacuation of the pleural air in the simple, uncomplicated spontaneous pneumothorax.

Chest tube drainage: for evacuation of the pleural air in recurrent pneumothoraces, complicated pneumothoraces, and cases with significant underlying lung disease; the chest tube should be left in until the majority of the air is reabsorbed and no reaccumulation of air is seen on sealing of the chest tube; this is usually 2–4 days.

Surgical removal of pulmonary blebs: pulmonary blebs have a high rate of rupturing with the development of a resultant pneumothorax; in patients with established pneumothoraces, the blebs should be removed or oversewn to prevent reoccurrence of the pneumothorax.

Pleurodesis: to prevent reoccurrence of a pneumothorax; the lung has its surface inflamed, which then adheres to the chest wall via the formation of scar tissue; pleurodesis is useful in cases of recurrent pneumothorax or if the pneumothorax is unresponsive to chest tube drainage (*ie*, in cases of cystic fibrosis or malignancy); pleurodesis can be done surgically (by mechanical abrasion of part of the lung) or chemically (chemicals such as tetracycline, quinacrine, or talc are used to cause the inflammation).

Other treatment options
• Chemical pleurodesis has the advantage over mechanical pleurodesis in that no surgery or general anesthesia is required; however, it is less effective than surgery (has a higher rate of pneumothorax reoccurrence), is not site specific (making future thoracic surgery more difficult), and can be very painful.

Treatment aims
To remove the pleural air with reexpansion of the lung.

Prognosis
For a simple, spontaneous pneumothorax: excellent.
For a tension pneumothorax: cardiopulmonary collapse can rapidly develop if treatment is not quickly instituted.
In cystic fibrosis: pneumothoraces are associated with increased morbidity and mortality.

Follow-up and management
• Symptomatic relief should occur within seconds of the air being evacuated.
• A bronchopulmonary fistula should be considered if unable to remove the chest tube without reaccumulation of air. Surgical exploration should be considered if there is no improvement after 7–10 days.

Risk for recurrence
Spontaneous pneumothorax
Thoracentesis performed: 25%–50%.
Chest tube drainage performed: 38%.
Cystic fibrosis
No drainage attempted: 60%.
Thoracentesis performed alone: 79%.
Chest tube drainage alone: 63%.
Chemical pleurodesis
Tetracycline administered: 86%.
Quinacrine administered: 12.5%.
Surgical pleurodesis: 0%.

General references

Jantz MA, Pierson DJ: Pneumothorax and barotrauma. *Clin Chest Med* 1994, **15:**75–91.

McLaughlin FJ, Matthews WJ, Streider DJ, *et al.*: Pneumothorax in cystic fibrosis: management and outcome. *J Pediatr* 1982, **100:**863–869.

Pagtakhan RD, Chernick V: *Kendig's Disorders of the Respiratory Tract in Children.* Philadelphia: WB Saunders Co.; 1990:545–556.

Schidlow DV, Taussig LM, Knowles MR: Cystic Fibrosis Foundation Consensus Conference Report on pulmonary complications of cystic fibrosis. *Pediatr Pulmonol* 1993, **15:**187–198.

Warick WJ: *Pediatric Respiratory Disease: Diagnosis and Treatment.* Philadelphia: WB Saunders Co.; 1993:575–578.

Diagnosis

Signs and symptoms

Alcohols
Ethanol: inebriation, coma, respiratory depression, hypothermia, hypotension.
Ethylene glycol: inebriation, emesis, hyperventilation, coma, seizures.
Methanol: inebriation, emesis, blindness, hyperventilation, coma, seizures, papilledema.

Caustics
Oral sores; dysphagia; chest or abdominal pain, respiratory distress.

Hydrocarbons
Oral irritation, respiratory distress; lethargy, coma, seizures.

Pesticides
Carbamates, organophosphates:
Muscarinic: salivation, lacrimation, urination, defecation, gastric cramping, emesis (SLUDGE); bronchorrhea, miosis.
Nicotinic: muscle fasciculations, tremor, weakness.
Central nervous system (CNS): agitation, seizures, coma.

Plants
• Six different toxidromes predominate.
Gastrointestinal irritant (philodendron, diffenbachia, pokeweed, daffodil).
"Digitalis-like" (lily-of-the-valley, foxglove, oleander, yew).
Nicotinic (wild tobacco, poison hemlock).
Atropinic (jimson weed, deadly nightshade).
Epileptogenic (water hemlock).
Cyanogenic (many fruit pits and seeds).

Investigations

Alcohols (ethanol, ethylene glycol, methanol)
Serum glucose: to check hypoglycemia.
Osmolar gap: may be elevated early after ingestion.
Anion gap (and acidosis): will increase with metabolism.
Toxic levels of alcohols:
Ethanol levels >100 mg/dL cause intoxication; >300 mg/dL cause coma.
Ethylene glycol levels above 20–50 mg/dL considered dangerous.
Methanol levels above 20–40 mg/dL are dangerous.

Caustics
Radiographs: evaluate airway, lung parenchyma, and esophagus.
Endoscopy: confirms degree of esophageal injury.

Hydrocarbons
Radiographs: may demonstrate pneumonitis; findings may be delayed 8–12 hours; obtain radiographs if patient becomes symptomatic.
Oximetry (or blood gas determination): to evaluate oxygenation.

Pesticides
Cholinesterase levels: rarely helpful in acute management.

Plants
Serum chemistries: may demonstrate acidosis or electrolyte abnormalities.
Electrocardiogram: may show "digitalis-like" conduction delays.

Etiology
The most common nonpharmaceutical poisoning exposures (from reports of the American Association of Poison Control Centers): cosmetics, caustics/cleaners, plants, foreign bodies, hydrocarbons, insecticides/pesticides.
The most common pediatric nonpharmaceutical ingestion fatalities: hydrocarbons, insecticides/pesticides, alcohols and glycols, caustics/cleaners (including gun-bluing agents).

Household products with minimal toxicity
• Nonsuicidal ingestions rarely require medical intervention.
Air fresheners, ant traps, antiperspirants/deodorants, bar soap, bleach (household), bubble bath, calamine lotion, candles, caulk, chalk, crayons (US manufacture), white glue, fingernail polish, ink pens, incense, latex paint, magic markers, makeup, mascara, matches (<2–3 books), pencils, modeling/play clay, shampoos/conditioners, shaving cream, silly putty, suntan lotion, thermometers, vitamins without iron.

Household plants with minimal toxicity
Aster, begonia, bougainvillea, christmas cactus, coleus, corn plant, crab apples, creeping Charlie/Jennie, dahlia, daisies, dandelion, dogwood, fern (asparagus, birdsnest, Boston), gardenia, hens and chicks, honeysuckle, impatiens, jade plant, lily (day, Easter, tiger), magnolia, marigold, petunia, prayer plant, rose, spider plant, violets, wandering Jew.

Complications
Alcohols: hypoglycemia, renal failure, blindness.
Caustics: airway obstruction, esophageal strictures, perforation.
Hydrocarbons: pneumonitis is primary toxicity; camphorated, halogenated, aromatic hydrocarbons; metals (eg, arsenic); pesticides.
Pesticides: shock, coma, respiratory arrest, seizures, encephalopathy (delayed peripheral neuropathy may occur).
Plants: complication vary by plant category.

Treatment

Pharmacologic and technologic treatment

Ethanol

Standard dosage	*For hypoglycemia:* dextrose, 2–4 mL/kg D$_{25}$W.
Special points	Dialysis is rarely necessary.

Ethylene glycol and methanol

• Ethanol slows metabolism and prevents organ damage while awaiting dialysis.

Standard dosage	Ethanol, loading dose 750 mg/kg; maintenance dose, 150 mg/kg/hour.
Special points	May be given intravenously or orally.
	Dialysis: indications include osmolar gap > 10 mosm/L, acidosis, renal failure, toxic levels.
	Adjust infusion as needed to maintain ethanol level of 100 mg/dL.
	Folate, pyridoxine, and thiamine may enhance clearance of formic and glycolic acids.

Caustics

Decontamination: wash skin and eyes with water or saline.

• Emesis, lavage, and charcoal are contraindicated.

Dilution: water or milk, 10–15 mL/kg, may reduce injury.

Special points	Controversial treatment: prednisolone, 2 mg/kg/day for 3 weeks plus taper (aim is to reduce esophageal stricture formation). Sparse evidence suggests benefit in circumferential second-degree burns.

Hydrocarbons

Decontamination: to prevent dermal absorption through irrigation.

Special points	Antibiotics: reserve for patients with discrete signs of superinfection, not used empirically.
	Steroids: no proven value.

Other: therapy exists for the systemic toxicity of some hydrocarbons; the regional poison center can be useful in this regard.

Pesticides (carbamates, organophosphates)

Standard dosage	Atropine, 0.01–0.05 mg/kg (minimum, 0.1 mg; maximum, 1 mg); repeat doses to effect; large total doses may be required.
	Pralidoxime, 20–40 mg/kg, repeated every 6 h for 24–48 h. Some advocate continuous infusion.
Special points	*Atropine*: reduces bronchorrhea and eases respiration.
	Pralidoxime: reverses and prevents fasciculations, weakness, and neuropathy.

Plants

Decontamination: ipecac and/or charcoal may be of benefit.

Special points	Specific antidotes are available for some plant poisons.

Other treatments

Alcohols: 4-methylpyrazole is an experimental drug that blocks alcohol dehydrogenase. It shows promise toward use to prevent metabolism of methanol and ethylene glycol.

Treatment aims

Alcohols: to prevent or reverse hypoglycemia and acidosis, to prevent renal failure, and to prevent optic injury.

Caustics: to reduce corrosive injury, maintain airway, identify perforation, and to prevent late stricture formation.

Hydrocarbons: to support respiration, and to prevent or treat systemic toxicity.

Pesticides: to support respiration and circulation, to treat acetylcholinesterase inhibition, and to prevent neuropathy and weakness.

Plants: to maintain circulation and pH balance, to prevent dysrrhythmia, and to support other organ systems.

Prognosis

Alcohols: prognosis is excellent if diagnosis and treatment occur early.

Hydrocarbons: patients asymptomatic at 6–8 h are unlikely to suffer significant morbidity; pneumonitis may resolve quickly, or progressively deteriorate.

Caustics: First-degree burns rarely form strictures, second-degree burns form strictures in 15%–40% of cases, third-degree burns form strictures in >90% of cases.

Pesticides: persistent effects may include peripheral neuropathy, memory impairment, personality changes, and weakness; early use of pralidoxime may reduce long-term effects.

Plants: most species are nontoxic; some may be life-threatening.

General references

Glaser D: Utility of the serum osmol gap in the diagnosis of methanol or ethylene glycol ingestion. *Ann Emerg Med* 1996, **27**:343–346.

Goldfrank L: Hydrocarbons. In *Goldfrank's Toxicologic Emergencies*, ed 5. Norwalk, CT: Appleton and Lange; 1994:1231–1244.

Howell J, et al.: Steroids for the treatment of corrosive esophageal injury: a statistical analysis of past studies. *Am J Emerg Med* 1992, 10:421–425.

Litovitz T, et al.: Comparison of pediatric poisoning hazards: an analysis of 3.8 million exposure incidents. *Pediatrics* 1992, **89**:999–1006.

Sofer S, et al.: Carbamate and organophosphate poisoning in early childhood. *Pediatr Emerg Care* 1989, **5**:222–225.

Diagnosis

Symptoms

• Acute poisoning can present with a broad spectrum of symptoms due to the potential for multiorgan system involvement. Nausea, vomiting, headache, malaise, and change in neurological well-being are common.

Signs

Physical signs seen after poisonings may be grouped into common recognizable syndromes known as "toxidromes." Special attention should be given to mental status, vital signs, pupil size and reactivity, skin moisture and flushing, and bowel sounds.

Agitation/delirium: alcohols, amphetamines and stimulants, anticholinergic agents, carbon monoxide, heavy metals, local anesthetics, lithium, lysergide (LSD), marijuana, phencyclidine, salicylates, withdrawal.

Coma: alcohols, anticholinergic agents, barbiturates, carbon monoxide, and cellular-hypoxia agents, clonidine, cyclic antidepressants, hypoglycemic agents, lithium, opiates, phenothiazines, sedative-hypnotics.

Hyperthermia: anticholinergics, drug-induced seizures, phenothiazines, quinine, salicylates, stimulants, thyroid hormones, withdrawal.

Hypothermia: alcohols, barbiturates, carbamazepine, carbon monoxide, hypoglycemic agents, narcotics, phenothiazines, sedative-hypnotics.

Hypertension: anticholinergic agents, monoamine oxidase inhibitors, phencyclidine, pressors, stimulants.

Hypotension: antihypertensives, cellular-hypoxia agents, disulfiram, heavy metals, membrane-depressants, opiates, sedative-hypnotics, sympatholytics.

Tachycardia: acidosis, anticholinergics, cellular-hypoxia agents, nicotine, stimulants, and sympathomimetics, vasodilators.

Bradycardia: antiarrhythmics, beta-blockers, calcium channel blockers, clonidine, digoxin, membrane-depressants, organophosphates, phenylpropanolamine.

Hyperpnea: acidosis, cellular-hypoxia agents, salicylates, stimulants.

Bradypnea: alcohols, anesthetics, barbiturates, benzodiazepines, clonidine, narcotics, paralytics, sedative-hypnotics.

Miosis: alcohols, clonidine, narcotics. organophosphates, phenothiazines, phencyclidine.

Mydriasis: anticholinergics, LSD, sympathomimetics.

Investigations

Serum chemistries: consider checking for hypoglycemia, acidosis, and anion gap, electrolyte imbalance.

ECG: consider checking for dysarrhythmia or conduction delays (atrioventricular block, long QRS, bundle branch block, or long QT).

Toxic screens: urine for qualitative screening of drugs of abuse, serum for specific levels of drugs, including acetaminophen.

Other: special circumstances may indicate tests of liver or renal function, urinalysis, creatine phosphokinase levels, carbon monoxide or methemoglobin determinations, radiographs, osmolar gap calculations, and/or other select tests.

Differential diagnosis

• Poisoning may manifest in varied and unusual ways. Suspect poisoning when the history is suspicious, when many organ systems are involved, or when signs and symptoms are confusing.

Etiology

• Toddlers, through exploration, ingest drugs that are attractive and available, and are typically poisoned by one agent only.

• Adolescent poisonings result from intentional abuse or misuse, and are often polypharmacy.

Child-related factors: age, impulsivity, pica.

Drug-related factors: availability, attractiveness, child-protective closures.

Environmental factors: household composition, family illness and stressors.

Epidemiology

• Over 3 million poisoning exposures occur yearly in the U.S.

• Two thirds of exposures occur in children under 18 y; one-half of exposures occur in children under 6 y; less than 10% of poisoning fatalities occur in children.

Most common medication exposures: analgesics, cough and cold preparations, topical agents, vitamins, antimicrobials.

Most common pharmaceutical ingestion fatalities: iron, antidepressants, cardiovascular medications, salicylates, anticonvulsants.

Complications

Respiratory failure: a common out-of-hospital cause of death.

Altered thermoregulation.

Hepatotoxicity.

Hypoxia.

Hypoglycemia and other metabolic derangements.

Hypertension, shock, and cardiac dysarrhythmias.

Nephrotoxicity.

Rhabdomyolysis.

Seizures, short- and long-term neurological dysfunction.

Treatment

Diet and lifestyle

• Environmental control measures can prevent poisoning events.

Pharmacologic treatment

Initial life support phase

Airway: maintain adequate airway, check protective reflexes.

Breathing: ensure adequate oxygenation and ventilation.

Circulation: cardiac monitors, attend to blood pressure and perfusion.

Drugs: O_2; dextrose (2–4 mL/kg D_{25}W); naloxone (1 mg for central nervous system depression, 2 mg for respiratory depression).

Other emergent conditions: stabilize using pediatric advanced life support or advanced cardiac life support guidelines.

Decontamination

Standard dosage	Ipecac-induced emesis: 10 mL in 6–12-month-old babies; 15 mL in toddlers; 30 mL in adolescents.
	Activated charcoal, 1–2 mg/kg (first dose usually given with sorbitol).
Contraindications	*Ipecac:* neurologic deterioration expected; caustics, hydrocarbons, and abrasives; aspiration risk (neonates included); uncontrolled hypertension.
	Activated charcoal: decontamination strategy of choice for most ingestions; drugs not bound by charcoal include iron, lithium, potassium, cyanide, alcohols, hydrocarbons.
Special points	*Ipecac:* for first-aid at home; rarely used in hospital setting.
	Activated charcoal: at least 10:1 ratio of charcoal to drug is optimal.

Whole-bowel irrigation (polyethylene glycol solution)

Dose: 500 mL/h in children; 2 L/h in adolescents; start slowly and advance.

Possible indications: sustained-release drugs; metals; massive ingestions; drugs that form concentrations; body packers/stuffers.

Nonpharmacologic treatment

Gastric lavage

Procedure: left side down, feet elevated; large-bore orogastric tube (>28 F) lavage with normal saline aliquots.

Indication: dangerous ingestions, in first hour, when charcoal alone is believed to be insufficient.

Contraindications: most caustics and hydrocarbons require cooperative, or sedated, patient.

• A cooperative or sedated patient is required in order to perform lavage.

General references

Henretig FM: Special considerations in the poisoned pediatric patient. *Emerg Med Clin North Am* 1994, 12:549–567.

Litovitz T, Manoguerra A: Comparison of pediatric poisoning hazards: an analysis of 3.8 million exposure incidents. *Pediatrics* 1992 89:999–1006.

McGuigan MA: Poisoning in children. *Pediatr Child Health* 1996, 1:121–127.

Diagnosis

Definition

Polycystic kidneys

Many cysts in both kidneys.

No renal dysplasia.

Continuity from nephron to urinary bladder.

Autosomal recessive polycystic kidney disease: bilateral cystic kidneys and congenital hepatic fibrosis (CHF).

CHF: periportal fibrosis; ductule proliferation.

Symptoms

Enlarged kidneys.

Protuberant abdomen.

Hematemesis.

Signs

Neonate: oligohydramnios, respiratory distress.

Infant: large abdomen, hypertension, hepatomegaly, splenomegaly.

Adolescent: portal hypertension, systemic hypertension.

Investigations

In utero **ultrasound:** diagnosis by 24 weeks.

Renal and liver ultrasound.

Biopsies rarely needed.

Hemoglobin, leukocyte count.

BUN, creatinine, electrolytes.

Liver enzymes, bilirubin: usually normal.

Complications

Respiratory distress.

Hyponatremia.

Portal hypertension.

Bleeding esophageal varices.

Hypersplenism.

Hypertension.

Growth failure.

Chronic renal failure.

Cholangitis.

Differential diagnosis

Multicystic kidney

No continuity between glomeruli and calyces.

Kidney does not function.

Opposite kidney is normal, absent, or dysplastic.

Bilateral multicystic kidneys cause oligohydramnios.

Complications include infection, injury; malignancy rare.

Autosomal dominant polycystic kidney disease (PKD): 1–3:100,000 liveborns.

Rarely presents with clinical findings at birth.

Four percent with the gene have clinical signs by 30 y.

PKD1 on 16p13.3; PKD2 on 4q13–q23.

Patients present with enlarged kidneys, hematuria, hypertension.

Berry aneurysm rupture rare in children.

Etiology

Autosomal recessive.

Linkage to 6p.

Epidemiology

Prevalence: one in 1:10,000–40,000.

Male and female gender equally affected.

Progression

End-stage renal failure.

Portal hypertension.

Autosomal recessive and autosomal dominant cystic kidney diseases

Autosomal recessive	Autosomal dominant
Autosomal recessive polycystic kidney disease	Autosomal dominant polycystic kidney disease
Meckel's syndrome	
Jeune's syndrome	PKD1
Renal–hepatic–pancreatic dysplasia	PKD2
Glutaric aciduria type II	Tuberous sclerosis
Zellweger syndrome	
Carbohydrate-deficient glycoprotein syndrome	

Treatment

Diet and lifestyle
Avoid contact sports.
No dietary manipulation.

Pharmacologic treatment
Hyponatremia: furosemide.
Hypertension: angiotensin-converting enzyme inhibitor.

Nonpharmacologic treatment
Psychosocial support.
Genetic counseling.
Bilateral nephrectomies to allow weaning from ventilator.
Dialysis.
Renal transplantation.
Portocaval shunts.
Liver transplantation.

Bioethical issues
Bilateral nephrectomies and dialysis in neonatal period.
In utero diagnosis and abortion.

Treatment aims
To control blood pressure.
To manage renal insufficiency.
To control portal hypertension.

Precautions
Avoid contact sports.
Immediate admission for gastrointestinal bleeding.
Treat infections.

Prognosis
•Neonates may die from respiratory and/or renal failure.
•Among those who survive the first year, 75% survive longer than 15 y.
Patients can survive to the third decade.

Follow-up and management
Blood pressure monitoring.
Serum creatinine, electrolytes.
Hemogram for anemia, leukopenia, thrombocytopenia caused by hypersplenism.
Esophageal varices.
Genetic counselling.

General references

Fick GM, Duley IT, Johnson AM, et al.: The spectrum of autosomal dominant polycystic kidney disease in children. *J Am Soc Nephrol* 1994, **4:**1654–1660.

Gabow PA, Kimberling WJ, Strain JD: Utility of ultrasonography in the diagnosis of autosomal dominant polycystic kidney disease in children. *J Am Soc Nephrol* 1997, **8:**105–110.

Guay-Woodford LM, Muecher G, Hopkins SD, et al.: The severe perinatal form of autosomal recessive polycystic kidney disease maps to chromosome 6p21.1-p12: implications for genetic counseling. *Am J Hum Genet* 1995, **56:** 1101–1107.

Kaplan BS, Kaplan P, Rosenberg HK, et al.: Polycystic kidney disease. *J Pediatr* 1989, 115:867–880.

Kaplan BS, Kaplan P, Ruchelli E: Hereditary and congenital malformations of the kidneys in the neonatal period. *Perinatol Clin North Am* 1992, 19:197–211.

Qian F, Germino FJ, Cai Y, et al.: PKD1 interacts with PKD2 through a probable coiled-coil domain. *Nature Genetics* 1997, **16:**179–183.

Diagnosis

Symptoms

Lack of breast development in girls older than 13 years.

Lack of testicular development and pubic hair in boys older than 14 years.

Inability to smell; color blindness.

Signs

Short stature and absence of signs of pubertal development.

Low weight or excessive weight.

Unable to distinguish odors.

Small, firm testes in males.

Phenotypic features of Turner's syndrome females.

Investigations

History: to evaluate familial delay, anorexia, or chronic illness.

Serum gonadotropins and gonadal steroids: elevation of gonadotropins indicate primary gonadal failure and indicate need for chromosomal analysis. Low gonadotropins and low gonadal steroids can be found in hypogonadotropic hypogonadism and constitutional delay.

Ovarian ultrasound.

MRI or CT of head if suspicious of brain tumor.

Complications

Infertility in both primary and secondary gonadal failure.

Psychosocial maladjustment.

Differential diagnosis

Primary gonadal failure.

Secondary gonadal failure.

Constitutional delay.

Delay secondary to chronic illness.

Etiology

Turner's, Noonan's, and Klinefelter's syndrome: primary gonadal failure.

Kallmann's, Prader-Willi syndrome: secondary gonadal failure.

Idiopathic hypogonadotropic hypogonadism.

Brain tumors and brain tumor treatment: eg, cranial irradiation.

Anorexia nervosa.

Chronic illness: eg, cystic fibrosis, Crohn's disease.

Epidemiology

• Constitutional delay is the most common cause of delayed puberty and reportedly more frequent in males (but this may be due to selection bias).

Turner's syndrome: 1:2000 females.

Klinefelter's syndrome: 1:600.

Treatment

Lifestyle

None except as directed to illnesses, such as anorexia nervosa.

Pharmacologic treatment

• Constitutional delay in males treated with low-dose testosterone (50–100 mg of depot testosterone i.m. once a month for 3–4 mo).

• Primary or secondary gonadal failure is treated with low-dose estrogen or testosterone, with gradually increasing dosing concentrations with age.

• Progesterone is added to estrogen therapy once the girl starts menstrual cycles.

Standard dosage

Males: testosterone esters at 50 μg i.m. for 6–12 mo. Increase at 50-mg increments yearly until 200 μg i.m. every 2–3 wk at age 18 y.

Females: conjugated estrogen, 0.3 mg daily for 6–12 mo. Then increase to 0.625 μg daily. If menses begin, cycle for 6 mo with ethinyl estradiol (20 μg daily for 21 d of 28-d cycles). After 6 mo, add progesterone (10 μg for last 7 d of 21-d cycle, *ie*, days 14–21).

Treatment aims

To develop secondary sexual characteristics to complete adult maturation without compromising final height.

Prognosis

• The development of secondary sexual characteristics is extremely good.

• The treatment of infertility in patients with secondary hypogonadism is more problematic.

Follow-up and management

• Follow-up at 6-mo intervals to monitor clinical sexual advancement.

• Bone age should be monitored at 6-mo intervals to evaluate skeletal maturation.

Other treatments

• Gonadotropins or gonadotropin-releasing hormone is used to treat infertility in those patients with secondary hypogonadism.

General references

Kulin HE: Delayed puberty. *J Clin Endocrinol Metab* 1996, **81**:3460–3464.

Styne DM: New aspects in the diagnosis and treatment of pubertal disorders. *Pediatr Clin North Am* 1997, **44**:505–529.

Diagnosis

Symptoms

Breast development in girls younger than 7.5 years.

Testicular development and pubic hair in boys younger than 9 years.

Headaches, nausea, vomiting, seizures, visual difficulties.

Signs

Excessive growth and physical signs of pubertal development.

Excessive weight gain.

Excessive hirsutism, androgen-dependent hair.

Skin: café-au-lait spots.

Neurologic abnormalities: *eg*, loss of visual fields, papilloedema.

Investigations

History: to evaluate familial early adolescence, steroid exposure, past history of central nervous system injury or exposure to steroids (ingestion or topical).

Bone age: relatively normal bone age suggests premature adrenarche or premature thelarche as opposed to advanced bone age, indicating precocious puberty.

Serum gonadotropin (ultrasensitive): if in the pubertal range, suggests central precocious puberty; low gonadotropins suggest gonadotropin-independent puberty.

Gonadotropin-releasing hormone stimulation test: to confirm central versus gonadotropin-independent puberty.

Ovarian ultrasound: to evaluate ovarian cysts associated with precocious puberty (*eg*, McCune–Albright syndrome).

MRI or head CT: if suspicious of brain tumor

Complications

Short stature.

Psychosocial maladjustment.

Infertility in children with late-onset congenital adrenal hyperplasia.

Differential diagnosis

Premature thelarche or premature adrenarche.

Central precocious puberty.

Gonadotropin-independent puberty.

Etiology

Premature therlarche and premature adrenarche

End-organ sensitivity.

Central precocious puberty

Idiopathic or familial early adolescence (especially girls).

Past history of brain injury (eg, cerebral palsy, hydrocephalus, meningitis).

Brain tumors and brain tumor treatment (eg, cranial irradiation).

Hypothalamic hamartoma.

Hypothyroidism.

Late-onset congenital adrenal hyperplasia.

Gonadotropin independent puberty

McCune-Albright syndrome.

Male familial precocious puberty.

Steroid-producing tumors.

Chorionic gonadotropin-producing tumors.

Exogenous gonadal steroids.

Congenital adrenal hyperplasia.

Epidemiology

Girls: idiopathic or familial precocious puberty accounts for close to 90% of cases.

Boys: only approximately 50% are idiopathic.

Treatment

Lifestyle

• Children with precocious puberty appear older and expectations (both in school and societal) are often higher. It should be recognized that these children are emotionally and intellectually younger than their appearance.

• Children with sexual precocity must be protected against sexual abuse.

Pharmacologic treatment

• There is no treatment for premature thelarche and adrenarche.

Central precocious puberty

Standard dosage   Depot gonadotropin-releasing hormone analogue, 7.5–11.5 mg i.m. once every 21–28 days.

Gonadotropin-independent puberty

• Treat the primary cause, *eg*, prevent ingestion of steroids, remove tumor or treat congenital adrenal hyperplasia

• In McCune–Albright syndrome or male familial precocious puberty, testolactone (40 mg/kg/d) alone or in conjunction with ketoconazole (400–800 mg/d).

Treatment aims

To prevent early maturation from compromising final height and to promote psychological well-being during childhood.

Prognosis

• The prognosis for prevention of early sexual development and achieving relatively normal adult height in children with central precocious puberty is good, except for those patients with brain tumors.

• The treatment of McCune–Albright syndrome and male familial precocious puberty is less effective.

Follow-up and management

• Follow-up at 6-mo intervals to monitor clinical sexual advancement.

• Bone age should be monitored at 6-mo intervals to evaluate skeletal maturation.

• Repeat gonadotropin-releasing hormone stimulation tests repeated after starting treatment to be sure dose is adequate to suppress hypothalamic–gonadotropin axis. Gonadotropin-releasing hormone testing can be repeated if clinical findings indicate inadequate suppression.

• Pharmacologic intervention should be discontinued when child reaches appropriate age for pubertal development.

Other treatments

• Use no treatment if height predictions are reasonable and psychosocial adaptation is good.

General references

Merke D, Cutler G: Evaluation and management of precocious puberty. *Arch Dis Child* 1996, **75:**269–271.

Styne DM: New aspects in the diagnosis and treatment of pubertal disorders. *Pediatr Clin North Am* 1997, **44:**505–529.

Diagnosis

Symptoms

Cough.

Hemoptysis.

Dyspnea.

Wheeze.

Chest pain.

Fever.

Malaise.

Fatigue.

Abdominal pain.

Recurrent otitis media.

Chronic rhinitis.

Diarrhea and vomiting: especially in relation to milk ingestion.

Gastrointestinal bleeding.

Consequences of adenoidal hypertrophy (snoring, obstructive apnea, rhinitis).

Growth retardation.

• Subclinical episodes of intrapulmonary hemorrhage may occur without overt hemoptysis.

• Additional features associated with Heiner's syndrome (pulmonary hemosiderosis with sensitivity to cow's milk) include:

Signs

Pallor.

Tachypnea.

Tachycardia, heart murmur.

Decreased air entry, wheeze, rales, rhonchi, asymmetric breath sounds.

Hepatosplenomegaly: occasionally.

Digital clubbing: occasionally; later phase of chronic disease.

Investigations

Pulse oximetry, arterial blood gas.

Chest radiograph, CT chest scan.

Pulmonary function testing: restrictive pattern, but obstruction may be present; altered diffusion capacity.

Lung biopsy.

Bronchoalveolar lavage.

Sputum evaluation and/or early morning gastric aspirates.

Sputum culture.

Electrocardiography: myocarditis may accompany idiopathic form.

Complete blood count, reticulocyte count.

Coombs test.

Serum bilirubin, blood urea nitrogen, creatinine, complete urinalysis.

Iron deficiency evaluation (serum Fe, total iron-binding capacity, free erythrocyte protorphyrin).

Stool for occult blood.

Coagulation studies.

Total serum hemolytic complement (CH_{50}), C3, C4.

Quantitative immunoglobulins: IgG, IgA, IgM, IgE; IgA often elevated.

Evaluate for Heiner's syndrome.

Evaluate for Goodpasture's syndrome.

Evaluate for cardiac cause of pulmonary lesion: *eg*, mitral stenosis.

Evaluate for collagen vascular diseases presenting as pulmonary hemosiderosis.

Evaluate for concurrent celiac sprue.

Complications

Acute, life threatening intrapulmonary hemorrhage.

Chronic anemia: secondary to iron deficiency and chronic disease.

Cor pulmonale.

Restrictive lung disease.

Differential diagnosis

• Consider conditions associated with hemoptysis.

Upper airway bleeding.

Trauma (blunt or penetrating).

Foreign body.

Bronchiectasis.

Cystic fibrosis.

Pneumonia.

Coccidioidomycosis, blastomycosis.

Hemorrhagic fevers.

Paragonimiasis.

Lung abscess.

Aspergillosis.

Pulmonary embolus.

Multiple pulmonary telangiectasias.

Ruptured arteriovenous fistula.

Sickle cell anemia (infarction).

Bronchogenic or enterogenous cysts.

Mediastinal teratoma.

Bronchogenic carcinoma.

Etiology

• Pulmonary hemosiderosis is the result of recurrent bleeding into the lung parenchyma. Certain cardiac and collagen-vascular disorders may cause this disorder as a secondary condition.

• A working classification scheme for pulmonary hemosiderosis includes: Idiopathic pulmonary hemosiderosis. Idiopathic pulmonary hemosiderosis associated with sensitivity to cow's milk (Heiner's syndrome), without and without upper airway obstruction. Pulmonary hemosiderosis secondary to another disease process: cardiac disease (eg, mitral stenosis) causing chronic left ventricular failure; Goodpasture's syndrome; collagen–vascular disorders; chronic bleeding disorders and hemorrhagic diseases.

Epidemiology

• The idiopathic forms most commonly occur in childhood, rarely in later life. Clusters of cases among infants have been reported (toxin?). Familial occurrence is rare. Heiner's syndrome presents in infancy and childhood.

Treatment

Lifestyle management

Patients must adapt to chronic illness, potential life-threatening episodes and to possible delays in definitive diagnosis.

There may be dietary exclusion (*eg*, milk or other protein implicated by challenge).

Patient should avoid environmental irritants and allergens.

Pharmacologic treatment

For severe, acute hemorrhage (respiratory distress and hypoxemia)

Standard dosage   Methylprednisolone pulses, 1 mg/kg every 6–8 h; corticosteroid dosage usually is decreased after 3 d of pulse therapy; taper is tailored to clinical response, usually 1 mg/kg/d for an intermediate period; attempt to establish alternate-day H2-blockers and antacids to protect gastric mucosa.

Consider as initial concurrent therapy: Cyclophosphamide, 1 mg/kg every 6 h (pulmonary hemorrhage may be presentation of vasculitic disorder or Goodpasture's syndrome)

Special points   *Cyclophosphamide*: as noted or azathioprine (2–4 mg/kg/d) may be added later if plasmapheresis has been successfully used to control refractory acute bleeding.

For subacute presentations

Standard dosage   Prednisone, 1 mg/kg/d orally until remission, followed by alternate-day regimen, depending on clinical course.

• Intravenous immunoglobulin has been successfully used to treat an exacerbation (400 mg/kg/d for 5 d followed by same dose every 2 wk for 3 mo [1]).

Maintenance therapy

Oral prednisone: decreasing daily morning doses for 3–12 months to prevent recurrences and progressive lung fibrosis.

Inhaled steroids: may be useful.

Azathioprine: may be added as a steroid sparing agent if long term therapy is warranted.

Nonpharmacologic treatment

For severe, acute hemorrhage (respiratory distress and hypoxemia)

• Monitor in an intensive care setting oxygen

• Correct anemia with RBC transfusion

• Avoid fluid overload, monitor pulmonary venous pressure

• Eliminate milk from diet as empiric trial regardless of laboratory test results (milk-specific IgE or precipitins). If associated with remission, consider challenge to determine role as trigger.

• Treat iron deficiency

• The role of desferoxamine is not established.

• Address potential environmental issues (*eg*, toxin exposure).

Treatment aims

To manage acute bleeding episodes (mild to life-threatening).
To monitor for side effects of therapy.
To evaluate for primary disorders that may cause secondary pulmonary hemosiderosis.
To treat anemia.
To monitor disease progression (lung function).
To monitor for potential late appearance of collagen–vascular disease in idiopathic cases.

Prognosis

• Outcomes are varied due in part to diverse etiologies. Many idiopathic cases enter prolonged remissions. Progressive pulmonary fibrosis is possible. In secondary cases, the primary disease usually determines the outcome.

Follow-up and management

• Even after discontinuation of immunosuppressive drugs, patients should be monitored for progressive pulmonary disease (pulmonary function testing) and the appearance of collagen–vascular disease (physical examinations and laboratory monitors of systemic disease).

Key reference

1. Case records of the Massachusetts General Hospital: case 16-1993. *N Engl J Med* 1993, **328:**1183–1190.

General references

Levy J, Wilmott RW: Pulmonary hemosiderosis [review]. *Pediatr Pulmonol* 1986 **2:**384–391.

Pfatt JK, Taussig LM: Pulmonary disorders. In *Immunologic Disorders of Infants and Children*, ed 4. Edited by Stiehm ER. Philadelphia: WB Saunders Co.; 1996:659–696.

Streider DJ, Budge EM: Idiopathic pulmonary hemosiderosis. In *Current Pediatric Therapy*, ed 15. Edited by Burg FD, Ingelfinger JR, Wald ER, Polin RA. Philadelphia: WB Saunders Co.; 1995:154–155.

Diagnosis

Signs and symptoms

• The term *maculopapular* refers to a rash that has discrete erythematous, tan or pink lesions, that may be flat or slightly raised.

Common conditions associated with maculopapular rash

• Maculopapular rashes are common in pediatric patients. They are found in a range of different conditions, some serious and some trivial.

Scarlet fever: characterized by a diffuse erythroderma and a very fine papular or sandpaper-like rash. There should be some identifiable site for the group A beta-hemolytic *Streptococcus* infection either in the throat, nose, or in a skin lesion. In the classic case there may be circumoral pallor and an accentuation of the skin folds of the antecubital fossa (Pastia's lines). The tongue may also have a papular eruption in the form of accentuated papillae (strawberry tongue). Because scarlet fever is a toxin-mediated disease, there is often conjunctival infection.

Roseola infantum: generally occurs in children who have a fever for several days with no apparent source of infection; as the fever breaks, a diffuse maculopapular rash erupts. The causative agent is herpes simplex virus (HSV)-6.

Erythema infectiosum (fifth disease): is caused by parvovirus B-19 and appears as a mild systemic febrile illness. The child has a "slapped cheek" erythema of the face followed by a diffuse lacy macular rash on the extremities.

Rubeola (measles): has many varied presentations but the classic is a child with cough, coryza, and conjunctivitis accompanied by a high fever. At the height of the febrile response, a rash erupts over the face and spreads down the trunk. Reaction to the live attenuated vaccine may appear similar, although the systemic reaction is less.

Rubella: this disorder is all but disappearing, but is noted to have morphologic characteristics similar to a mild case of measles. Often there is posterior auricular and suboccipital adenopathy and the complaint of arthralgias.

Pityriasis rosea: is presumed to be caused by a virus and is characterized at the outset by a single ovoid scaly lesion (the herald patch) that is often confused with tinea corporis. The subsequent stage is marked by a diffuse papular rash with many small ovid silver lesions that lie in a "Christmas tree" pattern on the back and chest. There is mild pruritis.

Epstein-Barr virus (EBV) infection (mononucleosis): is often associated with a maculopapular rash (5%–15%), particularly erupting after the administration of antibiotics (*eg*, ampicillin). The rash is usually distributed on the trunk and proximal extremities.

Rocky Mountain spotted fever: is noted to have a maculopapular rash that appears on the wrists and ankles and then becomes more generalized and petechial. Other signs and symptoms include fever, headache, myalgia, and periorbital edema.

Kawasaki disease: is now the most common cause of acquired heart disease and must be diagnosed early in order to minimize cardiac complications. Syndrome includes high fever for 5 days, erythema of the lips, palms, and soles, conjunctivitis, mucous membrane lesions, and a maculopapular rash.

Syphilis: in the adolescent, secondary syphilis may appear similar to pityriasis rosea. Infants may have a diffuse maculopapular rash with involvement of the palms and soles.

Differential diagnosis

• The pattern of distribution, timing of lesions, location, and presence and sequencing of other signs and symptoms will help to determine the diagnosis and subsequently the proper therapy.

• Examine more than the skin. Look at mucus membranes, the oropharynx, the conjunctiva, and all other parts of the examination.

• Always ask about recent and chronically used medications and immunizations.

• Scarlet fever, measles, and Kawasaki disease are difficult to differentiate because they are toxin mediated.

Investigations

Throat culture or skin culture for *Streptococcus*.

Titers of antibody specific for measles or rubella or parvovirus.

Monospot or EBV titers for mononucleosis.

Venereal Disease Reseach Lab (VDRL) for syphilis.

• The finding of thrombocytosis is suggestive of Kawasaki syndrome. In Rocky Mountain spotted fever there is often thrombocytopenia and hyponatremia. Other laboratory tests may be ordered to support specific diagnoses.

Treatment

General information

- Treatment depends on the diagnosis.
- Other therapies will be indicated for symptomatic relief or specific therapy. Parents will often excessively wash the child who has a rash. This will lead to excessive drying of the skin and the production of iatrogenic dermatoses.

Scarlet fever: penicillin, 25–50 mg/kg/d divided in 6-hourly or 8-hourly doses for 10 days; local moisturizers may help dry and peeling skin.

Roseola, rubella, and erythema infectiosum: require no specific treatment, but the use of antipyretics and pain medications will help comfort the child.

Rubeola: measles may have serious complications such as pneumonitis, dehydration, and thrombocytopenia. Children with measles must be closely monitored often hospitalized for observation.

Pityriasis rosea: requires control of itching and local skin care with moisturizers.

Epstein-Barr virus infection: although there is no specific treatment for mononucleosis, some of the symptoms of mononucleosis, such as the pharygitis and upper airway obstruction, may be modified by corticosteroids, 1–2 mg/kg/d.

Rocky Mountain spotted fever: in minor form, may be treated with tetracycline, 40 mg/kg/d for children older than 7, or chloramphenicol, 50–75mg/kg/d for younger children. When there are signs of systemic infection or encephalitis, then treatment should be given intravenously along with hospitalization.

Kawasaki disease: when the diagnosis is suspected, treatment with intravenous gamma-globulin (IVIG) should be administered at a dose of 2 gm/kg i.v. aspirin should be given to achieve a serum level of 20—30 mg/dL.

Drug reactions: should be managed by stopping the offending agent; in some cases, administration of corticosteroids may be indicated

Treatment aims
To alleviate symptoms.

Other information
Drug reaction: may have a maculopapular rash with a number of different patterns. Some are associated with a serum sickness, eg, reaction with fevers, arthralgias, and hepatomegaly.

Nonspecific viral exanthem: many other viral infections have been associated with rash, including those in the enterovirus and adenovirus families.

Other conditions: there are some uncommon causes of maculopapular rash, including tinea versicolor, varicella (prevesicular), dengue, Gianotti–Crosti syndrome, and papular urticaria. These all have their own characteristic patterns of eruption and patterns of location.

General references

Jaffe DM, Davis AT: Rash: maculopapular. In *Synopsis of Pediatric Emergency Medicine*. Edited by Fleisher GA, Ludwig S. Baltimore: Williams & Wilkins; 1996.

Ruiz-Maldonado R, Parish LC, Beare JM: *Textbook of Pediatric Dermatology*. Philadelphia: Grune & Stratton; 1989.

Rash, vesiculobullous

Diagnosis

Signs and symptoms

Acute eruptions

Varicella: the vesicular lesions are often preceded by systemic symptoms. Small papular lesions start on the head and trunk and evolve into vesicular lesions that cover the body and can also be found in the scalp and on the mucous membranes. The skin is pruritic. The lesions erupt over a 3- to 4-day period and then crust. Reactions to the varicella immunization appear identical to those caused by the wild virus and erupt about 2 to 3 weeks after the immunization.

Herpes zoster: the vesicular lesions are often painful and are found in a dermatome distribution.

Bullous impetigo: the bullae and vesicles vary in size and usually cluster in one area. Often an insect bite initiates the process by causing a nidus for scratching and inoculation with bacteria.

Staphylococcal scalded skin syndrome (SSSS): the bacteria may reside in a skin lesion or in the nares or other locations. The staphylococcus toxin produces a diffuse erythroderma and then blistering and peeling of the skin. Peeling characteristically starts around the mouth. This usually occurs in children < 6 years of age.

Herpes simplex: this viral illness may cause a cluster of skin lesions with or without mucosal lesions being present. The vesicles are usually red at their base and are painful.

Stevens-Johnson syndrome: often induced by infectious agents or by drugs. There is an erythema multiforme that may blister and there is mucous membrane involvement in the mouth, conjuctiva, and genital mucosa.

Hand-foot-and-mouth disease: caused by coxsackie A-16 virus, which produces vesicular lesions on hands, feet, and on oral mucosa. Fever and other systemic symptoms are often present. Other viruses and *Mycoplasma pneumoniae* may produce similar patterns of illness.

Drug-induced toxic epidermal necrolysis (TEN): may appear very similar to SSSS but can be differentiated by the level of blister formation on the skin biopsy.

System lupus erythematosus (SLE): the skin lesions of SLE are very variable and one form is a blistering lesion. Other systemic signs and symptoms are usually present.

Contact dermatitis: the prototype is poison ivy or rhus dermatitis, in which there are small vesicles filled with honey-colored fluid. They are often pruritic and, in the case of rhus, distributed in a linear pattern.

• Other rare conditions include blistering forms of Henoch-Schönlein purpura, syphilis, Kawasaki syndrome, insect bites, and friction blisters. These entities are all recognized by other signs and symptoms.

Chronic eruptions

Epidermolysis bullosa: this congenital condition manifests as blisters that occur in areas of the skin that are traumatized by rubbing or contact; hands and feet are common locations; disease ranges from minor peeling of the hands and feet to life-threatening forms.

Incontinentia pigmenti: effects girls and appears as a linear row of blister lesions in young infants; later, other changes occur in the form of whirls of hyperpigmentation.

Urticaria pigmenti: blistering lesions caused by mast cells in the peripheral extremities.

Dyshidrotic eczema: small recurrent crops of blistering skin on the palms and soles and adjacent areas of skin of atopic individuals.

Investigations

• If an infectious cause is suspected, cultures of the fluid within a bulla may be helpful. When considering herpetic lesions, a Tzanck smear showing multinucleated giant cells is supportive of the diagnosis. Ultimately, a skin biopsy may be necessary to determine the layer of blistering in the involved lesions.

Differential diagnosis

• Children who have vesiculobullous eruptions should be evaluated for a number of possible conditions: some acquired and some congenital.

• Determine the size, location, pattern of eruption, and pattern of distribution of the lesions. Also determine if there are other systemic signs and symptoms at the time, including fever, malaise, itching, pain, or other symptoms.

• Determine any ingestion or topical exposure to drugs or chemicals or other agents.

• Examine the entire body, paying attention to the mucous membranes, underlying nonbullous skin, the palms and soles.

Treatment

General information

Varicella: treatment involves control of fever with acetaminophen; avoidance of aspirin, use of antipruritics such as oatmeal baths and diphenhydramine, 5 mg/kg/day. Avoid concomitant use of topical and oral diphenhydramine.

Herpes zoster: may be treated with acyclovir and good pain control.

Bullous impetigo: may be treated with topical mupirocin 3 times daily if the lesions are few or with oral antibiotics, *eg*, cefadroxil, 30mg/kg/day divided every 12 hours for 10 days.

Staphylococcal scalded skin syndrome: children with this condition are usually admitted to the hospital and treated with i.v. oxacillin, 150 mg/kg/day divided every 6 hours; local skin care is important as there may be large area of skin loss and the possibility of fluid and electrolyte disturbances.

Herpes simplex: may be treated with topical acyclovir or i.v. acyclovir, 15 mg/kg/day every 8 hours for 5–7 days and good pain control. Be cautious regarding lesions in the genital area, which may have been sexually transmitted and thus child sexual abuse procedures must be followed.

Other conditions: require prompt referral to a dermatologist for more specialized diagnostic procedures and treatment.

Drugs: drugs that are possible etiologic agents must be stopped as soon as possible.

Heat or cold exposure: causes some bullous lesions; these must be treated according to protocols for burns or frostbite.

Treatment aims
To alleviate symptoms.

General references

Eichenfield LF, Honig PJ: Blistering disorders in children. *Pediatr Clin North Am* 1991, **38:**959–968.

Honig PJ: Rash, vesiculobullous. In *Synopsis of Pediatric Emergency Medicine*. Edited by Fleisher GA, Ludwig S. Baltimore: Williams & Wilkins; 1996.

Schachner L, Press S: Vesicular, bullous and pustular disorders of infants and children. *Pediatr Clin North Am* 1983, **30:**609–629.

Diagnosis

Symptoms and Signs

Humoral (B-cell) immunodeficiency.
Cough, chest pain, sputum production, fever.
Headache, fever, purulent nasal discharge.
Earache, fever.
Joint pain, swelling.
Headache, meningismus, mental status changes.
Nausea, vomiting, abdominal cramping, diarrhea.
Cell-mediated (T-cell) immunodeficiency.
Skin rashes.
Failure to thrive.
Fever, acute and "fever of unknown origin."
Sepsis.
Skin infections, pyoderma.
Headache, meningismus, mental status changes.
Collagen vascular disorders.
Phagocyte disorders.
Complement deficiency.
• *See* Granulomatous disease, chronic (CGD), Hyperimmunoglobulinemia E syndrome, immunodeficiency, severe combined.

Investigations

Initial history: include gestational and birth history; immunizations; age of onset; number, type, and course of infections with both normal or unusual organisms; autoimmune phenomena; past surgical history (note histology).
Detailed physical examination.
Screening laboratory evaluation for immune functions.
Complete blood count.
Antibody response to vaccines.
Total hemolytic complement (CH_{50}) activity.
Cultures, radiologic studies, erythrocyte sedimentation rate.
Evaluate for allergy, malabsorption, malnutrition, metabolic disease (*eg,* cystic fibrosis), autoimmune disorders.
Chest radiograph.
Detailed evaluation of specific immune system components.
IgG subclass quantitation.
Histology (B-cells, plasma cells).
Serum protein electrophoresis.
In vitro antibody production.
Mutation analysis.
Delayed hypersensitivity skin tests: tetanus, candida, trichophyton, mumps.
Enumerate circulating T-cells (flow cytometry: CD2, CD3, CD4, CD8).
Enzyme activity analysis.
In vitro T-cell activation.
Biopsy: bone marrow, thymus, lymph node, skin, gastrointestinal.
Chromosome analysis.
HL-A typing.
Natural killer cell enumeration and functional assays.
Detection of circulating immune complexes.
Assessment for collagen-vascular disorders.
Evaluation of oxidative metabolism.

Complications

Persistent infections.	Chronic lung disease.
Overwhelming infections, death.	Chronic liver disease.
CGD.	Periodontal disease.
Collagen vascular disorders.	Growth retardation.
Adverse reactions to vaccines.	

Differential diagnosis

• Primary immunodeficiencies are rare. Recurrent upper respiratory infections in 1–6 year olds.
Allergic disorders: recurrent sinusitis more often due to combination of natural infection/allergic inflammation/anatomic obstruction; asthma may pose as a recurrent pneumonia or bronchitis.
Immaturity of immune system in neonates.
Disorders with increased susceptibility to infections
Circulatory disorders.
Obstructive disorders.
Ciliary defects.
Interruption of skin (burns, eczema) or mucosa (trauma, sinus tracts).
Foreign bodies, aspiration, implanted devices.
Bacterial overgrowth secondary to antibiotics.
Chronic infection with resistant organism.
Continuous reinfection: eg, foods, pet contact.
"Secondary" immunodeficiencies
Malnutrition.
Metabolic disorders.
Inherited disorders.
Immunosuppression.
Infection.
Surgery and trauma.
Infiltrative diseases.
Malignant disorders.
Hematologic disorders.

Etiology

Extremely heterogeneous groups of disorders ranging from defects in a single-gene product in a specific cell type to systemic disorders. Etiologies include single or multi-gene defects, drug- or toxin-induced immunosuppression, nutritional, and metabolic.

Epidemiology

• The overall incidence of primary immunodeficiency is 1:10,000, resulting in ~ 400 new cases per year in the US. In general, ~ 40% of cases are diagnosed in the first year of life, 40% more by 5 years, and another 15% by 16 years.
• Among patients referred for immunodeficiency evaluation, Conley [1] has estimated that 50% of the patients were normal, 30% had allergic nonimmunologic disorders, 10% had serious but nonimmunologic disorders, and only 10% had immunodeficiency.

Treatment

Lifestyle management

• Full activity and diet should be encouraged with limitations dictated by medical and surgical plans specific to disorder.

• Patients must adapt to chronic disease, the threat of recurrent infection, and the work necessary for management.

• Active avoidance of new infection may be necessary for some patients.

Pharmacologic treatment

Preventative regimens

• Blood products for transfusion should be screened for viral infections (cytomegalovirus, hepatitis B and C, HIV) and irradiated if T-cell immunodeficiency is suspected.

• For prophylaxis against *Pneumocystis carinii* infection:

Standard dosage Trimethoprim (TMP)–sulfamethoxazole (SMX), 150 mg TMP/m², orally, in divided doses twice daily for 3 consecutive d/wk (maximum dose, 320 mg TMP/d); alternatives are pentamidine and dapsone.

For phagocyte disorders: long-term prophylaxis with TMP–SMX or dicloxacillin.

For chronic infections: long-term antimicrobial treatment.

For fungal infections: prolonged treatment with ketoconazole or itraconazole.

For management of varicella contact or infections: varicella immunoglobulin acyclovir.

For chronic candidal infections: topical or oral nystatin.

Immunization with killed vaccines (routine) for diagnosis and protection if patient is responsive.

IgA-deficient patients should not receive i.v. immunoglobulin because it may cause sensitization or reaction to contaminating IgA; blood transfusion from IgA-deficient donor may be indicated.

Immunoglobulin replacement

Standard dosage 400 mg/kg/mo i.v.; dose adjustments may be necessary up to 800 mg/kg/mo.

Special points Monitor trough levels; some patients may require preinfusion antipyretics/antihistamine prophylaxis.

Alternative dosage Monthly i.m. injections or subcutaneous infusions daily or every other day.

Growth factors

For patients with neutropenia or cyclic neutropenia: granulocyte colony-stimulating factor (CSF) or granulocyte-macrophage CSF.

For rare interleukin-2–deficiency: replacement therapy.

For "immunostimulant" in chronic granulomatous disease:

Standard dosage Interferon-γ, 50 μt/kg 3 times weekly.

Reduced dose of 1.5 μg/kg, if body surface area is less than 0.5 m².

Enzyme replacement

Bovine adenosine deaminase conjugated with polyethylene glycol usually administered weekly.

White blood cell transfusions

• Obtained via leukopheresis after pretreatment of donor with prednisone. May be administered systematically or intralesionally (*eg*, abscesses) for infections unresponsive to other management strategies.

Bone marrow transplantation

• Definitive therapy has been used for reconstitution in severe combined immunodeficiency, the Wiskott–Aldrich syndrome, CGD, and leukocyte adhesion deficiencies.

Treatment aims

To arrive at accurate diagnosis.
To prevent infection.
To effectively treat infection.
To constitute immune function or provide supplementation of defective component, if possible.
To provide genetic counseling, promote understanding of molecular and genetic testing, and detect carrier status (some X-linked disorders).

Follow-up and management

• Regularly monitor infection, immune function, and adverse effects of treatment.
• Monitor for potential disease associations: eg, collagen-vascular disease.
• Provide patient/parent education.
• Assure access to new treatment modalities.
• Ensure effective communication (another cornerstone of chronic disease management).
• Provide access to other needed subspecialty care.
• Guide patient and family through the transition from pediatric-oriented sphere to adulthood responsibilities for self-care and effective adaptation to adult-oriented routines.

Key references

1. Conley ME, Stiehm ER: Immunodeficiency disorders: general considerations. In *Immunologic Disorders in Infants and Children*, ed Edited by Steihm ER. WB Saunders Co.: Philadelphia; 1996:201–252.

General references

Johnston RB Jr: Recurrent bacterial infections in children. *N Engl J Med* 1984, **310:**1237–1243.

Rosen FS, Cooper MD, Wedgwood RJP: The primary immunodeficiencies. *N Engl J Med* 1995, **333:**431–440.

Schaffer FM, Ballow M. Immunodeficiency: the office work-up. *J Resp Dis* 1995, **16:**523–541.

Shearer WT, Buckley RH, Engler RJ, et al.: Practice parameters for the diagnosis and management of immunodeficiency. *Ann Allergy Asthma Immunol* 1996, **76:**282–294.

Stiehm ER: New and old immunodeficiencies. *Pediatr Res* 1993, **33 (suppl):**52–58.

Diagnosis

Definition

Rapidly progressive, and potentially reversible, cessation of renal function that results in the inability of the kidney to control body homeostasis manifest by the retention of nitrogenous waste products and fluid and electrolyte imbalance.

Symptoms

Lethargy, anorexia, nausea, vomiting: are symptoms seen in most patients.

Abdominal pain: may be expressed in children with obstructive uropathy.

Bloody diarrhea: a precursor to the most common form of hemolytic uremic syndrome.

Signs

Oliguria, hematuria: in many but not all cases; patients with acute interstitial nephritis might have polyuria and nocturia.

Edema and signs consistent with congestive heart failure (crackles, gallop, hepatomegaly, jugular venous distention): may be present in children with acute glomerulonephritis.

Abdominal mass: in cases of obstructive uropathy.

Pallor, jaundice, petechia: seen in children with hemolytic uremic syndrome.

Fever, rash: in acute interstitial nephritis.

Investigations

Urinalysis: will demonstrate erythrocyte casts and proteinuria in cases of acute glomerulonephritis and pyuria with eosinophils in acute interstitial nephritis. The specific gravity will be low in obstructive uropathy, acute interstitial nephritis, and acute tubular necrosis, and elevated in hemolytic uremic syndrome, acute glomerulonephritis, and in prerenal azotemia.

Serum chemistries: will demonstrate hyponatremia, hyperkalemia, metabolic acidosis, hypocalcemia, hyperphosphatemia, and azotemia.

Complete blood count: may show a normocytic anemia except in cases of hemolytic uremic syndrome, in which there will be a microangiopathic hemolytic uremia and thrombocytopenia.

Renal ultrasound: essential for diagnosing obstructive uropathy, in which hydronephrosis will be present; otherwise the kidney is enlarged and echogenic.

Electrocardiogram, echocardiography: to monitor for changes seen in hyperkalemia and for pericardial changes.

• The specialist studies include C3 (decreased in acute glomerulonephritis and lupus), antinuclear antibodies (lupus), and antineutrophil cytoplasmic antibodies (Wegener's granulomatosis).

The fractional excretion of sodium: ($[C_{Na}/C_{creatinine}] \times 100$): <1 in prerenal azotemia and >2 in acute tubular necrosis.

Renal biopsy: in patients with prolonged or unexplained acute renal failure when definitive therapy may be necessary.

Complications

Congestive heart failure: secondary to fluid overload or anemia.

Hypertension: secondary to fluid overload.

Cardiac dysfunction: secondary to hyperkalemia.

Uremia: manifest by pericarditis, increased risk of bleeding, infection.

Severe metabolic acidosis.

Tetany: secondary to hypocalcemia.

Malnutrition: secondary to decreased appetite and dietary restrictions.

Differential diagnosis

• Chronic renal failure is usually insidious and associated with poor growth, polyuria, and anemia.

• An elevated BUN can also be seen in patients with upper gastrointestinal bleeding or in hypercatabolic states.

• An elevated creatinine can be caused by specific medications (trimethoprim-sulfamethoxazole, cimetidine).

Etiology

• Prerenal azotemia occurs as a result of decreased perfusion to the kidney secondary either to decreased intravascular volume or diminished cardiac output.

• Postrenal (obstructive) renal failure should especially be considered in newborns; the obstruction can occur in the lower tracts (posterior urethral valves) or in the upper tracts in children with a single kidney.

Intrinsic renal disease: acute tubular necrosis (commonly follows hypoxic or nephrotoxic injury); glomerulonephritis (most commonly postinfectious acute glomerulonephritis); vascular lesions such as hemolytic uremic syndrome, renal venous thrombosis; and acute interstitial nephritis (may be idiopathic or secondary to medications [nonsteroidal anti-inflammatory drugs, penicillin] or infection).

Epidemiology

• The most common form of acute renal failure is prerenal azotemia.

• Acute renal failure secondary to acute tubular necrosis is commonly encountered in the hospital setting, especially in intensive care units. The combination of ischemia plus nephrotoxic agents such as aminoglycosides, amphotericin B, contrast or chemotherapeutic agents place these individuals at risk.

Treatment

Diet and lifestyle

• Patients with acute renal failure are usually hospitalized and require meticulous fluid management; fluid intake should not exceed insensible fluid losses plus urine output if the patient is euvolemic.

• A "renal diet" (low protein, potassium, sodium, and phosphorous, high carbohydrate) should be instituted.

Pharmacologic treatment

Preventive

• Mannitol or furosemide to prevent acute renal failure is controversial; they can be used prior to the initiation of known nephrotoxic agents such as amphotericin B, cisplatin or contrast as prophylaxis or in cases of acute tubular necrosis secondary to myoglobinuria as a method to augment urine flow.

• The conversion from an oliguric state (<0.5 mL/kg/h) to a nonoliguric state may improve the prognosis.

Supportive therapy

• Maximize the presence of an effective circulatory volume; patients in shock require large infusions of crystalloid (normal saline, lactated Ringer's solution) even if there is not urine output; patients with fluid overload may respond to fluid restriction and diuretic therapy (furosemide 1–4 mg/kg/dose, depending on renal function) to manage congestive heart failure.

• Monitor serum potassium levels frequently. Calcium gluconate (0.5–1 mL/kg over 2–10 min), glucose (0.5 g/kg), and insulin (0.1 U/kg), sodium bicarbonate (1–2 mEq/kg over 10–30 min) and Kayexolate (1 g/kg p.o. or p.r.) are effective therapy for hyperkalemia.

• Severe acidosis (pH <7.2) may require therapy with sodium bicarbonate. However, this may precipitate symptomatic hypocalcemia and cause hyponatremia and fluid overload. Hypertension may require aggressive treatment if encephalopathy is present.

• Administer ulcer prophylaxis.

• Adjust drugs according to renal failure.

Specific therapy

• In some forms of glomerulonephritis, corticosteroid and cytotoxic therapy may be indicated.

• Acute interstitial nephritis is managed by removing the offending agent and possibly corticosteroids.

• Surgery may be indicated in obstructive causes of renal failure; a postobstructive diuresis may develop after relief of the obstruction.

Treatment aims

To prevent the development of acute tubular necrosis by providing adequate renal perfusion and avoiding nephrotoxic agents.

To identify forms of acute renal failure amenable to treatment.

To provide supportive therapy until the return of renal function or as the patient enters a chronic stage of the disease.

Other treatments

• Dialysis is indicated in cases of fluid overload refractory to diuretic therapy, severe hyperkalemia, refractory metabolic acidosis, and uremia; conventional dialysis (peritoneal or hemodialysis) as well as continuous arteriovenous hemodiafiltration or pump-assisted continuous venovenous hemodiafiltration can be considered.

Prognosis

• Many children with isolated acute renal failure have a good prognosis with return of renal function.

• Children with multiorgan failure have a high mortality rate despite good supportive care.

• Nonoliguric renal failure is associated with a lower mortality rate than oliguric renal failure.

Follow-up and management

• Patients with prolonged anuria should be followed for associated sequelae including hypertension, proteinuria, and chronic renal failure.

General references

Sehic A, Chesney RW: Acute renal failure: diagnosis. *Pediatr Rev* 1995, **16:**101–106.

Sehic A, Chesney RW: Acute renal failure: therapy. *Pediatr Rev* 1995, **16:**137–141.

Siegel NJ, van Why SK, Boydstrun II, *et al.:* Acute renal failure. In *Pediatric Nephrology,* ed 3. Edited by Holliday MA, *et al.* Baltimore: Williams & Wilkins; 1994:1176–1203.

Diagnosis

Definition
Irreversible, progressive decline in renal function.
Defined as a creatinine clearance ≤75 mL/min/1.73 m² (Schwartz formula).

Symptoms
Often nonspecific.
Listlessness, failure to thrive, growth retardation, nausea, vomiting, anorexia.
Edema.
Polydipsia, polyuria, enuresis.
School failure.

Signs
Pallor, sallow complexion.
Growth failure.
Hypertension.
Dysmorphic features of underlying disorder.

Investigations
Urine analysis: protein, blood, casts, specific gravity.
24-hour urine protein determination: if dipstick test >2 plus positive.
Serum sodium, potassium, chloride, bicarbonate, calcium, phosphate creatinine, BUN.
Hemoglobin: iron and erythropoietin studies if severely anemic.
Renal and bladder ultrasound.
Further imaging studies predicated on ultrasound findings.
Creatinine clearance: unreliable and unhelpful.
Serum parathyroid hormone (PTH); alkaline phosphatase.
Bone age: if growth retarded; finger and wrist radiography for osteodystrophy.
Kidney biopsy: if a treatable glomerulopathy suspected; rarely needed if approaching end-stage renal failure.

Complications
Anemia.
Osteodystrophy.
Growth failure.
Hypertension.
Tetany.
Depression.
School failure.
Pruritis.
End-stage renal failure.

Differential diagnosis
Acute renal failure: symptoms more severe, oligoanuria, bloody diarrhea (hemolytic uremic syndrome), sore throat, more active urine sediment (poststreptococcal glomerulonephritis).

Etiology
Obstructive uropathy (23.7%).
Aplasia/dysplasia/hypoplasia (18.8%).
Reflux nephropathy (9.7%).
Focal segmental glomerulosclerosis (7.4%).

Epidemiology
Of 649 patients in the North American Pediatric Transplant Registry, 65.9% male, 63.9% white.

Progression
• Varies according to underlying cause: chronic renal failure secondary to posterior urethral valves tends to progress more slowly than glomerular diseases.
• May remain stable, and in some cases may improve, for variable periods.
• More rapid declines during midgrowth spurt and puberty (but not affected by growth hormone treatment).
• Predict by plotting reciprocal of serum creatinine against time.

Treatment

Diet and lifestyle
Intrude as little as possible on lifestyle.

Salt supplementation if salt-losing nephropathy.

Salt restriction if edematous, hypertensive.

Hyperkalemia: potassium restriction, Kayexalate, may be indication for chronic dialysis.

Protein and phosphate restriction: difficult in growing children.

Supplement calorie intake.

Pharmacologic treatment
Anemia: erythropoietin, folate, iron.

Osteodystrophy: calcitriol, monitor serum PTH, phosphate binders (calcium citrate preferred).

Metabolic acidosis: sodium bicarbonate.

Hypertension: calcium channel blockers; angiotensin-converting enzyme (ACE) inhibitors also useful but monitor serum creatinine and potassium.

Growth below fifth centile: growth hormone.

Nonpharmacologic treatment
Educate child and family.

Psychosocial support for psychosocial problems.

Surgical treatment of obstructive uropathy.

Peritoneal dialysis, hemodialysis if symptoms.

Preemptive renal transplantation preferred.

Bioethical issues
Chronic dialysis and/or transplantation in neonates, infants with multiorgan failure.

Serum creatine level for dialysis or transplanting.

Precautions
Avoid nonsteroidal anti-inflammatory agents.

Treat urinary tract infections.

Avoid aluminum- and magnesium-containing compounds.

Avoid, if possible, potentially nephrotoxic antibiotics.

Treatment aims
To control hypertension, treat urinary tract infections.
To manage obstructive uropathy.
To avoid nephrotoxins.
• Use ACE inhibitors where indicated.
To maintain normal lifestyle.
To treat anemia.
To treat growth failure.
To prevent osteodystrophy.

Prognosis
Depends on underlying cause.

Follow-up and management
Regular serum creatinine, electrolytes, calcium, phosphate, intact PTH, hemoglobin, height, weight, blood pressure.
Support: by telephone, social worker, psychologist.
Regular evaluation of nutrition, medication compliance.

General references
Fine RN, Kohaut EC, Brown D, Perlman AJ: Growth after recombinant human growth hormone treatment in children with chronic renal failure: report of a multicenter randomized double-blind placebo-controlled study. Genentech Cooperative Study Group. J Pediatr 1994, 124:374–382.

Krmar RT, Gretz N, Klare B, et al.: Renal function in predialysis children with chronic renal failure treated with erythropoietin. Pediatr Nephrol 1997, 11:69–73.

Sedman A, Friedman A, Boineau F, et al.: Nutritional management of the child with mild to moderate chronic renal failure. J Pediatr 1996, 129:13–18.

Warady BA, Hebert D, Sullivan EK, et al.: Renal transplantation, chronic dialysis, and chronic renal insufficiency in children and adolescents: the 1995 Annual Report of the North American Pediatric Renal Transplant Cooperative Study. Pediatr Nephrol 1997, 11:49–64.

Diagnosis

Definition

Full or incomplete manifestations of renal tubular disorders may present *in utero*, in the neonate, or in infancy.

Laboratory abnormalities are specific indicators of particular renal tubular defects.

Symptoms

Irritability, poor feeding, unexplained vomiting, dehydration, failure to thrive, drowsiness, tetany, seizures.

Polydipsia, polyuria: nephrogenic diabetes insipidus.

Signs

Growth retardation.

Rickets: bowing, splayed wrist, rosary.

Hypotonia.

Dehydration.

Developmental delay.

Cataracts, jaundice: galactosemia.

Investigations

Hyperchloremic metabolic acidosis plus increased anion gap: renal tubular acidosis.

Hyponatremia with renal salt wasting: renal adysplasias, pseudohypoaldosteronism, Bartter's syndrome.

Hyperkalemia: renal adysplasia, pseudohypoaldosteronism, renal tubular hyperkalemia syndromes.

Hypouricemia: Fanconi's syndrome.

Hypophosphatemia: Fanconi's syndrome, X-linked hypophosphatemic rickets.

Glucosuria: Fanconi's syndrome, hereditary glucosurias.

Hematuria: renal calculi, nephrocalcinosis.

Hypercalciuria.

Polyuria plus low urine serum glucose: nephrogenic diabetes insipidus, Fanconi's syndrome.

Acidosis plus high urine pH: distal renal tubular acidosis.

Lactic acidosis: mitochondrial disorders plus Fanconi's syndrome.

Fructose intolerance: molecular analysis of aldolase B gene in blood.

Galactosemia: galactose ("reducing substances") in blood and urine; deficient erythrocyte galactose-1 phosphate uridyl transferase.

Pseudohypoaldosteronism: hyponatremia, hyperkalemia, elevated plasma aldosterone, and renin.

Nephrogenic diabetes insipidus: serum sodium, chloride, creatinine elevated; serum vasopressin are normal/increased; no antidiuretic response to exogenous vasopressin.

Complications

Dehydration.

Tetany.

Differential diagnosis

Fanconi's syndrome:generalized proximal tubule dysfunction; vitamin D–resistant rickets; metabolic acidosis.

X-linked hypophosphatemic rickets: failure to thrive; bowing of legs, waddling gait.

Renal glycosuria: isolated renal glycosuria is uncommon and benign.

Type I distal renal tubular acidosis ("classic" dRTA): growth failure, osteodystrophy, high-frequency deafness, nephrocalcinosis, renal calculi.

Bartter's syndrome: hyperkaliuria, hypokalemia, metabolic alkalosis, hyperaldosteronism, resistance to the pressor effect of angiotensin, juxtaglomerular apparatus hyperplasia, increased renal renin production.

PHA: salt-wasting tubular unresponsiveness to aldosterone.

Renal tubular hyperkalemia: inappropriately low urine potassium concentration, renal salt wasting, and metabolic acidosis; serum creatinine concentration is often increased.

NDI: irritability, poor feeding, failure to gain weight, unexplained dehydration and fever.

Etiology

Fanconi's syndrome: cystinosis, hereditary fructose intolerance, galactosemia, Wilson's disease (all with autosomal recessive inheritance); cytochrome-c oxidase deficiency, iphosphamide.

PHA: autosomal dominant or recessive.

dRTA: failure to excrete sufficient NH^4 when there is impaired trapping of NH^4 in the collecting duct as a result of low rates of H^+ secretion.

Bartter's syndrome: idiopathic.

RTH: marked prematurity, renal adysplasia, urinary tract obstruction/infection, PHA, congenital adrenal hypoplasia, tubulointerstitial diseases.

NDI: X-linked with abnormal gene on Xq28.

Epidemiology

Each of these conditions is extremely rare.

Treatment

Diet and lifestyle

Fructose intolerance: withdraw all fructose-containing foods.

Galactosemia: withdraw milk-containing foods.

PHA: sodium chloride.

NDI: copious solute-free water intake.

X-linked hyperphosphatemic rickets: phosphate, calcitriol.

dRTA: sodium bicarbonate or sodium citrate.

Pharmacologic treatment

Fanconi's syndrome: calcitriol, bicarbonate, phosphate.

Bartter's syndrome: indomethacin.

NDI: indomethacin plus thiazide diuretic.

Cystinosis: treat Fanconi's syndrome; cysteamine for specific treatment of cystinosis; treat hypothyroidism; renal transplant for chronic renal failure.

Nonpharmacologic treatment

Genetic counseling.

Cystinosis: *in utero* diagnosis.

Precautions

Vigilant care.

Careful follow-up.

Avoid noxious foods.

Galactosemia: newborn screening programs for early detection; prenatal diagnosis is unreliable.

Prognosis

Chronic.

Decompensations likely.

Guarded and variable.

Death may occur.

Follow-up and management

Careful, frequent assessments.

Ensure compliance.

General references

Carlisle EJF, et al.: Renal tubular acidosis (RTA): recognize the ammonium defect and pHorget the urine pH. *Pediatr Nephrol* 1991, **5:**242.

Kaplan BS, Kaplan P: Renal tubular disorders in the neonate. In *Intensive Care of the Fetus and Neonate.* Edited by Spitzer A. St. Louis: Mosby–Year Book Inc.; 1996.

Rheumatic fever (acute rheumatic heart disease)

Diagnosis

Definition
• Rheumatic heart disease (RHD) occurs after acute rheumatic fever (ARF), which is a postinfectious immune disease secondary to a streptococcal infection [1].
• RHD affects the valves of the heart, with the mitral and aortic being the most commonly affected valves. RHD is more likely to occur with recurrent episodes.

Diagnosis
• Diagnosis of ARF is made from the modified Jones criteria [2] (*see* table), with a positive diagnosis requiring two major or one major and two minor criteria.

Modified Jones criteria for the diagnosis of acute rheumatic fever		
Major manifestations	**Minor manifestations**	**Supporting evidence**
Carditis	Arthralgia	Positive throat culture for group
Polyarthritis	Fever	A *Streptococcus* or positive, rapid
Chorea	Elevated acute phase reactants:	streptococcal test
Erythema marginatum	ESR and C-reactive protein	Elevated or rising streptococcal
Subcutaneous nodules	Prolonged PR interval	antibody titer

Symptoms
Carditis: chest pain, shortness or breath, cough, palpitations with sensation of elevated or irregular rate or rhythm, anorexia, fatigue, and exercise intolerance.

Arthritis: occurs in 70% of patients with ARF; symptoms include joint pain.

Sydenham's chorea: affects 15% of patients with ARF; reflects involvement of basal ganglia of central nervous system; appears ~3 months after streptococcal infection; symptoms include emotional liability and loss of attention span.

Signs

Carditis
Tachycardia; murmur: mitral insufficiency (MI), relative mitral stenosis, or aortic insufficiency (AI); **congestive heart failure (CHF); arrhythmias.; pericarditis; arthritis:** large joints (knees, ankles, wrists, elbows); asymmetric and migratory; **Sydenham's chorea:** involuntary and purposeless movements and muscular incoordination; **erythema marginatum:** 5%; **subcutaneous nodules:** <5%.

Investigations
Chest radiography: cardiomegaly when carditis is present or marked MI or aortic insufficiency (AI); pulmonary venous congestion and/or pulmonary edema may be present when congestive heart failure occurs.

ECG: with carditis or CHF, sinus tachycardia; PR prolongation with myocarditis; 1°, 2°, and 3° atrioventricular block; nonspecific ST-T abnormalities or T wave inversion; premature atrial or ventricular contractions; with chronic RHD, left atrial enlargement or left ventricular hypertrophy; atrial fibrillation uncommon in children.

Echocardiography: used to evaluate the presence and degree of myocardial dysfunction, specific chamber enlargement, presence of MI and AI, and pericardial effusion; with chronic RHD, echocardiography can determine the degree of mitral regurgitation or stenosis as well as transvalvar gradients and measurement of valve area.

Laboratory studies (for diagnosis of acute rheumatic fever)
Acute phase reactants: elevated WBC, ESR, CRP.

Streptococcal infection: elevated streptozyme; anti-streptolysin O, anti-streptokinase, anti-hyaluronidase, anti-DNAseB, anti-NADase titers.

Differential diagnosis
Collagen vascular diseases: juvenile rheumatoid arthritis, systemic lupus erythematosus, mixed collagen vascular diseases, poststreptococcal arthritis, serum sickness, infectious arthritis (gonococcal), sickle cell disease, leukemia.

Pericarditis: bacterial, viral, myoplasma infections; collagen vascular disease.

Congenital heart disease with mitral insufficiency, mitral valve prolapse.

Endocarditis: may be superimposed on congenital mitral valve defect.

Kawasaki disease.

Etiology
• Rheumatic fever and subsequent RHD are a consequence of an infection with group A hemolytic streptococcus (*Streptococcus pyogenes*), with the initial infection being a pharyngitis. This infection in a susceptible host results in an immune reaction that causes inflammation of the heart, joints, brain, and vascular and connective tissue. There is a period of latency of ~3 weeks between the infection and appearance of rheumatic fever.

Epidemiology
• Acute rheumatic fever occurs most commonly between the ages of 4–15 y. Only 2%–3% of infected untreated children will develop rheumatic fever after a streptococcal pharyngitis. Once a patient has had their first episode of rheumatic fever, 50% of those patients will have a recurrence of rheumatic fever with a new streptococcal infection.

• Current incidence in the U.S. is 0.5–3.1 per 100,000 population, which is a progressive decline over the past 50–60 y [3]. This decline relates to early treatment of streptococcal infections, improved economic standards with less crowded living conditions, and/or a change in the virulence of the organism.

Complications
Congestive heart failure.

Recurrent ARF.

Chronic rheumatic valvular heart disease.

Treatment

Diet and lifestyle

• With AFR, bed rest is recommended until all signs of inflammation have subsided, usually 4–6 weeks. Gradual resumption of activity is advised. Competitive activity or vigorous physical activity should be avoided for approximately 3 months or longer if significant cardiac involvement is present. Amount of activity eventually allowed will depend on type and degree of RHD.

• No specific dietary restrictions. Good nutrition should be maintained. If CHF is present, a low-salt diet should be followed. If arrhythmias present, caffeine should be avoided.

Pharmacologic treatment

For primary infections

Standard dosage   *Treatment*:Benzathine penicillin G, 1.2 Mu i.m.

Penicillin V, 250 mg 3 times daily p.o. for 10 d.

Erythromycin, 50 mg/kg/d p.o. in 3–4 divided doses for 10 d.

Prophylaxis: Benzathine penicillin G, 1.2 MU i.m. every 3–4 wk.

Penicillin V, 250 mg p.o. twice daily.

Erythromycin, 250 mg p.o. twice daily.

Sulfadiazine, 1 g p.o. daily.

Special points   Patients allergic to penicillin require prophylaxis with erythromycin.

For carditis (mild to moderate)

Standard dosage   Aspirin, 90–100 mg/kg/day.

Special points: Monitor serum level: 25–30 mg/dL; continue dose for 4–8 wk and wean over 4–6 wk; monitor acute phase reactants as guide to therapy.

Main drug interactions

Main side effects

For severe carditis with congestive heart failure

Standard dosage   Oral prednisone, 2 mg/kg/d for 2 wk with wean over following 2–3 wk; start aspirin 1 week prior to stopping steroid therapy.

Digoxin to treat CHF, either acutely or in patients with chronic valve insufficiency. (*See* Myocarditis for dosage.)

Furosemide, 1 mg/kg twice daily.

For significant myocardial infarction or aortic insufficiency and left ventricular dysfunction

Standard dosage   *Infants and children*: Enalapril, 0.1 mg–0.5 mg/kg/d in 2 divided doses.

Adolescents:Enalapril, 2-5 mg/d increased to 10–40 mg/day as tolerated in 1–2 divided doses.

Infants: Captopril, 0.05–0.3 mg/kg/dose every 6–8 hours initially titrated to maximum of 6 mg/kg/d.

Children and adolescents: 6.25–12.5 mg/dose every 8 hours; increase to 25 mg/dose and by 25 mg/dose to maximum of 450 mg/d.

Special points: Lower dosage in patients with renal impairment, severe congestive heart failure. Administration in volume-depleted patients may cause severe hypotension.

Treatment aims

To relieve symptoms by treating strepto-coccal infection.

To prevent recurrences of ARF.

Other treatments

• Surgical treatment of severe valvular insufficiency or stenosis. Use balloon valvuloplasty to treat mitral stenosis.

• Bed rest with limited activity.

• Subacute bacterial endocarditis prophy-laxis is indicated for any valvar involve-ment. Second-line drug should be used as flora may become resistant to penicillin used for chronic rheumatic prophylaxis.

Prognosis

Excellent for a single episode of ARF.

• Resolution of signs of valvar involve-ment occurs in 70%–80% with mild mitral valvular involvement in those who do not develop recurrent ARF and remain appropriately on prophylaxis. With significant valvar involvement, prog-nosis depends on extent of cardiac com-promise and the need for surgery. If valve repair is not possible, valve replacement is well tolerated, with new bioprosthetic valves and procedures such as the Ross procedure for aortic valve involvement.

Follow-up and management

Patients require close follow-up, monthly prophylaxis injections (or equivalent). If cardiac involvement remains, 3–12 monthly visits to cardiologist to follow degree of valve involvement is indicated. Periodic chest radiography, ECG, Holter monitoring. Echocardiography and car-diac catheterization may be indicated to follow progression of cardiac lesions.

Key references

1. Kaplan MH: Rheumatic fever, rheumatic heart disease, and the streptococcal con-nection: the role of streptococcal antigens cross reactive with heart disease. *Rev Infect Dis* 1979, 1:988–996.

2. Dajani AS, Ayoub EM, Bierman FZ, *et al.*: Guidelines for the diagnosis of rheumatic fever: Jones criteria (updated 1992). *Circulation* 1992, 87:302–307.

3. Gordis L: The virtual disappearance of rheumatic fever in he United States: lessons in the rise and fall of disease. *Circulation* 1985, 72:1155–1162.

Seizures, febrile and acute

Diagnosis

Definition

Febrile seizure (FS): a convulsion occurring during a febrile illness—but in the absence of intracranial infection—in an infant between roughly 6 months and 5 years of age.

• FSs are classified as simple if all of the following criteria are met (otherwise they are termed complex): brief (<15 minutes), generalized, single event within a febrile illness, otherwise normal neurodevelopmental status.

Acute symptomatic seizures: are precipitated by acute illness (either systemic or involving the central nervous system directly), but exclude FS as defined above.

Convulsive status epilepticus: may occur with both FS and acute symptomatic seizures, and is defined as continuous seizures for ≥30 minutes, or recurrent seizures for ≥30 minutes without recovery of consciousness between fits.

Symptoms

• Acute symptomatic seizures are usually convulsive, with or without disturbance in consciousness. Convulsive activity may be generalized or lateralized.

• Individual seizure types are discussed in the next section.

• Aura is occasionally present but is unusual in FS and acute symptomatic seizures.

• Postictal focal paralysis (Todd's paralysis) is usually brief but may last for hours.

• Postictal lethargy is generally related to the duration of a convulsion but is highly variable.

• Other symptoms are attributable to underlying acute illness.

Signs

• Patients should be thoroughly examined and checked carefully for the following signs:

Mental state; source of infection; focal neurologic deficit; systemic evidence of intoxication; evidence of raised intracranial pressure; nuchal rigidity; cardiovascular abnormalities; chronic neurologic disorder; skin and eye lesions; evidence of trauma; other signs attributable to underlying illness.

Investigations

• Investigation may be deferred in simple FS if the source of the fever is known, and intracranial infection can be confidently excluded (this implies that the duration of fever prior to the FS is very brief).

• Investigation may be necessary to exclude intracranial infection in FS and is usually indicated to define the cause of acute symptomatic seizures. It may include the following investigations:

Neuroimaging (cranial CT, MRI, or MRA): for tumor, abscess, encephalitis, stroke, hemorrhage, trauma; should generally be performed prior to lumbar puncture.

Electroencephalography: for epilepsy, encephalitis, metabolic encephalopathy.

Lumbar puncture and cerebrospinal fluid analysis: for meningoencephalitis or hemorrhage.

Complete blood count: for a variety of infectious and hematologic disorders.

Metabolic studies: for electrolyte derangement (especially hyponatremia and hypocalcemia), hypoglycemia, and so on.

Toxin screens of urine or blood: for suspected poisoning or drug abuse.

Differential diagnosis

• FS must be distinguished from intracranial infection causing seizures.

• An acute seizure (febrile or nonfebrile) may be the presenting symptom of epilepsy, which is defined as recurrent, afebrile seizures. However, the distinction is often difficult, and it is wise to start with the assumption that seizures result from underlying acute illness until this possibility is excluded with reasonable confidence.

• Syncope, especially if complicated by brief tonic posturing or a few generalized jerks ("convulsive syncope"), may mimic an acute symptomatic seizure.

• Other paroxysmal disorders include breathholding spells, movement disorders, dystonic reactions to drugs, pseudoseizures, narcolepsy/cataplexy, night terrors.

Etiology

• Recurrent, simple FS are commonly familial (ie, they are triggered by fever in individuals with polygenically determined susceptibility).

• Acute symptomatic seizures include seizures due to intracranial infection, trauma, hemorrhage, stroke, electrolyte disturbance, poisoning, hypertensive crisis, and so on.

Epidemiology

• FS occurs in roughly 2%–3% of children by age 6.

• Acute symptomatic seizures are especially common in the first postnatal year.

Complications

Transient respiratory depression: common, but generally not serious in the absence of status epilepticus.

Aspiration pneumonia.

Physical injury.

Status epilepticus.

Treatment

Pharmacologic treatment

• For acute seizures and status epilepticus, ensure adequate airway and circulation, administer supplemental oxygen by mask if available.

• Identify and treat underlying cause of acute symptomatic seizures. Use caution in correcting electrolyte imbalance, especially hyponatremia.

• Control fever with antipyretic agents, sponge bath, cooling blanket.

• Drug treatment is generally not indicated for brief febrile convulsions and may not be necessary in acute symptomatic seizures if the cause (eg, hypoglycemia) can be eliminated.

• For prolonged seizures or status epilepticus, administer intravenous benzodiazepine (diazepam or lorazepam).

• For multiple seizures or status epilepticus, consider administration of intravenous phenobarbital (especially for recurrent FS), phenytoin, or phosphenytoin.

Standard dosage Phenobarbital, 20 mg/kg i.v.

Phenytoin, 20 mg/kg i.v. (must be administered slowly).

Diazepam, 0.2–0.3 mg/kg i.v. or 0.3–0.5 mg/kg rectally.

Lorazepam, 0.05–0.10 mg/kg i.v.

Special points *Benzodiazepines*: cause transient respiratory depression, which is potentiated by phenobarbital

Phenytoin: produces less sedation than other agents, but it may be difficult to change to a maintenance regimen in young children.

Prophylaxis of febrile seizure

• The great majority of children with FS do not require drug prophylaxis.

• Antipyretics may help to terminate prolonged fits, but do not necessarily prevent subsequent fits within an illness.

• Consider prophylaxis if attacks are prolonged or frequent, especially in a young child (eg, <2 y of age).

• Consider features that increase the risk for recurrence or subsequent epilepsy (*see* Prognosis). The presence of a single factors should not necessarily prompt prophylaxis, but multiple factors tend to increase risk dramatically.

• Consider one of the following regimens:

Standard dosage Continuous oral phenobarbital, 5 mg/kg/d; adjust to obtain serum level of 15–20 mug/mL.

Intermittent oral diazepam (during febrile illness), 0.3 mg/kg every 8 hours.

Intermittent rectal diazepam for prolonged fits, 0.3–0.5 mg/kg as necessary.

Special points *Continuous oral phenobarbital*: reasonably effective; prophylaxis is continuously present.

Intermittent oral diazepam (during febrile illness): treatment limited to period of highest risk; long-term cognitive side effects avoided.

Intermittent rectal diazepam (for prolonged fits): requires motivated parents; treatment is aimed at shortening rather than eliminating seizures.

Main side effects *Continuous oral phenobarbital*: cognitive and behavioral side effects.

Intermittent oral diazepam: sedation.

Intermittent rectal diazepam: sedation; transient respiratory suppression.

Treatment aims

To prevent or limit status epilepticus and other complications.

To provide appropriate reassurance.

Prognosis

• Only one third of children with a first FS experience recurrence.

• Only 2% of children with a first FS go on to have epilepsy by age 7.

• Risk factors for FS recurrence or subsequent epilepsy are similar and include underlying neurologic disease or developmental delay, multiple seizures within a single febrile illness, focality, family history of FS or epilepsy, and febrile status epilepticus.

Follow-up and management

• Monitor neurodevelopmental status.

• Reconsider decision regarding FS prophylaxis in light of recurrence, side effects, and so on.

General references

Aicardi J: *Epilepsy in children*, ed 2. New York: Raven Press; 1994.

Hirtz DG: Generalized tonic-clonic and febrile seizures. *Pediatr Clin North Am* 1989, **36**:365–382.

Diagnosis

Symptoms

Seizures: usually abrupt onset, stereotyped, variably preceded by aura.

Loss of or altered awareness.

Abnormal posture, tone, movements.

Sensory: visual, auditory, gustatory, visceral, or tactile sensations.

Psychic: deja vu, derealization, macropsia or micropsia, fear, anxiety, rage.

West syndrome

Seizure type: infantile spasms (with developmental regression).

Age of onset: 3–12 months.

EEG: hypsarrhythmia.

Response to treatment: Often poor.

Childhood absence epilepsy

Seizure type: frequent absences (one fifth of patients have tonic-clonic seizures).

Age of onset: 4–9 years.

EEG: 3 Hz spike-and-wave.

Response to treatment: usually excellent.

Benign Rolandic epilepsy:

Seizure type: focal motor seizures in sleep (may generalize).

Age of onset: 3–11 years.

EEG: central-midtemporal spikes.

Response to treatment: usually excellent.

Juvenile myoclonic epilepsy

Seizure type: myoclonic and tonic–clonic on awakening.

Age of onset: 9–15 years.

EEG: Generalized 4–6 Hz spike-and-wave.

Response to treatment: usually excellent.

Signs

- Signs may be absent or relate to underlying chronic neurological disorder.
- Patients should be checked for the following:

Abnormal mental state, focal neurologic deficit, raised intracranial pressure.

Evidence of adverse effects from antiepileptic drugs.

Cardiovascular abnormalities, cutaneous lesions, evidence of systemic illness.

Investigations

Interictal electroencephalography (EEG): may help to support the clinical diagnosis and suggest a particular electroclinical seizure syndrome.

Ambulatory EEG monitoring or continuous inpatient video-EEG monitoring: mey be necessary for analysis of ictal events.

Neuroimaging: is usually indicated but may be deferred in certain settings.

CSF analysis: is sometimes indicated in the evaluation of acute seizures.

Antiepileptic drug concentration measurement: is helpful in monitoring compliance and assessing role of medication in symptoms and seizure control.

Blood chemistries: to detect underlying systemic disease associated with the epilepsy or its treatment.

Differential diagnosis

Breath-holding spells: these are invariably provoked by minor trauma or situationally induced anger or upset.

Pseudoseizures: may occur in isolation or in patients with proven epilepsy.

Hyperekplexia (startle disease).

Cardiac arrhythmia, especially when associated with convulsive syncope.

Paroxysmal torticollis or vertigo.

Narcolepsy and other sleep disorders.

Paroxysmal movement disorders (eg, paroxysmal choreoathetosis/dystonia).

Alternating hemiplegia.

Recurrent transient ischemic attacks.

Migraine.

Etiology

Idiopathic (and presumably genetic) or symptomatic (ie, associated with a diverse array of underlying brain abnormalities or insults).

Epidemiology

- Prevalence of active epilepsy is roughly 4–8:1000 children.
- Idiopathic epilepsies predominate (55%–90% of cases) in most studies.

Complications

Accidents and trauma.

Status epilepticus.

Sudden unexpected death, atrial arrhythmias.

Psychosocial handicap.

Treatment

Diet and lifestyle

• Sleep deprivation, alcohol use/withdrawal, and intercurrent illnesses may precipitate seizures in individuals with epilepsy.

• Patients with uncontrolled seizures are generally not allowed to drive, swim, climb heights alone, or to operate dangerous tools.

• Ketogenic diet (in selected refractory patients).

Pharmacologic treatment

Infantile spasms: corticotropin injections, benzodiazepines, valproic acid.

Absence epilepsy: ethosuximide or valproic acid.

Rolandic epilepsy: carbamazepine or phenytoin. In some cases it may be appropriate to leave this disorder untreated.

Juvenile myoclonic epilepsy: valproic acid.

Temporal lobe epilepsy and other epilepsies with seizures of focal onset: carbamazepine or phenytoin; phenobarbital, mysoline, gabapentin, lamotrigine, or benzodiazepines may also be useful.

Primary generalized tonic-clonic epilepsy: valproate, carbamazepine, phenytoin, phenobarbital.

Standard dosage:	Carbamazepine (Tegretol), 15–30 mg/kg/d in two or three divided doses (serum level, 4–12 µg/mL).
	Phenytoin (Dilantin), 5–8 mg/kg/d in two divided doses (serum level, 10–20 µg/mL).
	Ethosuximide (Zarontin), 15–20 mg/kg/d in two divided doses (serum level, 50–100 µg/mL).
	Valproic acid, sodium valproate, sodium divalproex (Depakene, Depakote), 15–30 mg/kg/d in two or three divided doses according to preparation (serum level, 50–100 µg/mL).
	Phenobarbital, 3–6 mg/kg/d (serum level, 10–40 µg/mL).
	Chlorazepate (Tranxene), 1–3 mg/kg/d in three divided doses (serum level unclear).
	Gabapentin (Neurontin), possibly 100–400 mg 3 times daily (pediatric dose not established); serum level not established.
	Lamotrigine (Lamictal), pediatric dose and serum level not established.
	Corticotropin, ACTH (Acthar gel) for infantile spasms: 40 units i.m. daily for several weeks, then taper.
	Prednisone, 2–4 mg/kg/d for several weeks, then taper.
Main side effects	Bone marrow suppression, hepatic failure, pancreatitis, drug, rash, gingival hyperplasia, dose-related sedation, and ataxia.

Nonpharmacologic treatment

Surgical treatment

Temporal lobectomy or other focal resection: where clinical, electrophysiological, or neuroimaging evidence indicates consistent origin of seizures from a focus that is potentially resectable without unacceptable morbidity.

Anterior corpus callosotomy: performed in selected patients with refractory atonic seizures or generalized convulsions without a clear focus.

Treatment aims

To control seizures with minimal treatment morbidity.

To minimize functional impairment due to epilepsy.

Prognosis

A significant majority of children with epilepsy respond to antiepileptic therapy with complete control or substantial reduction in seizure frequency; the prognosis is strongly influenced by the particular syndrome.

The prognosis for remission after 2 y of excellent control on medication is roughly 70%, but varies according to syndrome and individual risk factors, including EEG, neurodevelopmental status, family history, and so on.

Patients with infantile spasms or the Lennox-Gastaut syndrome are frequently refractory to treatment, and evolution to other seizure types often occurs.

Follow-up and management

Staged treatment strategy:

Eliminate provocative factors (especially sleep deprivation) to the extent possible.

Start with monotherapy with agent of choice at gradually increasing doses (corticotropin and prednisone are exceptions) until control is achieved or dose-related toxicity appears. If necessary, repeat trial of monotherapy with another agent.

Combination therapy is reserved for patients not responding to monotherapy.

Reevaluate diagnosis and appropriateness of therapy periodically.

Withdrawal of therapy in patients with excellent control for 1–3 y.

Consider ketogenic diet or surgery in refractory cases.

General references

Aicardi J: *Epilepsy in Children*, ed 2. New York: Raven Press; 1994.

Mizrahi EM: Seizure disorders in children. *Curr Opin Pediatr* 1994, **6**:642–646.

Morton LD, Pellock JM: Diagnosis and treatment of epilepsy in children and adolescents. *Drugs* 1996, **51**:399–414.

Serum sickness

Diagnosis

Symptoms
Pruritis, fever, arthralgia: common.

Signs
Periarticular swelling.
Lymphadenopathy.
Rash: urticaria and angioedema most common.
Mobilliform, purpuric: less common.

Investigations

To aid in diagnosis
Urinalysis: aluminumuria and casts possible.
Complete blood count: can be slight-to-moderate leukocytic.
C3, total serum hemolytic complement (CH$_{50}$): can be reduced.
Sedimentation rate: can be elevated.

To assess cause
• Investigate exposure to 1–14 days prior to onset of symptoms (usually medication).

Complications
Renal disease: glomerulonephritis.
Respiratory distress.
Neurological symptoms: Guillain–Barré, peripheral neuritis.
• Complications are rare.

Treatment

Pharmacologic treatment
• Stop offending agent.

Antihistamines
Standard dosage   Hydroxyzine, 2 mg/kg/d every 6 h.

Diphanhydromine, 5 mg/kg/d every 6 h.

Nonsteroidal
Standard dosage   Ibuprofen, 30–50 mg/kg/d every 6 h

Nuproxen, 10–20 mg/kg/d every 12 h.

Corticosteroids
Standard dosage   1–2 mg/kg/d divided in 3 doses with taper over 7–10 d.

General guidelines
• Most patients can be followed as outpatients.

• Patients can require hospitalization if renal involvement, respiratory distress, or change in mental status.

Prophylaxis
• Administer antihistamines and/or steroids if there is a need to administer foreign serum or proteins.

Treatment aims
To resolve symptoms rapidly.

Prognosis
Usually self-limited; resolves within 2–3 wk; can rarely recur.

Follow-up and management
• Once symptoms resolve, no further testing is indicated.
• Avoid future use of offending agent.

General references:

Effmeyer JC: Serum sickness. *Ann Allergy* 1986, 156:105–109.

Herbert A: Serum sickness: reactions from Cef in children. *J Am Acad Derm* 1991, **25**:805–808.

Lauley T: A prospective clinical and immunologic analysis of patients with serum sickness. *N Eng J Med* 1984, 311:1407–1412.

Diagnosis

Symptoms

Failure to thrive and growth retardation.

Intractable or recurrent pneumonia: cough, fever, shortness of breath (frequently respiratory viral infections and opportunistic infections).

Persistent oropharyngeal thrush or stomatitis.

Recalcitrant candidal diaper dermatitis.

Persistent or recurrent diarrhea, vomiting: *eg*, rotavirus, adenovirus.

Bacterial sepsis: *eg*, gram-negative sepsis.

Persistent skin rash: erythematous, eczematoid dermatitis is a clue to graft-versus-host (GVH) disease; *in utero* transfusion of maternal cells or transfusion of unirradiated blood product.

Skin infections and or lesions.

Chronic conjunctivitis.

Adverse reactions to vaccines.

Signs

Failure to thrive, wasting, growth retardation.

Fever.

Evidence for pneumonia: tachypnea with wheeze, rhonchi, rales, or consolidation; normal chest examination possible.

Tachycardia: fever, systemic illness.

Oropharyngeal thrush.

Frequent absence of lymphoid tissue: tonsillar, lymph nodes.

Hepatosplenomegaly: infection, GVH disease.

Skin infection: bacterial, fungal, viral.

Eczematoid skin rash: GVH disease.

Investigations

Complete history and physical examination: Family history for immunodeficiency (*Note*: family history can often be negative in X-linked lethal disorders because many cases are new mutations).

Culture sites of suspected infection: surveillance cultures for persistent infection or colonization (oropharynx, trachea, stool, urine, blood, and skin) as appropriate for viral, fungal, bacterial, and mycobacterial agents.

Complete blood count with differential and platelets.

Chest radiograph.

Ancillary imaging studies: as indicated to evaluate infection.

Pulse oximetry: and arterial blood gas determination as appropriate.

Electrocardiography.

Ophthalmologic examination: infection.

Survey blood chemistry: electrolytes; hepatic and renal function.

Urinalysis.

Skin biopsy for suspected GVH disease.

Chromosome analysis.

HLA typing.

Complications

Death: uniformly fatal by 2 years of age if untreated.

Overwhelming infections.

GVH disease.

Differential diagnosis

HIV infection, AIDS

• Entities that express either predominantly cell-mediated defects or variable combinations of both T- and B-cell dysfunctions include:

CD8 lymphocytopenia (ZAP-70 deficiency).

Defective expression of the T-cell receptor–CD3 complex.

Major histocompatability complex class I or II antigen deficiency.

Reticular dysgenesis.

Omenn syndrome.

Primary CD4 or CD7 deficiency.

Interleukin-2 (IL-2) deficiency.

Multiple cytokine deficiency.

Signal transduction deficiency.

Di George syndrome (thymic hypoplasia).

Wiskott–Aldrich syndrome.

Ataxia telangiectasia.

Cartilage hair hypoplasia.

Common variable immunodeficiency.

Protein-losing enteropathy.

Etiology

• There are two categories of more severely immunodeficient SCID phenotypes.

1. Group with severely decreased numbers of both T- and B-cells: these patients often have normal or increased natural killer cell function; all of the disorders in this group exhibit autosomal recessive inheritance and include a) ADA deficiency, b) PNP deficiency, and c) a heterogenous subgroup whose members' molecular defects remain to be defined but account for ~50% of this group.

2. Group with severely decreased T-cell numbers but with the presence of variable numbers of B-cells: included here are a) defects in the common gamma chain of the IL-2 receptor, which are shared with the receptors for other interleukins, inherited as an X-linked recessive characteristic, and the most common in this subgroup; b) Jak3 deficiency, which is inherited as an autosomal recessive defect and is critical to signaling by the IL-2 receptor; and c) a heterogenous subgroup whose members' molecular defects remain to be elucidated.

Epidemiology

• Frequency ranges from ~1:50,000–500,000 births; genetically acquired as either X-linked (most common) or autosomal recessive; cases maybe sporadic or familial.

Treatment

Diet and lifestyle

• Prior to transplantation, patients should be a) placed in protective isolation until transplant completed and engrafted, b) irradiated, c) transfused with only cytomegalovirus (CMV)-negative blood products, and d) vaccinated with no live virus.

• After transplantation, lifestyle is expected to be essentially normal. Routine follow-up with immunologist recommended (monitor for infection and immunologic function).

Bone marrow transplantation

• Bone marrow transplantation should be performed as soon as possible. Preferred donors include 1) HLA-matched sibling; 2) parent (one haplotype match) stem cells after removal of mature T-cells (prevent GVH disease); and 3) unrelated, HLA-matched donor. Consider cytoreduction in recipient with remaining T-cell activity.

Pharmacologic treatment

Prophylaxis against *Pneumocystis carinii*: trimethoprim-sulfamethoxazole, pentamidine.

IVIG infusions: prevent of infection; supplement frequently dysfunctional or delayed B-cell function post-transplantation.

Oral IVIG: for management of viral-induced persistent diarrhea.

Replacement therapies: as appropriate (*eg*, ADA, IL-2 infusions).

• Aggressively identify and manage all infections.

• Avoid transmission of CMV and other viruses and prevent GVH through careful blood banking procedures.

• Avoid exposure to agents in live viral vaccines. Defer immunization of patient and close, intrafamilial contacts who may transmit the virus to the patient.

Other therapies

Thymus transplantation.
Gene therapy: strategies are evolving.

Treatment aims

To reconstitute immunologic function.
To prevent infections and GVH disease.
To treat ongoing and new infections.

Prognosis

90% survival for HLA-identical (BMT) recipients.
70% survival for haploidentical (BMT) recipients.

Follow-up and management

Routine follow-up physical examination and immunologic studies.
Monthly intravenous gamma globulin therapy.
Monitor for complications of infection, treatment, and onset of GVH disease.
Genetic counseling, including carrier detection.

References

Bonilla FA, Oettgen HC: Normal ranges for lymphocyte subsets in children [editorial]. *J Pediatr* 1997, **130**:347–348.

Buckley RH, Schiff RI, Schiff SE, *et al.*: Human severe combined immunodeficiency: genetic, phenotypic, and functional diversity in one hundred eight infants. *J Pediatr* 1997, **130**:378–387.

Hague RA, Rassam S, Morgan C, Cant AJ: Early diagnosis of severe combined immunodeficiency syndrome. *Arch Dis Child* 1995, **70**:260–263.

Hong R: Disorders of the T-cell system. In *Immunologic Disorders in Infants and Children*, ed 4. Edited by Stiehm ER. WB Saunders: Philadelphia; 1996:343–360.

Rosen FS. Severe combined immunodeficiency: a pediatric emergency. *J Pediatr* 1997, **130**:345–346.

Diagnosis

Symptoms

• Sexually transmitted diseases (STDs) present with a multitude of symptoms that are dependent on the site of infection. Infection of the lower genital tract in young women results in dysuria, vaginal discharge, and abnormal menstrual bleeding. With infection of the upper genital tract, lower abdominal pain and tenderness is present. Occasionally, this may present with right upper quadrant pain due to perihepatitis. Young men, if symptomatic, most often present with dysuria or penile discharge. They may also have testicular pain. Symptoms consistent with proctitis, conjunctivitis, pharyngitis, genital ulcers or warts, inguinal adenitis, rash or arthritis may all be manifestations of sexually transmitted diseases.

Signs

Uncomplicated disease: vaginitis (local inflammation, abnormal discharge, type varies with the infecting agent); cervicitis (friable cervix, discharge from the cervical os); urethritis (inflamed mucosa, discharge).

Complicated disease: pelvic inflammatory disease (lower abdominal, cervical motion and/or adenexal tenderness/enlargement, right upper quadrant tenderness, fever); epididymitis (pain/swelling over the epididymis).

Investigations

In females

External genital examination for discharge, warts, ulcerative lesions.

Internal examination for appearance of cervix, uterine, adenexal and cervical motion tenderness.

Cervical cultures for *Neisseria gonorrhoeae, Chlamydia trachomatis.*

Vaginal wet mount for *Trichomonas vaginalis, Gardnerella vaginalis.*

Urine or serum pregnancy test.

In males

External genital examination.

Urethral cultures for *N. gonorrhoeae, C. trachomatis.*

Urinalysis/culture.

Other investigations

Cultures for herpes simplex virus, chancroid as determined by physical examination.

Rapid plasma reagin (RPR), hepatitis B, and HIV serology.

Complications

Reinfection.

Increased risk of contracting other STDs.

Involuntary infertility, ectopic pregnancy, and chronic pelvic pain.

Differential diagnosis

Urogenital: appendicitis, ectopic pregnancy, ovarian cyst, endometriosis, urinary tract infection (UTI), pyelonephritis.

Gastrointestinal: gastroenteritis, hepatitis, cholecystitis, inflammatory bowel disease (IBD).

Etiology

• Bacterial, viral and protozoal infections spread via sexual contact or during the delivery of a newborn.

Bacterial: *N. gonorrhoeae, C. trachomatis, G. vaginalis, Treponema pallidum, Haemophilus ducreyi, Calymmatobacterium granulomatosis.*

• Viral: *herpes simplex virus, human papilloma virus, HIV.*

Protozoal: *T. vaginalis.*

Epidemiology

• Estimated prevalence rates of infection with *N. gonorrhoeae* or *C. trachomatis* in teens <19 y is 25%.

• Over one-third of STD cases occur in young adults <19 y.

Other information

• Define confidentiality to parent and teen at the beginning of the interview. Respect the teens' right of confidentiality.

• Obtaining sexual history, including number/sex of partners, type of sexual contact, previous pregnancy, or STD helps to identify the teen at risk.

• A teen infected with one STD is likely to have another. Look for multiple STDs and have a low threshold for treating.

Treatment

Lifestyle management

Encourage routine screening for STDs in high-risk teens.

Provide safe-sex counseling.

Provide partner treatment.

Pharmacologic treatment

For urethritis/cervicitis

Standard dosage	*N. gonorrhoeae*: cefixime, 400 mg p.o. once.
	Ciprofloxacin, 500 mg once p.o.
	C. trachomatis: azithromax, 1 g p.o. once; or doxycycline, 100 mg twice daily for 7 d.
Special points	Consider treating for both *N. gonorrhoeae* and *C. trachomatis* unless culture results are available or follow-up is assured.

For pelvic inflammatory disease or perihepatitis

Standard dosage	Ceftriaxone, 250 mg i.m. once plus doxycycline, 100 mg twice daily for 14 d.
	Cefoxitin, 2 g i.v. every 6 h plus doxycycline, 100 mg twice daily for 14 d (i.v therapy for 48 h after clinical response).
Special points	Polymicrobial: gonoccoci, chlamydia, anaerobes, facultative gram-negative aerobes.

For epididymitis

Standard dosage	Ceftriaxone, 250 mg i.m. once plus doxycycline, 100 mg twice daily for 14 d.

For proctitis

Standard dosage	Ceftriaxone, 125 mg i.m. once plus doxycycline, 100 mg twice daily for 14 d.

For vaginitis

Standard dosage	*Gardnerella vaginalis*: metronidazole, 2 g p.o. once or 500 mg twice daily for 7 d.
	T. vaginalis: metronidazole, 2 g p.o. once or 500 mg twice daily for 7 d.

For genital ulcers

Standard dosage	*HSV (primary):* acyclovir, 200 mg p.o. 5 times daily for 10 days.
	HSV (recurrent): acyclovir, 200 mg p.o. 5 times daily for 5 days.
	Syphilis (primary): benzathine penicillin, 2.4 MU once i.m.
	Chancroid: azithromax, 1 g p.o. once.
	Ceftriaxone, 250 mg once i.m.
Contraindications	*Azithromax*: contraindicated in pregnant patients and patients < 15 years of age.
	Ciprofloxazin: contraindicated in pregnant patients and patients < 17 years of age.

Treatment aims

To eradicate disease and prevent sequelae.

To prevent spread through patient follow-up, routine screening programs, partner treatment.

Prognosis

• Rates of clinical cure are excellent with the above regimens.

• Patients with upper genital tract disease have a sixfold increase in ectopic pregnancy and 20%–70% chance of involuntary infertility depending on the infective agent and number of episodes.

Follow-up and management

• Patient with complicated disease should be reevaluated within 48–72 h.

• Teens with uncomplicated disease may be reevaluated at 6–8 wk to screen for reinfection.

• All sexual partners in the 8 wk preceding the onset of symptoms should be referred for treatment.

Other treatments

Consider hospitalization in patients with upper genital tract disease and treat with i.v. therapy for 48 h following clinical response.

General references

Hammerschlag MR, Golden NH, OH MK: Single dose of azithromax for the treatment of genital chlamydia infections in adolescents. *J Pediatr* 1993, **122:**961–965.

Sexually transmitted diseases treatment guidelines. *MMWR Morb Mortal Wkly Rep* 1993, **42:**1–102.

Shafer MA, Sweet RL: Pelvic inflammatory diseases in adolescent females. *Pediatr Clin North Am* 1989, **36:**:513–532.

Weber JT, Johnson RE: New treatments for *Chlamydia trachomatis* genital infection. *Clin Infect Dis* 1995, **20(suppl 1):**S66–S71.

Zambrano D: Recent advances in antibiotic regimens for the treatment of obstetric-gynecologic infections. *Clin Ther* 1996, **18:**214–227.

Shock

Diagnosis

Definition

• Inability of the circulatory system to provide sufficient oxygen and nutrients to meet the metabolic demands of the tissue.

Symptoms

• Fatigue, dizziness, confusion, irritability, agitation, lethargy, shortness of breath.

Signs

Early (compensated)

Tachycardia, prolonged capillary refill (2 s), cool or mottled extremities.

Tachypnea.

Decreased activity.

Normal to increased pH due to respiratory compensation.

Uncompensated (end-organ compromise and cellular ischemia)

Increased tachycardia, delayed capillary refill (>4 s), pallor or cyanosis.

Hyperpnea, dyspnea, grunting.

Hypotension.

Oliguria.

Signs of congestive heart failure (cardiogenic shock).

Decreased level of consciousness or altered mental status.

Uncompensated metabolic acidosis decreased pH, other laboratory abnormalities due to multiple organ system ischemia.

Late or prearrest

Increasing hypotension, thready or absent peripheral pulses, cold extremities.

Bradypnea, bradycardia.

Decreased level of consciousness to coma.

Anuria.

Investigations

Physical examination (*see* Signs).

Laboratory: complete blood count, platelets, prothrombin time (PT), partial thromboplastin time (PTT), electrolytes, blood urea nitrogen, creatine, glucose, ionized calcium, blood culture, arterial blood gas (ABG), toxicology screens if indicated, urinalysis (UA).

History: short or long history of lethargy, poor feeding, fluid losses, decreased urine output; trauma; congenital heart disease; preexisting conditions; fever, recent infections or exposures; immunodeficiency; medications and potential ingestions.

Chest radiography (CXR): heart size, pulmonary vascularity, pulmonary edema, liver and spleen size, tension pneumothorax.

Complications

• Multisystem organ failure after inadequate circulation leads to anaerobic metabolism, increasing metabolic acidosis, cell dysfunction, damage, and/or cell death.

Etiology

Clinical picture fairly similar despite variable cause, but determination of type of shock will assist in treatment.

Three main types of shock: hypovolemic, cardiogenic, and distributive.

Rarely, two other types: dissociative (carbon monoxide poisoning, methemoglobinemia) and obstructive (pericardial tamponade, tension pneumothorax).

Hypovolemic

Most common cause in children.

Decreased circulating intravascular volume due to blood loss (trauma, gastrointestinal, intracranial), plasma loss (burns, hypoproteinemia), or water loss (vomiting, diarrhea, glucosurin, etc.)

Distributive

Most often due to vasodilation and peripheral pooling caused by anaphylaxis, central nervous system injury, toxic ingestion.

(May see flushing, bounding pulses, hyperdynamic precordium, wide pulse pressure, warm extremities, fever)

Cardiogenic

Less common cause of shock in children; most often due to decreased contractility.

Can usually be distinguished by signs of CHF and by history.

Caused by congenital heart disease, postcardiac surgery, dysrhythmias, cardiomyopathy, myocarditis, hypoxic–ischemic injury, drug intoxication, hypoglycemia, acidosis, hypothermia.

Other information

• Hypotension is a *late* sign signaling cardiovascular decompensation.

• Estimation of lower limit (5th percentile) of normal systemic blood pressure (BP) in children >1 y: 70 mm Hg + (2 × age in y). Minimum normal systolic BP in neonates is 55–60 mm Hg. In infants, it is 70 mm Hg.

• Estimated normal diastolic BP is two-thirds of systolic.

Treatment

Pharmacologic treatment: inotropes

• Consider use after 80 mL/kg of fluids, cardiogenic shock, or at anytime for signs of volume overload with persistent shock.

• Start with standard dose and titrate up to effect.

Dopamine

• First choice to improve contractility and increase splanchnic and renal blood flow for persistent hypotension after fluid resuscitation.

Standard dosage   2 µg/kg/min to increase renal blood flow.

5–10 µg/kg/min to increase cardiac output (β effect).

>10 µg/kg/min for a pressor effect (α effect).

Maximum dose: 20 µg/kg/min.

Dobutamine

• First choice in cardiogenic shock; selective β_1-receptor; increases CO, not HR or SBP.

Standard dosage   2–5 µg/kg/min. Maximum: 20 µg/kg/min.

Epinephrine

• Useful for profound septic shock and hypotension unresponsive to fluid resuscitation, or if unresponsive to dopamine or dobutamine.

• See β_1, β_2, and α effect of increased SBP, CO, HR.

Standard dosage   0.1 to 0.3 µg/kg/min. Maximum: 1.0 µg/kg/min.

Main side effects   Arrhythmias, excessive afterload (may need vasodilator), hyperglycemia, hypokalemia.

Nonpharmacologic treatment

Oxygenate/ventilate

100% Oxygen: assist ventilation, if needed, via bag-valve-mask.

• Consider orotracheal intubation (after initial fluid resuscitation if possible due to potential adverse effects of intubation and positive pressure ventilation in hypovolemic patient.

• Monitor by ABG or pulse oximetry.

Vascular access

• Large bore, two sites; obtain blood for laboratory work-up, if possible.

• Attempt peripheral first, then central or intraosseous, cutdown last resort.

• Obtain laboratory results if possible.

Fluid administration/guidelines

Crystalloid: normal saline (NS), lactated Ringer's.

Colloids: 5% albumin, fresh frozen plasma (FFP), whole blood (WB) or packed red blood cells (pRBC).

Guidelines

• Give first 40–60 mL/kg as crystalloid in rapid (10–20 min) 20-mL/kg boluses.

• Reassess after each bolus.

• Maintain hematocrit >33%.

• pRBC or WB for hematocrit (Hct) <33% or persistent signs of hypovolemia after 40 mL/kg crystalloid in patients with suspected blood loss (10 mL/kg, type specific or O-negative uncrossmatched).

• Consider 5% albumin (10 mL/kg) after crystalloids for Hct >30% or if blood is not available.

• Continue volume expansion beyond 60–80 mL/kg if circulation remains unsatisfactory with no signs of volume overload.

Treatment aims

• Rapid recognition and treatment is needed to prevent further injury by optimizing oxygenation, ventilation, and organ perfusion.

Other treatments

• Avoid/treat hypothermia.
• Treat documented hypoglycemia.
• Treat documented hypocalcemia.
• Presumptive administration of antibiotics if septic or unclear cause.
• Treat acidosis (<7.2) persisting after volume resuscitation and establishment of adequate ventilation.
FFP: for prolonged PT/PTT (10 mL/kg).
Platelets: for diffuse bleeding or count <50,000 (0.2 U/kg).
Inadvertent use of D_5NS or D_5 LR for fluid resuscitation will lead to hyperglycemia and an osmotic diuresis.

Prognosis

• Shock is a continuum that if untreated is progressive and uniformly fatal.
Treated hypovolemic shock has mortality of <10% if uncomplicated. Treated septic shock has a varying mortality depending on age, underlying diseases, and microorganisms (from 10% to >60%).

Follow-up and management

• Frequent and thorough reassessment.
• After initial stabilization, transport to appropriate intensive-care setting as soon as possible.

General references

American Heart Association: Fluid therapy. In Textbook of Pediatric Advanced Life Support. 1994:1–18.

Aoki BY, McCloskey K: Cardiovascular system. In Evaluation, Stabilization, and Transport of the Critically Ill Child. St. Louis: Mosby; 1992.

Bell LM: Shock. In Textbook of Pediatric Emergency Medicine, ed 3. Edited by Fleisher G, Ludwig S. Philadelphia: Williams & Wilkins; 1993:44–54.

Blumer JL: Shock in the pediatric patient. In Current Concepts in Critical Care Medicine. 1995:1–20.

Zaritsky AL, Moorman SN: Shock. In Pediatric Transport Medicine. Edited by McClosky K, Orr R. New York: Mosby; 1995:200–218.

Sickle cell disease

Diagnosis

Symptoms

Newborn screening: identifies the majority of infants affected with sickle cell disease before symptoms appear.

Fever, lethargy, coma: may be presenting symptoms of life-threatening sepsis episodes; peak incidence during first 4 years of life.

Pallor, lethargy: due to acute exacerbation of anemia due to aplastic crisis or splenic sequestration crisis.

Painful episodes (vaso-occlusive crises): infants present with swollen, painful hands and feet (hand–foot syndrome). Pain in older children occurs in abdomen and extremities; in adolescents in back, chest, and legs. Chest pain may herald serious acute chest syndrome. Painful episodes account for >90% of hospital admissions.

• Patients with sickle cell (SC) disease and Sβ° thalassemia are generally more severely affected than those with SC or Sβ+ thalassemia who have milder courses.

Signs

• Patients in mild crisis have no signs. **Jaundice:** may worsen with fever, infection, or painful episode.

Fever: infection may precipitate crises, crisis may mimic infection.

Pallor, tachycardia: worsening anemia may be due either to sequestration in spleen or marrow aplasia.

Localized swelling, tenderness, or redness of bone, joint, or muscle: may indicate vaso-occlusion or infection.

Investigations

General investigations

Complete blood count: to establish degree of anemia and leukocytosis.

Reticulocyte count: to establish degree of hemolysis.

Hemoglobin electrophoresis: to determine variant hemoglobins.

"Sickle prep": to confirm presence of hemoglobin S (not necessary if electrophoresis performed).

Hemoglobin F estimation: high concentrations diminish severity.

Extended erythrocyte antigen typing: to ensure appropriate erythrocytes for transfusion; should be performed before transfusion.

Blood urea nitrogen, creatinine, electrolytes analysis: to monitor renal function.

Liver function tests: to monitor degree of hemolysis and for hepatitis.

In crises

• The results should be compared with those from the stable state.

Complete blood count: hemoglobin raised with dehydration; falls in sequestration and aplasia.

Reticulocyte count: falls in aplastic crisis (due to parvovirus B19).

Blood urea nitrogen, creatinine, electrolytes: to detect dehydration.

Liver function tests: to measure dysfunction.

Cultures and viral screening: urine, blood, sputum, throat swab; to exclude infection (before antibiotic treatment); screening for parvovirus (not routine unless reticulocytopenic and anemic).

Differential diagnosis

• Distinguishing vaso-occlusive episode from infection of bone, joint, or chest may be difficult.

Etiology

• Sickle cell disease is inherited in an autosomal recessive pattern.

• Clinical problems also occur when hemoglobin S interacts with other variant hemoglobins (eg, SC) and with a β-thalassemia gene (β° or β+).

Epidemiology

• Symptoms rarely manifest before the age of 4–6 months because of the presence of fetal hemoglobin due to the late switching off of the fetal hemoglobin gene.

Complications

Stroke: occurs in 8% of patients, median age 7 years. Recurrence rate is 50% but can be prevented with routine erythrocyte transfusions.

Sequestration crisis: infants and young children are susceptible to acute episodes of pooling of erythrocytes in spleen (splenic sequestration), causing rapid development of severe anemia, which may be followed by hypotension, shock, and sometimes death.

Other manifestations of vaso-occlusion

Acute chest syndrome: a triad of chest pain, fever, dyspnea that mimics or may be accompanied by acute pneumonia; patient may deteriorate quickly; simple or exchange transfusion may be necessary.

Repeated episodes of priapism: may result in impotence.

Proliferative retinopathy: common in SC patients.

Aplastic crisis: infection with parvovirus B19 causes temporary cessation of erythrocyte production. Sickle cell patients develop symptomatic anemia due to shortened erythrocyte survival and preexisting degree of anemia. May require erythrocyte transfusion if severe.

Infection: increased susceptibility to serious, life-threatening infection due in part to splenic hypofunction from early age. High risk for infection with encapsulated organisms, *Streptococcus pneumoniae, Haemophilus influenzae, Salmonella.*

Cholecystitis and cholelithiasis: risk increased by long-term chronic hemolysis.

Treatment

Diet and lifestyle

• Patients should avoid factors that precipitate painful crisis, *eg*, infection, dehydration, exhaustion, cold, marked temperature changes, smoking, high altitude, and unpressurized aircraft; in some patients, stress is reported to be a precipitant.

Pharmacologic treatment

Analagesia

Standard dosage	*For mild to moderate pain*: acetaminophen, 12–15 mg/kg every 6 hours.
	Codeine phosphate, 1–2 mg/kg every 4–6 hours (up to 3 mg/kg in 24 hours), or nonsteroidal anti-inflammatory drugs, all orally.
	For severe pain: morphine, 0.1 mg/kg i.v. loading dose, then 1–2 mg/kg i.v. infusion over 24 hours using patient-controlled analgesia system.
	Hydromorphone hydrochloride, 0.05 mg/kg i.v. every 3–4 hours.
Contraindications	*Oral drugs*: hepatic and renal impairment, peptic ulceration, asthma.
	Parenteral drugs: raised intracranial pressure.
Special points	*Narcotics*: respiratory rate must be monitored carefully.
Main drug interactions	*Codeine, morphine, and hydromorphone*: other central nervous system depressants, tricyclic antidepressants.
Main side effects	*Oral drugs*: rashes, blood dyscrasias, acute pancreatitis, constipation, respiratory depression.
	Morphine: respiratory depression, nausea, bronchospasm, severe pruritus.
	Hydromorphone: same as morphine, biliary or urinary tract spasm.

Antibiotics

• Infants and young children are all placed on penicillin prophylaxis.

Standard dosage	Penicillin VK, 125 mg twice daily (<10 kg), 250 mg twice daily (>10 kg).
Contraindications	Penicillin allergy.
Main drug interactions	Anticoagulants, antacids, oral contraceptives.
Main side effects	Nausea, diarrhea, rashes, pseudomembranous colitis.

Nonpharmacologic treatment

Rehydration

• Oral fluids increased in patients with mild pain; i.v. $D_5 0.5NSS$ fluids in patients with severe pain at 1.0–1.5 times maintenance.

Blood transfusion

Simple transfusion: when hemoglobin < 4–5 g/dL and patient is symptomatic from anemia; for aplastic crisis, sequestration, bleeding (*eg*, renal papillary necrosis). Dose of packed red blood cells is 3–10 mL/kg.

For preparation for surgery: simple transfusion to 10 g/dL.

Exchange transfusion: when hemoglobin >5 g/dL but improved oxygen transport needed for rapidly progressive acute chest syndrome.

Overall goal of exchange transfusion: hemoglobin S < 30%, total hemoglobin 10–13.0 g/dL.

Long-term transfusion: to maintain hemoglobin at 10–13.0 g/dL, with hemoglobin S < 30%; for prevention of recurrence of stroke transfusions are given indefinitely, for sickle chronic lung disease, prevention of recurrence of splenic sequestration, or priapism (usually up to 1 year).

Treatment aims

To provide early, effective pain relief.
To prevent and treat infection.
To maintain hydration and tissue oxygenation.

Prognosis

• Sickle cell disease variants have different clinical manifestations; no markers exist to predict severity for a particular patient.
• Eighty-seven percent of patients are alive at 20 y, 50% at 50 y. Deaths in childhood are most commonly due to infection.
• Deaths in adolescents and young adults are most commonly due to neurological and lung complications.
• In one-third of adults who die prior to 50 y of age, death occurs during an acute sickle crisis (pain, acute chest syndrome, stroke).
• Bone marrow transplantation has been successful in some and is a potential cure for selected patients.
• Drugs that raise hemoglobin F levels, thus decreasing vaso-occlusion, are in clinical trials.

Follow-up and management

• Full education and counseling must be provided, with family screening and genetic advice.
• Penicillin prophylaxis must be ensured for children; pneumococcal and hemophilus B vaccination should be given.
• Children should be carefully checked for growth and development.

General references

Embury SH, Hebbel RP, Mohandas N, Steinberg MH: *Sickle Cell Disease: Basic Principles and Clinical Practice.* New York: Raven Press; 1994.

Gill FM, Sleeper LA, Weiner SJ, et al.: Clinical events in the first decade of life in a cohort of patients with sickle cell disease. *Blood* 1995, **86:**776–783.

Platt OS, Brambilla DJ, Rosse WF, et al.: Mortality in sickle cell disease: life expectancy and risk factors for early death. *N Engl J Med* 1994, **330:**1639–1644.

Vichinsky EP, Haberkern CM, Neumayr N, et al.: A comparison of conservative and aggressive transfusion regimens in the perioperative management of sickle cell disease. *N Engl J Med* 1995, **33:**206–213.

Diagnosis

Symptoms

Cough, postnasal drip, congestion: common.

Pain, headache, fever, fatigue, irritability: less common.

Signs

Sinus tenderness or fullness: less common in subacute or chronic disease.

Malodorous breath.

Purulent drainage: may or may not be thick or discolored.

Rhinorrhea with nasal edema.

Investigations

• Sinusitis is usually diagnosed clinically.

Rhinoscopy: performed by otolaryngologist.

CT scan: to confirm diagnosis; coronal views without contrast, usually done if consideration of surgery.

Plain films: much less reliable; rarely performed.

Maxillary sinus aspiration: to assess cause; performed by otolaryngologist if complicated.

• If episodes are repeated, suggest allergy evaluation or immunological evaluation if other frequent infections.

Complications

Exacerbation of underlying reactive airways: in patients with asthma.

Periorbital cellulitis, orbital cellulitis, intracranial abscess, cavernous sinus thrombosis.

• Above all, complications are very unusual in immunocompetent host with the exception of exacerbation of asthma.

Differential diagnosis

Viral upper respiratory infection.
Allergic rhinitis with postnasal drip.
Immunodeficiency (antibody).
Ciliary dyskinesia.
Cystic fibrosis.
Anatomical abnormality.

Etiology

Streptococcus pneumonia.
Hemophilus influenza (nontypable).
Branhamella catarrhalis.
Viral isolates.
• In chronic disease, consider anaerobes (*Staphylococcus*).

Epidemiology

Complications in 1%–5% of upper respiratory infections.
• More common in patients with allergies or underlying immune dysfunction.
• Usual cause of repeat sinusitis is failure to eradicate initial episode.

Classification

Acute: symptoms that last 10 d but <30 d.
Subacute: symptoms 30–90 d.
Chronic: symptoms >90 d.
Recurrent: acute sinusitis with resolution between episodes.

Treatment

Diet and lifestyle
• No changes are necessary.

Pharmacologic treatment

Standard dosage   Amoxicillin, 40 mg/kg/d divided in 3 doses.

Amoxicillin claulanate, 40/10 mg/kg/d divided in 3 doses.

Sulfamethoxazole-trimethoprim, 40/8 mg/kg/d divided in 2 doses.

Cefaclor, 40 mg/kg/d divided in 3 doses.

Cefadroxil, 30 mg/kg/d divided in 2 doses.

Cefuroxine axetil, 30 mg/kg/d divided in 2 doses.

Cefixime, 8 mg/kg/d.

Cefprozil, 30 mg/kg/d divided in 2 doses

Cefpodoxine proxetil, 20 mg/kg/d divided in 2 doses.

Loracarbef, 30 mg/kg/d divided in 2 doses.

Clarithromycin, 15 mg/kg/d divided in 2 doses.

Ceftibuten, 9 mg/kg/d.

Special points   Treat long enough to eradicate infection.

Initial episode: if symptoms improve dramatically a minimum of 10 d.

Other patients: at least 7 d beyond resolution of symptoms.

Chronic: minimum of 3–4 wk, may require a second course of antibiotics.

Main Side Effects   Prolonged antibiotic treatment may be associated with vaginitis in female adolescents.

Prolonged antibiotic therapy can be associated with increased bacterial resistance.

Main drug interactions Penicillin can interfere with contraceptive effect of birth control pills in female adolescents.

Macrolide antibiotics will interfere with theophylline metabolism.

Macrolide antibiotics will increase blood levels of tefenadine and artemizole.

Treatment aims
To minimize symptoms of pain and rhinorrhea.
To avoid development of complications.

Prophylaxis
Not shown to prevent future episodes in immunocompetent host.

Other treatments
Antihistamine and/or decongestants.
Nasal steroids.
Nasal irrigation.
Mucolytics.
Fiberoptic endoscopic sinus surgery: if unresponsive to prolonged medical therapy at least 3 mo before consideration of surgical referral.

Prognosis
• 30% will respond spontaneously without treatment.
• 95% will respond fully to initial course of antibiotics.
• If immunocompetent host, prognosis is excellent.

Follow-up management
• If symptoms do not respond to initial course of therapy, a second course of antibiotics should be administered of larger duration.
• If unresponsive to protracted courses of therapy, consider CT scan and/or ear, nose, and throat referral.
• Treat underlying allergies when present.

General references

Wald ER: Sinusitis in children. *N Eng J Med* 1992, **326:**319–323.

Wald ER: Subacute sinusitis in children. *J Pediatr* 1989, **115:**28–31.

Ott N: Childhood sinusitis. *Mayo Clinic Procedures* 1991, **66:**1238–1247.

Goldenhersh MJ: Sinusitis: early recognition, aggressive treatment. *Contemp Pediatr* 1989, **6:**22–42.

Diagnosis

Symptoms

Hypersomnia: excessive or inappropriate sleep; includes narcolepsy.

Insomnia: impaired ability to initiate or maintain sleep.

Parasomnia: abnormal behavior during sleep.

Night terrors

Represent incomplete arousal from non–rapid eye movement (REM) sleep.

Onset usually before age 4–6.

Nocturnal episodes of partial awakening with intense fear and agitation: often with moaning or screaming with autonomic arousal; tachycardia, rapid respirations, dilated pupils, perspiration.

Confused and unresponsive appearance: typically, patient cannot be awakened.

Attacks last 10–30 minutes: may occur weekly or more for months or years.

Nightmares

Represent awakening during disturbing dreams.

Awakenings associated with vivid recall of content of dream.

Child is fearful and agitated but readily calmed.

Somnambulism (sleepwalking)

Repeated episodes of rising from bed during sleep, walking about with blank, staring face and relative unresponsiveness.

When patient is awakened initial confusion rapidly clears.

Sleep apnea

Usually obstructive and associated with snoring, partial awakening, and excessive daytime somnolence.

Narcolepsy

Irresistible daytime sleep attacks, typically brief (10–20 minutes), plus one or more of the following conditions:

Cataplexy: daytime attacks of sudden loss of muscle tone precipitated by sudden intense emotions.

Sleep paralysis: inability to move or speak upon awakening or falling asleep.

Hypnogogic hallucinations: intense, often frightening, dreamlike sleep imagery on falling asleep or awakening.

Signs

In sleep apnea, obesity or evidence of airway obstruction (*eg*, enlarged tonsils, retro- or micrognathia or other craniofacial anomaly, macroglossia, tumor) may be present.

Investigations

Airway examination: laryngology consultation.

HLA typing: in narcolepsy (association with DR2 and Dqw1 alleles).

Neuroimaging (cranial CT, MRI, or MRA): if epilepsy is suspected; rarely, hypothalamic lesions produce hypersomnolence. In addition, "Ondine's curse" (central apnea during sleep) has been associated with brainstem neoplasms.

Electroencephalography (routine or following sleep deprivation): for seizures.

Multiple sleep latency test: uses EEG to measure latency to sleep onset and to REM-sleep onset following sleep deprivation (reduced in narcolepsy).

Polysomnography: for suspected sleep apnea, or to exclude epilepsy; includes combined monitoring of oxygen saturation, nasal airflow (via thermistor), respiratory effort (via strain gauge or chest impedance monitor), ECG, EEG.

Differential diagnosis

Epilepsy.

Physiologic myoclonus of sleep (hypnic jerks).

Depression.

Drug-related sleep disturbance.

Hysteria.

Etiology

• There is strong evidence for a genetic cause in narcolepsy.

• The origin of most other sleep disorders is obscure.

• Except in premature infants, sleep apnea is more commonly obstructive rather than central.

• Disorganized sleep patterns are common in autistic and mentally retarded children.

Epidemiology

• The prevalence of sleep disorders varies widely according to the population studied, diagnostic criteria, and vigor of ascertainment.

• Narcolepsy is relatively common in whites (roughly 1:1000–4000 individuals) but is rarely seen in Jews.

• Narcolepsy rarely appears before adolescence but is probably underdiagnosed in that age group.

Complications

Diminished academic performance.

Cor pulmonale or sudden death in sleep apnea.

Accidents (especially in narcolepsy).

Treatment

Diet and lifestyle

• For circadian rhythm shifts, adjustment of sleep schedule is indicated.

• Regular bedtime, often with a period of quiet and ritualized relaxation, is often helpful in syndromes of insomnia or sleep avoidance. Encouraging attachment to a specific toy, blanket, and so on will often enhance the child's sense of security.

• Frequent "checking" on children with sleep avoidance often exacerbates the situation.

• Regular, scheduled short naps may help to reduce the frequency of sleep attacks in narcolepsy; long naps should be avoided.

• In selected children (especially autistic patients) with severe, longstanding, refractory sleep disturbance, consideration should be given to the purchase of an enclosed, padded crib to ensure the safety of the patient, reduce parental reinforcement, and to improve parental sleep.

Pharmacologic treatment

Insomnia

• Chloral hydrate or benzodiazepines (eg, lorazepam) may provide short-term benefit but tolerance usually develops rapidly. When used intermittently, they are sometimes helpful in the management of sleep problems in autistic or mental retarded individuals. A variety of other agents, including melatonin, have been used anecdotally, but controlled trials in children are generally lacking and safety is not clearly established.

Narcoleptic sleep attacks

Standard dosage	Methylphenidate, maximum 60 mg/d (adults), dosed and titrated according to symptoms. Other stimulants (dexedrine, pemoline) sometimes helpful.
Main side effects	Insomnia, anorexia, end-of-day "rebound" symptoms as dose wears off, dysphoria, moodiness, agitation, possible growth impairment (controversial); rare, idiosyncratic hepatic failure with pemoline.

Narcoleptic cataplexy

Standard dosage	Imipramine or clomipramine, 10–50 mg once daily (adult dose).
Special points	Cataplexy does not respond to stimulants, but these can be used in combination with clomipramine.
Main side effects:	appetite changes, orthostasis.

Night terrors

Pharmacologic treatment should generally be avoided, although nightly sedation with benzodiazepines has been reported to be successful.

Nonpharmacologic treatment

Appropriate surgical intervention (eg, tonsillectomy/adenoidectomy, resection of tumor, mandibuloplasty, and so on) or nocturnal continuous positive airway pressure in selected patients with obstructive sleep apnea.

In children with night terrors, a nightly planned awakening prior to the usual time of the attack may be helpful.

Treatment aims

To eliminate daytime hypersomnolence or sleep attacks, and other symptoms of narcolepsy.

To protect patients from injury (especially in somnambulism and narcolepsy)

Prognosis

• Narcolepsy is typically a lifelong disorder.

• Night terrors generally resolve spontaneously within a few months, but occasionally persist for several years.

Follow-up and management

• Driving should be restricted in uncontrolled narcolepsy or other syndromes with disabling hypersomnolence.

• Consider sleep diary for long-term management.

General references

American Thoracic Society: Standards and indications for cardiopulmonary sleep studies in children. Am J Respir Crit Care Med 1996, 153:866–878.

Mitler MM, Aldrich MS, Koob GF, Zarcone VP: Narcolepsy and its treatment with stimulants: ASDA standards of practice. Sleep 1994, 17:352–371.

Potsic WP, Wetmore RF: Sleep disorders and airway obstruction in children. Otolaryngol Clin North Am 1990, 23:651–663.

Woody RC: Sleep disorders in children. Semin Neurol 1988, 8:71–77.

Diagnosis

Symptoms

Soreness and Difficulty swallowing.
Concurrent coryza, laryngitis, productive cough: suggesting viral cause.
Malaise, fever, headache: common.

Signs

General

Injected mucous membranes of pharynx, tonsils, conjunctivae, and tympanic membranes.
Enlarged tonsils: sometimes with exudates.
Enlarged cervical lymph nodes.

Streptococcal infection

Gray exudates in tonsillar follicles.
Enlarged injected tonsillar and peritonsillar area.
Coated tongue with fetor.
Enlarged, tender cervical nodes.
Occasional meningismus.
Diffuse punctate erythema, flushed cheeks, circumoral pallor, reddened mucous membrane, white then red strawberry tongue: scarlet fever signs.

Infectious mononucleosis

Prolonged fever: often for 10–14 days.
Nasal voice/"fish mouth" breathing.
Enlarged lymph nodes and splenomegaly.
Palatal petechiae and clean tongue.
Enlarged tonsils: sometimes almost meeting with confluent white exudates.
Faint maculopapular rash.

Streptococcal follicular tonsillar exudates (top) and confluent exudates (bottom) in infectious mononucleosis.

Coxsackie A virus

5–10 small aphthoid ulcers: scattered over oral cavity.
Firm vesicular lesions: along sides of fingers and on feet (usually few).
Papular lesions: especially on feet and lower legs, occasionally up to buttocks.

Diphtheria

Toxic, listless, tachycardia due to myocarditis: low-grade or nonexistent fever.
Adherent whitish membrane: spreading from tonsils to oropharynx or oral cavity.
Enlarged anterior cervical lymph nodes: with surrounding edema.

Investigations

Throat swab: to check for streptococcal infection and diphtheria; usually not needed for viral infections. Rapid streptococcal test.
Differential leukocyte count: elevated neutrophil leukocytosis indicates streptococcal infection; elevated, many atypical mononuclear cells indicate infectious mononucleosis.
Serology: for Epstein–Barr virus, mycoplasma.

Complications

Peritonsillar abscess, reactive phenomena: rheumatic fever, glomerulonephritis, erythema nodosum, Henoch–Schönlein purpura; with streptococcal infection.
Respiratory obstruction, hepatitis, splenic rupture: with infectious mononucleosis.
Nerve palsies, myocarditis: with diphtheria.
Erythema multiforme: with *Mycoplasma pneumoniae* infection.

Differential diagnosis

• Differential diagnosis depends on the underlying cause.

Etiology [1]

• Causes include the following:
Pharyngitis with nonspecific features
Viral infection, especially adenoviruses, enteroviruses, influenza or parainfluenza virus, Epstein–Barr virus, coronavirus.
Beta-hemolytic *Streptococcus pyogenes* group A, C, or G.
M. pneumoniae, Corynebacterium diphtheriae, Neisseria gonorrhoeae.
Pharyngitis with clinically recognizable features
Streptococcus pyogenes infection: cause of follicular tonsillitis, scarlet fever.
Epstein–Barr virus infection: cause of infectious mononucleosis.
Coxsackievirus infection: cause of hand, foot, and mouth disease (A16), herpangina (A).
C. diphtheriae infection: cause of diphtheria.

Epidemiology

• Very common disease of children.
• Adenoviral infection is the most common viral type identified in children with respiratory illnesses, which are more prevalent in crowded conditions.
• Enteroviral infection usually occurs in late summer or early autumn, with one or two types dominating (out of >70).
• Some influenza virus activity is usual each winter, with some larger outbreaks.
• Epstein–Barr virus circulates throughout childhood but is usually only manifest symptomatically in teenagers and young adults.
• Streptococcal infection occurs in late winter and early spring, especially in school children.
• Very few cases of diphtheria occur in the United States each year.

Treatment

Diet and lifestyle
• Infants should be breast-fed and subsequently provided with adequate nutrition throughout childhood.
• Respiratory secretions must be disposed of hygienically.

Pharmacological treatment [2]
• Immunization should be given as nationally recommended: *eg*, against diphtheria, influenza A.
• Symptomatic treatment is indicated for presumed viral infections: *eg*, throat lozenges, acetaminophen.

Antibiotics
• Penicillins are effective against streptococcal and diphtherial infections [3,4].

Standard dosage	Benzathe penicillin 50,000 U/kg/M i.m. Phenoxymethylpenicillin, 25–50 mg/kg/d in divided doses every 6 h.
Contraindications	Hypersensitivity.
Special points	Erythromycin, 40 mg/kg/d in divided doses every 6 h, or new macrolides are other options.
Main drug interactions	None.
Main side effects	Sensitivity reactions, diarrhea.

Antitoxin
• Antitoxin should be given immediately on clinical suspicion of diphtheria.

Standard dosage	Antitoxin 20,000–100,000 U i.v. (depending on disease severity).
Contraindications	Hypersensitivity (epinephrine should be available).
Special points	Test dose is needed before full dose because of equine origin of antitoxin.
Main drug interactions	None.
Main side effects	Sensitivity reactions, including serum sickness.

Treatment aims
To provide symptomatic relief.
To reduce infectivity.
To prevent rheumatic fever (in streptococcal infections).
To neutralize circulating toxins of diphtheria promptly.

Other treatments
Drainage of peritonsillar abscess, indicated by marked inferior and posterior displacement of tonsil.
Tracheostomy for respiratory obstruction.
Tonsillectomy in children with recurrent tonsillitis more than five times per year.

Prognosis
• Full rapid recovery is usual.
• Occasionally, patients suffer from post-viral fatigue, especially after influenza, Epstein–Barr, or enteroviral infections.
• Mortality from diphtheria is 5%–10%; survivors usually recover completely.

Follow-up and management
• Patients who have apparently recovered from streptococcal tonsillitis may continue to have enlarged and tender cervical nodes that subsequently spread infection as cellulitis or septicemia.
• Patients with diphtheria should be followed up after 2–6 wk for late nerve palsies and myocarditis.

Notification
• Diphtheria and scarlet fever are legally notifiable diseases in the United States.

Key references
1. Denny FW: Tonsillopharyngitis. *Pediatr Rev* 1994, **15:** 185–191.
2. Goldstein MN: Office evaluation and management of the sore throat. Otolaryngol Clin North Am 1992, 25:837–842.
3. Kline JA, Runge JW: Streptococcal pharyngitis: a review of pathophysiology, diagnosis, and management. J Emerg Med 1994, 12:665–680.
4. Klein JO (ed): Proceedings of a symposium: group A steptococcal infections: an era of growing concern. *Pediatr Inf Dis J* 1991, 10:53–78.

Diagnosis

Signs and symptoms

• The child who requires interfacility medical transport may have any diagnosis.

• There is limited opportunity for diagnostic assessment during transport due to limited space, personnel, and resources.

• Signs and symptoms should be assessed prior to transport and a working diagnosis established.

• Signs, symptoms, and issues necessitating transport include:

Cardiovascular, respiratory, neurologic, or other compromise requiring acute stabilization, intervention, or therapy.

Need for pediatric specialist such as pediatric surgeon or neonatologist.

Higher level of care or different services than can be provided at referring institution.

Investigations

• Preparation of the child is the most important part of transport.

• Adequate pretransport interventions, stabilization, and anticipation of potential disease or injury process progression is imperative.

• Contact appropriate receiving physicians and collate all available pretransport information [1].

Complications

• Problems regarding the transport of an ill or injured child occur when 1) inadequate detail is paid to pretransport stabilization, and 2) inappropriate prioritization is given to the speed of the transport.

• COBRA/OBRA legislation holds the referring physician responsible for initiating appropriate care and ensuring its continuance during the transport period.

Basic life support unit
For stable children.
Does not allow for significant interventions if the patient deteriorates.
Ensures direct and safe transportation.

Paramedic ambulance
Paramedics are trained for acute intervention and stabilization.
Not for prolonged monitoring or diagnosis assistance.
The level of pediatric training and experienced skill set of the paramedics vary greatly.

Critical care ambulance (air or ground)
Includes a critical care nurse and paramedic or respiratory therapist.
Excellent general acute interventional and monitoring skills.
Explore pediatric expertise, training, and experience.

Transport physician
May be more or less as effective as the critical care team without a physician.
Physicians may add diagnostic expertise, but vary in their familiarity with the transport environment. The most important aspects of pediatric interfacility transport include familiarity with all aspects of the transport environment, significant pediatric experience, and the ability to intervene as indicated during the process.
The specific title of the transport personnel is less important than their pediatric experience and skills and their familiarity with all aspects of the transport environment [2].

Determination of mode of transport (air or ground)
Consult the specialized transport service to help determine appropriate mode of transport.
Ensure appropriate staff and transportation for each individual patient.

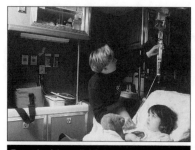

Example of the pediatric transport environment.

Treatment

- The main treatment issues for pediatric transport are those required to ensure stabilization during transport [3].
- The patient's airway, breathing, and circulation must be stabilized prior to transport.
- Tubes and lines should be quite secure.
- Plan for the worst scenario that could be reasonably expected given the disease process, length and mode of transport.
- Medications should be given prior to transport if possible to decrease the intratransport work load.
- Immobilization, if indicated, should be initiated and reassessed routinely.
- If specific therapy or personnel are needed at the receiving hospital, these should be arranged prior to the transport [4].
- Copies of all records and radiographs should be available for the transport personnel on their arrival.
- Changes in the patient's condition or unexpected results from interventions should be communicated to the transport team and receiving hospital to allow for a seamless transition of care [1].
- Although almost all intervention can be accomplished in the transport environment, the limited personnel and space dictate that whatever can be accomplished prior to the transport be done. This may involve a transport team spending extra time at the referring institution preparing the patient for the transport. Assistance from referring hospital staff can be invaluable in this process.

Other information

- Explore the interfacility transport options in your environment prior to the need for transport.
- Ask transport service representatives to review their available level of care and pediatric expertise.
- Understand how to directly contact a transport team.
- The fastest care is sometimes not the most appropriate. Understanding the different philosophies of bringing tertiary care to the patient versus bringing the patient to tertiary care is important.
- A sophisticated pediatric transport service should be able to offer immediate advanced pediatric assessment, intervention suggestions, and experienced transport personnel [4].
- If an acutely ill patient presents to the office environment, consider immediate transfer to the closet emergency department via the emergency medical system (911) for stabilization. Arrange interfacility transport from that location [5].

Key references

1. Bolte RG: Responsibilities of the referring physician and referring hospital. In *Pediatric Transport Medicine.* Edited by McCloskey K, Orr R. St. Louis: Mosby; 1995:33–40.

2. McCloskey K, Hackel A, Notterman D, et al.: Guidelines for Air and Ground Transport of Neonatal and Pediatric Patients: Task Force on Interhospital Transport. Elk Grove Village: American Academy of Pediatrics; 1993.

3. Aoki BY, McCloskey K: *Evaluation, Stabilization, and Transport of the Critically Ill Child.* St. Louis: Mosby Year-Book; 1992.

4. Woodward GA: Responsibilities of the Receiving Hospital. In *Pediatric Transport Medicine.* Edited by McCloskey K, Orr R. St. Louis: Mosby; 1995:41–49.

5. Woodward GA: Patient transport and primary care. In *Pediatric Primary Care: A Problem-Oriented Approach,* ed 3. Edited by Schwartz MW, Curry TA, Sargent AJ, et al. St. Louis: Mosby-Year Book, Inc.; 1997: 41–49.

General references

Jaimovich DG, Vidyasagar D, eds.: *Handbook of Pediatric and Neonatal Transport Medicine.* Philadelphia: Hanley & Belfus, Inc.; 1996.

McCloskey KA, Orr RA, eds. *Pediatric Transport Medicine.* St. Louis: Mosby; 1995.

Diagnosis

Definition

• Strabismus is defined as misaligned or "crossed" eyes.

• The danger of strabismus is the development of amblyopia, which is the loss of vision in one or both eyes with an otherwise normal eye examination. One of the major causes of amblyopia is strabismus, when one eye is preferentially used for fixation while the other eye is allowed to deviate off of the visual axis.

Signs and symptoms

"Crossed eyes" appearance: is the major finding in strabismus. The eyes may be seemingly fixed in one direction, called tropia; this tropia may occur as esotropia (nasal deviation), exotropia (outward deviation), hypertropia (deviation upward), or hypotropia (deviation downward).

Phoria: a tendency to move toward misalignment if the eyes are not kept in position by active fusion.

Pseudostrabismus: occurs in infants who have a flat nasal bridge, which gives the appearance of strabismus; upon testing, the eyes are found to be aligned.

• All newborns should be checked for proper eye alignment by noting the position of a reflected pen light on the corneal surface. The light should fall in the same position on each eye. Newborns should also be tested for a red reflex.

• When asymmetry of the eyes is found on physical examination, a cause should be determined. Frequently, this will require consultation with an ophthalmologist.

• If the eye seems red, painful, tearing, or has a white light reflex (leukokoria), immediate consultation should be obtained.

Investigations

Physical examination techniques: most often used in the office setting; he corneal light reflex test should be performed on every visit.

The cover–uncover test: also checks for fusion and determines both tropias and phorias. A refixation of the uncovered eye means that there had been malalignment and is diagnostic of a tropia. With a phoria there will be deviation of the eye when fusion is broken, *ie*, when the eye is covered. When the eye is subsequently uncovered it will move back into position to maintain fusion.

Worth Four Dot test: for children 3 years of age and older.

Complications

• The complication from missing the diagnosis of strabismus is the development of amblyopia and the ultimate loss of stereoscopic three-dimensional vision.

• Other complications may result from missing underlying diagnoses that could be treated.

Differential diagnosis

• Anything that impairs or imbalances binocular vision is likely to produce strabismus and resultant amblyopia.

• The causes of esotropia include infantile esotropia, sixth nerve palsy, Duane's syndrome, accommodative esotropia, and sensory deprivation esotropia (due to retinoblastoma, cataract or eyelid hemangioma that blocks vision).

• Exotropia, hypertropia, and hypotropia all have their own differential diagnosis list, but these forms of strabismus are much more rare.

Etiology

• The cause of amblyopia is the lack of visual stimulation of the brain during the critical period of visual development. This period is usually the first 6 y of life.

• When two visual images are sent to the brain simultaneously, suppression occurs and there is "shut off" of one image. When suppression occurs over a long period, amblyopia ensues.

• The earlier the process of suppression begins, the more profound it is likely to be. Thus, defects in the first year of life are likely to be more refractory.

Epidemiology

• Amblyopia is the most common cause for visual loss in the U.S.

• ~ 5% of the population is affected.

• Esotropia accounts for 75% of the cases of strabismus.

Treatment

General treatment

• The main issue in treatment is referral to an ophthalmologist as soon as the condition is diagnosed.

• The ophthalmologist has several modes of treatment available depending on the age of the child and the underlying pathology.

• For accommodative esotropia, glasses are given to correct the hyperopia. Focusing problems are also treated with glasses, and if amblyopia is present, patching therapy may help the weak eye to strengthen. Cataracts, if present, may require surgical removal. Other forms of strabismus may require other therapies, including use of drops that weaken eye muscles or surgical repair of muscles.

Treatment aims

• The goals of therapy are to end amblyopia and realign the eyes to restore binocular vision.

• Screen all newborns, infants, and children for strabismus.

• Diagnose the condition early.

• Refer to a pediatric ophthalmologist.

Prognosis

• The prognosis will depend on early diagnosis and close follow-up by the ophthalmologist.

Follow-up and management

• The indications for referral include any alteration in the red reflex, asymmetric or diminished visual acuity, constant strabismus, acute onset of strabismus, presence of family history of retinoblastoma or congenital cataracts, or simply parental concern about the observation of strabismus.

General references

Magramm I: Amblyopia: etiology, detection and treatment. *Pediatr Rev* 1992, **13**:7–14.

Nelson LB, Wagner RS, Simon JW, et al.: Congenital esotropia. *Surv Ophthalmol* 1987, **31**:1321–1324.

Quinn G: The crossed eye. In *Pediatric Primary Care*, ed 2. Edited by Schwartz W, Charney EB, Curry TA, Ludwig S. Chicago: Yearbook; 1987:393–397.

Diagnosis

General information

This section relates to neurally mediated syncope (NMS), vasodepressor syncope (VDS), and the cardiovascular conditions associated with syncope, including arrhythmias (supraventricular tachycardia, ventricular tachycardia, long QT syndrome, atrioventricular block, sinus node disease, postoperative atrial flutter, ventricular tachycardia, atrioventricular block, structural heart disease), left ventricular outflow tract obstruction (especially aortic stenosis, idiopathic hypertrophic subaortic stenosis); severe pulmonic stenosis; dilated cardiomyopathy; pulmonary artery hypertension (Eisenmenger's syndrome) [1].

Definition

• Sudden loss of consciousness and postural tone with spontaneous recovery.

Symptoms

• Symptoms associated with vasodepressor or NMS are usually not associated with exercise, but may be precipitated by warm surroundings, dehydration secondary to prolonged exercise, prolonged sitting or standing, frightening or surprising occurrences.

Dizziness, lightheadedness; headache, nausea, vomiting; chronic fatigue; sensation of warmth; visual blurring or blackout; loss of hearing.

Symptoms associated with other cardiovascular causes of syncope: **chest pain, palpitations, dizziness, lightheadedness, visual or hearing loss:**

Signs

Loss of consciousness.

Bradycardia, tachycardia, hypotension, pallor, diaphoresis, seizure activity.

Marked orthostatic hypotension: with decrease of systolic blood pressure of >10–20 mm Hg from supine to standing position and increase of heart rate of >20–30 bpm.

Investigations

ECG: normal in NMS. May show baseline sinus or junctional bradycardia, or sinus arrhythmia. With other types of syncope, ECG reflects underlying condition. In long QT syndrome, QTc is prolonged. Other arrhythmias such as supraventricular tachycardia, ventricular tachycardia, or atrioventricular block may be noted.

Echocardiography: not indicated in clear cut-neurally mediated syncope unless an associated congenital heart defect such as mitral valve prolapse is suspected. Indicated in other forms of syncope to look for structural or functional heart disease.

Electrophysiologic study: indicated if syncope associated with ventricular tachycardia, supraventricular tachycardia, Wolff-Parkinson-White (WPW) syndrome, atrial flutter, or atrial fibrillation with WPW syndrome.

Catheterization: indicated to evaluate structural heart disease, *eg*, determine gradient in aortic stenosis.

Head-upright tilt table test [2]: to document presence of NMS in questionable cases or those associated with prolonged syncope or seizure activity. Helps to direct therapy by defining type of NMS [3]: cardioinhibitory (abrupt fall in heart rate < 40 bpm or prolonged pause of >3 seconds) mixed (hypotensive and bradycardic response), or vasodepressor response (gradual or abrupt fall in blood pressure).

Holter monitoring: to evaluate arrhythmic causes of syncope.

Exercise stress testing: to evaluate syncope occurring with exercise, which may be vasodepressor, but is more often secondary to an arrhythmia, especially long QT syndrome.

Differential diagnosis

Noncardiac causes of syncope: hypoglycemia, seizure disorders, migraines, drugs, dehydration, sychological disorders.

Etiology

Neurally mediated syncope.

Congenital heart defects

Preoperative lesions: aortic stenosis, coarctation of the aorta, hypertrophic cardiomyopathy, Ebstein's anomaly, Marfan syndrome, mitral valve prolapse, coronary artery anomalies.

Postoperative lesions: complete or D-transposition of the great arteries, single ventricle complexes/Fontan repair, tetralogy of Fallot, ventricular septal defect, atrioventricular canal defect, aortic stenosis/hypertrophic cardiomyopathy, pulmonary artery hypertension, and other defects.

Acquired heart disease

Myocarditis, dilated cardiomyopathy, kawasaki disease.

Arrhythmias

Long QT syndrome, Wolff–Parkinson–White syndrome/supraventricular tachycardia: atrial fibrillation, ventricular tachycardia, bradycardia: sick sinus syndrome, complete atrioventricular block.

Epidemiology

• Neurally mediated syncope is the most common cause of syncope in children [4]; up to 50% of adolescents may have an episode of syncope. Recurrent problem in 5%–10% of adolescents. 1%–3% of emergency room visits are for syncope. Incidence of syncope associated with arrhythmias and structural heart disease is unknown.

• Sudden death is known to occur in 2%–5% of postoperative patients after surgery for congenital heart disease and in 10-20%/y of long QT syndrome patients after presentation with syncope.

Complications

Injury: fracture of skull, teeth, long bones in automobile, bicycle, or swimming accidents.

NMS generally not associated with life-threatening complications.

Other cardiovascular causes of syncope can result in cardiac arrest and sudden death.

Treatment

Diet and lifestyle

Neurally mediated syncope [5]

• Increase fluid intake to 10–12, 8 oz glasses of fluid per day including some (approximately four glasses) of electrolyte replacement fluid or water with NaCl tablet.

• Increase salt intake by salting foods and eating salty, nonfat snacks or foods.

• Avoid caffeine and diuretics.

Pharmacologic treatment

For neurally mediated syncope [5]

Standard dosage   Fludrocortisone acetate, 0.05–0.2 mg/d in 1–2 divided doses.

Nadolol (β-blocker), 1 mg/kg/d in 2 divided doses

Atenolol (β-blocker), *older children and adolescents*: 25–75 mg daily.

Disopyramide, *older children and adolescents*: 200 mg every 12 h of continuous release formulation.

Fluoxetine (serotonin uptake inhibitor), 20 mg/d to maximum of 80 mg/d.

Sertraline, 50–200 mg/d.

Contraindications

Special points   *Fludrocortisone acetate*: with refractory NMS, may titrate to 0.6 mg/d.

Disopyramide: avoid in patients with decreased ventricular function; acts by negative inotropic effect.

Fluoxetine: may require 6 wk before fully effective.

Sertraline: may require 6 wk before fully effective.

Main drug interactions   *Fludrocortisone acetate*: effects of anticholinesterase antagonized.

Fluoxetine: monoamine oxidase inhibitors, tricyclic antidepressants.

Sertraline: monoamine oxidase inhibitors.

Main side effects   *Fludrocortisone acetate*: cardiovascular: hypertension, edema, congestive heart failure; central nervous system: headache, convulsions; metabolic: hypokalemia.
Fluoxetine: asthenia, fever, headache, pharyngitis, dyspnea, rash, nausea.
Sertaline: Nausea, diarrhea, tremor, dizziness, insomnia, somnolence, increased sweating, dry mouth.

For other causes of syncope

• Appropriate treatment for specific arrhythmia or congenital heart defect.

Treatment aims
To prevent episodes of syncope.
To treat underlying causes

Other treatments
Pacemaker: rarely indicated in NMS in children. Even prolonged asystolic form of NMS can be treated with fluids, salt, and pharmacologic methods.
Support stockings.
Elevate head of bed.

Prognosis
Excellent with NMS.
• Most adolescents will have resolution of condition as they age. Most will be controlled by simple means. Less than 25% require long-term medication.

Follow-up and management
For NMS, periodic office visits depending on symptoms and whether medicated.
For other causes of syncope, follow-up dependent on cause of syncope.

Key references
1. Hannon DW, Knilans TK: Syncope in children and adolescents. *Curr Probl Pediatr* 1993, 23:358–384.
2. Grubb BD, Temesy-Armos P, Moore J, et al.: The use of head-upright tilt table testing in the evaluation and management of syncope in children and adolescents. *PACE Pacing Clin Electrophysiol* 1992, 15:742–748.
3. Sutton R, Peterson M, Brignole M, et al.: Proposed classification for tilt-induced vasovagal syncope. *Eur J Pacing Electrophysiol* 1992, 2:180–183.
4. Pratt JL, Fleisher GR: Syncope in children and adolescents. *Pediatr Emerg Care* 1989, 5:80–82.
5. Grubb BO, Kosinski D: Current trends in etiology, diagnosis, and management of neurocardiogenic syncope. *Curr Opin Cardiol* 1996, 11:32–41.

Diagnosis

Symptoms and signs

Tiredness: indicating anemia; one of the most difficult and resistant symptoms in systemic lupus erythematosus (SLE).

Polyarthralgias and nonerosive symmetric arthritis: involving predominantly small joints (rarely deforming) [1,2].

Rashes: photosensitive, discoid, and, less often, classic facial butterfly rash [1].

Vasculitic lesions of extremities: leading to gangrene of digits (rare).

Oral or pharyngeal ulcers, which are painless.

Myalgia or myositis.

Pleuritic or pericardial pain: may have pleural or pericardial effusions.

Epistaxis, bleeding gums, menorrhagia, purpura: symptoms of thrombocytopenia.

Visual and auditory hallucinations or epilepsy: in patients with CNS involvement.

Edema or hypertension: *eg*, nephrotic syndrome or acute nephritic illness.

Alopecia [1].

Raynaud's phenomenon: a triphasic response of color change from white to purple to red with exposure to cold.

Lymphadenopathy.

Fever: usually low-grade.

Livedo reticularis: erythematosis vasculitis lesions usually on legs.

Criteria for diagnosis is at least 4 of 11 of the following:

Photosensitivity, malar rash, discoid rash, oral ulcers, hematologic involvement (hemolytic anemia, thrombocytopenia, or leukopenia), **arthritis, serositis (pericarditis or pleuritis), nephritis, ANA, CNS involvement** (psychosis, encepholopathey, infarct, etc.), **immunologic involvement** (false positive RPR, DS-DNA antismith, or LE cell).

Investigations

Laboratory tests

• These are useful in the diagnosis of SLE, but no single diagnostic test is available [1].

Complete blood count: may reveal anemia, leukopenia, neutropenia, lymphopenia, or thrombocytopenia; raised ESR common in active disease; evidence of hemolytic anemia requires further investigation, *eg*, Coombs' test [1].

Antinuclear antibody analysis: antibodies found in at least 95% of SLE patients but not disease-specific; antibodies to double-stranded DNA and Sm are relatively disease-specific but do not occur in all patients (~60% and ~30%, respectively); antibodies to Ro, La, and ribonucleoprotein helpful in defining disease subsets and overlap syndromes; positive antiphospholipid antibodies and lupus anticoagulant define patients at risk from major arterial and venous thromboses [1,2].

For markers of disease activity or organ involvement

ESR measurement: elevated with disease activity.

Plasma-complement analysis: low C3, C4, and CH50 indicate activity.

Anti–double-stranded DNA antibody analysis: antibodies can rise with disease flares, especially those involving the kidney.

Dipstick testing of urine: for proteinuria and hematuria.

Microscopic examination: for red cell casts, leukocyte casts.

Measurements of renal function and 24-hour urine protein loss.

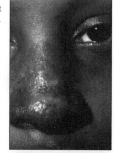

Discoid rash over nose and face.

Differential diagnosis

Other connective tissue diseases: e.g., rheumatoid arthritis, progressive systemic sclerosis.

Infection.

Malignancy: especially leukemia and lymphoma.

Etiology

• Causes include the following:

Genetic factors and inherited defects of the early components of the classic complement pathway.

Environmental factors: e.g., sunlight.

Drugs: e.g., hydralazine, procainamide, phenytoin.

Epidemiology

• The prevalence of SLE in children in the United States is approximately 0.5 per 100,000 children.

• The highest incidence is in adolescent girls.

• SLE is rare before age 5.

• Prevalence is 5 girls to 1 boy [4].

Complications

Severe renal involvement: resulting in renal insufficiency or renal failure.

Cerebral involvement: infarcts or neuropsychiatric disease [3].

Infections secondary to immunosuppression.

Major thrombotic events: especially when high-titer antiphospholipid antibodies are present [2].

Treatment

Diet and lifestyle

• Patients, especially those with photosensitivity, should avoid sunlight and should use high-factor sunscreen (ultraviolet A and B).

Pharmacologic treatment

Indications

Discoid lupus erythematosus rashes: topical steroids.

Joint and skin involvement: hydroxychloroquine; NSAIDs.

Systemic involvement: acute treatment by corticosteriods, introduction of cytotoxic agents, *eg*, azathioprine, methotrexate, and cyclophosphamide.

Vasculopathy (including cerebral involvement): pulse cyclophosphamide and methylprednisolone [5].

Nephritis: corticosteroids and cyclophosphamide.

Systemic treatment

Standard dosage	Hydroxychloroquine, 4–7 mg/Kg/d (usually 200 mg once or twice daily). Prednisone, 0.25–2.00 mg/kg/day (maximum 60 mg/day) and azathioprine, 1–3 mg/kg daily to allow subsequent steroid reduction. Pulse methylprednisolone, 1 g i.v. daily for 3 d and pulse cyclophosphamide, 500–1000 mg/m², adjusted downward for creatinine clearance <35 mL/min or myelosuppression. Cyclophosphamide is given i.v. monthly or 6 months, then i.v. every 3 months until clinical improvement or toxicity occurs. Cyclophosphamide dosing is complex and should be supervised by a specialist (*eg*, rheumatologist, nephrologist).
Contraindications	Known hypersensitivity, systemic infections.
Special points	*Cyclophosphamide*: infusions must be preceded by a complete blood count to check for bone-marrow toxicity, in particular evidence of neutropenia.
Main drug interactions	*Cyclophosphamide:* concurrent allopurinol should be avoided because of enhanced toxicity.
Main side effects	*Hydroxychloroquine:* retinopathy, skin rashes. *Azathioprine:* bone-marrow suppression, gastrointestinal disturbances, liver toxicity. *Cyclophosphamide:* nausea and vomiting, hair loss, hemorrhagic cystitis, premature menopause [5]. All cytotoxic agents: teratogenicity (adequate contraception essential) [5].

Treatment aims

To alleviate disease flares.

To alter outcome.

Prognosis

• Renal and cerebral involvement and the complications of treatment, especially infection, are the major contributors to mortality.

• The survival rate has improved in the past 2 decades and is now ~95% at 5 y.

Follow-up and management

• Close monitoring of lab data at least every 2–3 mo following CBC, urine analysis, as well as complement levels and DS-DNA.

• Prompt treatment of lupus flares is mandatory.

• The use of oral cytotoxic drugs requires monthly blood counts to check for bone-marrow suppression, liver function tests with methotrexate, and azathioprine.

Key references

1. Tan EM, Cohen AS, Fries JF, *et al.* The 1982 revised criteria for the classification of systemic lupus erythematosus. *Arthritis Rheum* 1982, **25**:1271–1277.

2. Seaman DE, Londino AV Jr, Kwoh K, *et al.*: Antiphospholipid antibodies in pediatric systemic lypus erythematosus. *Pediatrics* 1995, **96**: 1040–1045.

3. Yancey CL, Doughty RA, Athreya BH: Central nervous system involvement in childhood systemic lupus erythematosus.

4. Cassidy JT, Petty Ross E. (eds): Systemic lupus erythematosis. *Textbook of Pediatric Rheumatology*, ed 3. W.B. Saunders: Philadelphia; 1995:260–322.

5. Fox DA, McCune WJ: Immunosuppressive drug therapy of systemic lupus erythematosus. *Rheum Dis Clin North Am* 1994, **20**:265–291.

Diagnosis

Definition
• Rapid heart rate originating in or involving structures located above ventricular tissue. Supraventricular tachycardia (SVT) includes the following:

Atrioventricular (AV) nodal reentrant supraventricular tachycardia.

AV reentrant SVT (concealed accessory pathway with SVT and Wolff–Parkinson–White (WPW) syndrome with SVT); primary atrial tachycardia; junctional ectopic tachycardia; atrial flutter; atrial fibrillation.

Symptoms [1]
Palpitations: rapid regular heart rate with sudden onset and offset; throbbing in neck; sensation of fluttering in chest; **chest or abdominal pain:** discomfort in chest, often associated with nausea or abdominal discomfort; **syncope or presyncope:** loss of consciousness, dizziness or light-headedness at onset of rapid heart rate, due to hypotension.

Signs
Tachycardia: rapid heart rate of 150–320 bpm, greater than expected for age or activity level; **tachypnea:** secondary to pulmonary venous congestion from congestive heart failure (CHF); **hypotension:** associated with pallor and diaphoresis.

Congestive heart failure
• Unlikely to occur unless structural or functional heart disease present or tachycardia persists for >24 hours. **Infants:** poor feeding, irritability, lethargy, tachypnea, dyspnea, pallor, diaphoresis; **children and adolescents:** dyspnea, tachypnea, orthopnea, exercise intolerance, easy fatigability, pallor, diaphoresis.

Investigations
ECG: Regular, rapid rhythm usually with narrow QRS complex (*see* figure A). An ECG should be obtained immediately on conversion from SVT to sinus rhythm to look for the presence of delta waves confirming the WPW syndrome (*see* figure B).

Chest radiography: usually normal unless CHF or associated congenital heart disease or cardiomyopathy is present.

Echocardiography: to rule out the presence of associated congenital heart disease or functional heart disease: Ebstein's anomaly of the tricuspid valve or corrected L-transposition of the great arteries are the most common congenital lesions.

Electrophysiologic study: indicated in patients who present with syncope or cardiac arrest, those refractory to medication, or with medication side effects that cannot be tolerated. For risk assessment in WPW and to radiofrequency ablation.

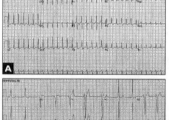

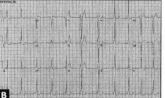

Complications
Congestive heart failure.

Cardiac arrest: associated with atrial fibrillation and WPW with rapid AV conduction.

Electrocardiograms (ECGs). A, ECG of supraventricular tachycardia. B, ECG showing Wolff–Parkinson–White anomaly.

Differential diagnosis
• The primary differential is between the various forms of SVT and VT
• Any wide QRS tachycardia should be considered VT until proven otherwise

Etiology [2]
Atrioventricular reentrant tachycardia
• The structural substrate is a congenital abnormality of the conducting system of the heart, whereby an extra electrical connection exists between the atria and the ventricles. A manifest accessory pathway appears as the WPW anomaly and conducts both forward and backward. A concealed accessory pathway only conducts backwards from the ventricle to atrium.
• Tachycardia arises when an electrical impulse passes from the atrium to the ventricle through the normal AV node but returns to the atria by the accessory pathway.

Atrioventricular nodal reentrant tachycardia
• Patients have two functionally separate pathways within or close to the AV node. Tachycardia arises in a similar way, arising in patients with AV reentrant tachycardia.

Atrial flutter: seen *in utero* and in infancy in structurally normal heart or after surgery for congenital heart defects involving atrial surgery, such as the intra-atrial repairs (Mustard or Senning) for complete D-transposition of the great arteries or the Fontan repair for functional single ventricle.

Atrial fibrillation: uncommon in children.

Epidemiology
Supraventricular tachycardia is estimated to occur in one in 250–1000 children. Most common at less than 4 months of age. Other common age groups include the years around puberty and 5–7 y of age. SVT is associated with infection, fever, or drug (decongestant or sympathomimetic amines) exposure in 20%–25%, WPW syndrome in 25%, congenital heart disease in 20%, concealed accessory pathways, and AV nodal reentry in the remainder. Atrial flutter occurs in 25%–40% of patients after atrial surgery, especially intra-atrial repair of complete transposition of the great arteries or the Fontan repair.

Treatment [3]

Diet and lifestyle
• Avoid caffeine, chocolate. Activity restriction generally not required.

Pharmacologic treatment

Acute treatment

Standard dosage Adenosine [4], i.v. bolus, 50–100 μg/kg followed by saline flush. Increase by 50 μg/kg increments every 2 min to 400 μg/kg or 12 mg maximal dose.

Digoxin, 30 μg/kg i.v. total digitalizing dose (TDD); maximum dose, 1 mg; initial dose, one-half TDD; second dose, one-quarter TDD; third dose, one-quarter TDD.

Propranolol (β-blocker), 0.05–0.1 mg/kg over 5 min every 6 h.

Esmolol (β-blocker), i.v. load: 500 μg/kg/min over 1 min followed by 50 μg/kg/min over 4 min; repeat in 5 min with 500 μg/kg/min over 1 min, 100 μg/kg/min over 4 min; maintenance infusion: 50–200 μg/kg/min.

Amiodarone, 5 mg/kg over 1 h i.v., followed by 5–10 μg/kg/min infusion.

Procainamide (class I antiarrhythmic), 5 mg/kg i.v. over 5–10 min or 10–15 mg/kg over 30–45 min; infusion: 20–100 μg/kg/min.

Special points *Adenosine*: emergency equipment should always be available when given to children.

Digoxin: second and third doses may be given every 2 h if SVT still present; usually given every 6–8 h; a fourth additional dose may be given if patient still in SVT.

Propranolol and esmolol: blood glucose should be checked initially in small infants and young children taking this drug; give with food to avoid hypoglycemia.

Amiodarone: long elimination half-life; increases pacing threshold.

Procainamide: may be proarrhythmic; is metabolized to *N*-acetyl procainamide (NAPA), which has antiarrhythmic activity.

• **Avoid verapamil in children <1 y of age; causes collapse and death [5].**

Long-term oral therapy

Standard dosage *Digoxin*: 40–60 μg/kg TDD p.o. (i.v. dose is 75% of p.o. dose); maintenance: 10–15 μg/kg/d divided every 12 h.

Propranolol: (β-blocker), 0.25–1 mg/kg/oral dose every 6 h.

Nadolol (β-blocker), 0.5–1 mg/kg/dose every 12 h.

Atenolol (β-blocker), 25–100 mg/d in single dose used for older children and adolescents.

Procainamide: 20–100 mg/kg/d every 4–12 h.

Flecainide (class I antiarrhythmic): 50–200 mg/m²/d every 12 h.

Propafenone: 200–300 mg/m² in 3–4 doses or 8–10 mg/kg.

Amiodarone, loading dose: 10 mg/kg/dose twice daily for 7–14 d; maintenance: 5–10 mg/kg/dose daily.

Sotolol, 135 mg/m²/d.

Contraindications *Flecainide*: avoid in CHF.

Special points *Flecainide*: more proarrhythmic than other class 1 agents, especially in presence of congenital heart defect or cardiomyopathy.

Treatment aims
Pharmacologic: to terminate paroxysm of tachycardia; to suppress recurrent tachycardia. For radiofrequency ablation: to cure tachycardia.

Other treatments
Vagal maneuvers: Valsalva maneuver, gagging, headstand.
Ice.
Radiofrequency ablation [6].
Surgical ablation.

Prognosis
Excellent for control and eventual cure; 75% controlled with first medication used; 10%–20% refractory.
1%–3% incidence of sudden death associated with WPW.
With radiofrequency ablation, 80%–95% cure achievable.

Follow-up and management
Periodic ECGs and office visits. Holter or transtelephonic monitoring to assess symptoms.
Aspirin after radiofrequency ablation for 4–6 wk. Follow-up ECGs after radiofrequency ablation.

Key references
1. Garson A Jr, Gillette PC, McNamara DG: Supraventricular tachycardia in children: clinical features, response to treatment, and long-term follow-up in 217 patients. *J Pediatr* 1981, **98**:875–882.
2. Ko JK, Deal BJ, Strasburger J, *et al.*: Supraventricular tachycardia mechanisms and their age distribution in pediatric patients. *Am J Cardiol* 1992, **69**:1028–1032.
3. Kugler JD, Danford DA: Management of infants, children, and adolescents with paroxysmal supraventricular tachycardia. *J Pediatr* 1996, **129**:324–338.
4. Ralston MA, Knilans TK, Hannon DW, Daniels SR: Use of adenosine for diagnosis and treatment of tachyarrhythmias in pediatric patients. *J Pediatr* 1994, **124**:139–143.
5. Epstein ML, Kiel EA, Victorica BE: Cardiac decompensation following verapamil therapy in infants with supraventricular tachycardia. *Pediatrics* 1985, **75**:737–740.

Tachycardia, ventricular

Diagnosis

Definition
• Rapid heart rate originating in or involving structures located in His–Purkinje or ventricular tissue.

Symptoms [1]
Palpitations: rapid regular heart rate with sudden onset and offset; throbbing in neck; sensation of fluttering in chest; **chest or abdominal pain:** discomfort in chest, often associated with nausea or abdominal discomfort; **shortness of breath; syncope or presyncope:** loss of consciousness, dizziness or light-headedness at onset of rapid heart rate, due to hypotension; **cardiac arrest; sudden death.**

Signs
Tachycardia: heart rate higher than expected for age or activity level.

Infants: heart rate 200–300 bpm; children and adolescents: heart rate 150–300 bpm; tachypnea; hypotension: associated with pallor and diaphoresis; **cannon waves in jugular vein and change in intensity of first heart sound:** secondary to AV dissociation.

Signs of congestive heart failure
• More likely to occur in the presence of structural or functional heart disease.

Infants: poor feeding, irritability, lethargy, tachypnea, dyspnea.

Children and adolescents: dyspnea, shortness of breath, orthopnea, exercise intolerance, easy fatigability.

Investigations
ECG: usually regular, rapid rhythm with wide QRS complex (*see* figure).

• An ECG should be obtained immediately on conversion from VT to sinus rhythm to look for evidence of ischemia (ST segment changes or T wave abnormalities), or ventricular hypertrophy. The QTc interval should be carefully measured by hand.

Chest radiography: usually normal unless congestive heart failure (CHF), associated congenital heart disease, or cardiomyopathy is present.

Echocardiography: to rule out the presence of associated congenital heart disease, tumors, right ventricular dysplasia, or functional heart disease, especially cardiomyopathies.

Electrophysiologic study (EPS): indicated in patients who present with syncope or cardiac arrest, those with pre- or postoperative congenital heart disease, or potentially life-threatening arrhythmias, either by appearance of arrhythmia, such as multiform or polymorphic VT or rapid VTs; exceptions would be VT associated with the long QT syndrome.

Adenosine: helpful in making definitive diagnosis of wide QRS tachycardia. Has little effect on VT, except in a special variety originating in the right ventricular outflow tract. Terminates most supraventricular tachycardia and results in atrioventricular block uncovering most atrial tachycardias.

Cardiac atheterization and angiography: used to determine the underlying hemodynamic status of the patient and further define anatomic defects. May identify coronary artery anomalies such as a coronary passing between the aorta and pulmonary artery or anomalous origin of the coronary.

Complications
Congestive heart failure (see descrption), pulmonary edema, shock.

Cardiac arrest.

Sudden death.

Differential diagnosis
• The primary differential is between the various forms of supraventricular tachycardia and VT. Any wide QRS tachycardia should be considered VT and treated as such until proven otherwise.

Etiology [2]
Congenital heart disease: most common in postoperative setting in tetralogy of Fallot, ventricular septal defect, AV canal defects, aortic stenosis and insufficiency, single ventricle. Also seen in unoperated CHD: aortic stenosis, aortic insufficiency, Ebstein's anomaly, mitral valve prolapse, Eisenmenger's syndrome.

Acquired heart disease: myocarditis, rheumatic heart disease, collagen vascular diseases, Kawasaki disease.

Cardiomyopathies: hypertrophic cardiomyopathy, dilated cardiomyopathy, right ventricular dysplasia, Marfan syndrome, neuromuscular disorders such as Duchenne muscular dystrophy.

Tumors and infiltrates: rhabdomyomas, oncocytic transformation, Purkinje cell tumors, hemosiderosis (thalassemia, sickle cell anemia), leukemia.

Ventricular tachycardia associated with structurally normal heart: this form of VT originates in the right ventricular outflow tract or left ventricular septum.

Other: electrolyte imbalance, drugs and toxins, anesthesia, central nervous system lesions, long QT syndrome.

Epidemiology
• Ventricular tachycardia occurs in 15% of postoperative tetralogy of Fallot patients and 10% of ventricular septal defect patients. Sudden death from VT/ventricular fibrillation occurs in 5% of postoperative patients who have had surgery involving the ventricle.

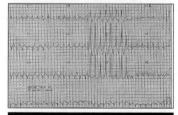

ECG of ventricular tachycardia.

Treatment

Diet and lifestyle

Avoid caffeine, chocolate. Activity restriction for competitive and vigorous sports activities required for long QT syndrome, myocarditis, and cardiomyopathies. For idiopathic VT or those with VT and normal cardiac function, activity may generally be allowed after the VT has been controlled for 6 months.

Pharmacologic treatment

Acute treatment

Standard dosage	Lidocaine, 1–2 mg/kg i.v. bolus every 5–15 min; infusion: 10–15 μg/kg/min.
	Esmolol (β-blocker), i.v. load: 500 μg/kg/min over 1 min followed by 50 μg/kg/min over 4 min; repeat in 5 min with 500 μg/kg/min over 1 min, 100 μg/kg/min over 4 min; maintenance infusion: 50–200 μg/kg/min.
	Propranolol (β-blocker), 0.05–0.1 mg/kg i.v. over 5 min every 6 h.
	Procainamide, 5 mg/kg i.v. over 5–10 min or 10–15 mg/kg over 30–45 min; infusion: 20–100 μg/kg/min.
	Amiodarone, 5 mg/kg over 1 h i.v., followed by 5–10 μg/kg/min infusion.
	Phenytoin, 3–5 mg/kg over 5 min, maximum 1 mg/kg/min.
	Bretylium, 5 mg/kg bolus every 15 min; infusion: 5–10 mg/kg over 10 minutes every 6 h.
	Magnesium, 0.25 mEq/kg over 1 min followed by 1 mEq/kg over 5 h to achieve Mg^{2+} level 3–4 mg/dL.
Special points	*Lidocaine:* may be repeated in 2–3 min; use lower dosage (one-half) for patients with hypoglycemia.
	Esmolol and propranolol: blood glucose should be checked initially in small infants and young children placed on this drug; give with food to avoid hypoglycemia.
	Procainamide: may be proarrhythmic; metabolized to *N*-acetyl procainamide, which has antiarrhythmic activity.
	Amiodarone: long elimination half-life; increases pacing threshold.

• **Avoid verapamil in children with VT.**

Long-term oral therapy

• Oral therapy should be supervised by a pediatric cardiologist with experience in treating VT. All anti-arrhythmics have arrhythmogenic properties, some more pronounced than others. It has not been determined that treatment with antiarrhythmics prevents sudden death in these patients.

Standard dosage	*Propranolol:* 0.25–1 mg/kg/p.o. dose every 6 h.
	Nadolol (β-blocker), 0.5–1 mg/kg/dose every 12 h.
	Atenolol (β-blocker), 25–100 mg/d in single dose used for older children and adolescents.
	Mexiletine, *infants and children:* 2–5 mg/kg/dose every 8 h; *older children and adolescents:* 150–300 mg/dose 3 times daily.
	Procainamide: 20–100 mg/kg/d every 4–6 h.
	Flecainide, 50–200 mg/m²/d every 12 h.
	Propafenone, 200–300 mg/m² in 3–4 doses or 8–10 mg/kg.
	Amiodarone: loading dose: 10 mg/kg/dose twice daily for 7–14 d; maintenance: 5–10 mg/kg/dose daily.
	Phenytoin, loading dose: 10–20 mg/kg/d every 12 h for 2 d.
	Sotolol, 135 mg/m²/d.

Treatment aims

Pharmacologic

To terminate paroxysm of tachycardia and prevent symptoms.

To suppress recurrent tachycardia.

For RFA or surgical ablation

To cure tachycardia.

Other treatments

DC cardioversion with 2–5 J for patients with hemodynamic compromise or those in mild distress and unresponsive to medications.

Radiofrequency ablation (RFA): has been shown to be effective in patients with structurally normal hearts and sites in the right ventricular outflow tract and left ventricular septal areas as well as some with postoperative congenital heart disease, such as tetralogy of Fallot or ventricular septal defect.

Surgical ablation: guided by electrophysiologic mapping.

Other surgery: surgery to remove tumors or correct hemodynamically significant lesions such as a residual ventricular septal defect, aortic stenosis, aortic insufficiency, or pulmonary insufficiency may help control VT.

Automatic internal cardioverter/defibrillator: used predominantly in hypertrophic cardiomyopathies or long QT syndrome.

Prognosis

Depends on underlying disease and presentation.

Long-term prognosis is good for those with normal hearts.

Key references

1. Davis AM, Gow RM, McCrindle BW, Hamilton RM: Clinical spectrum, therapeutic management, and follow-up of ventricular tachycardia in infants and young children. *Am Heart J* 1996, **131:**186–191.

2. Vetter VL: Ventricular arrhythmias in pediatric patients with and without congenital heart disease. In *Current Management of Arrhythmias.* Edited by Horowitz LN. Ontario: B.C. Decker Inc.; 1990.

Diagnosis

Symptoms

• β-Thalassemia is manifest during the first year of life in 90% of patients; a few present at 3–4 years (late-onset β-thalassemia major).

• Ten percent of patients with β-thalassemia major have a mild course (not dependent on transfusion). Referred to a β-thalassemia intermedia patients.

• Detection can result from antenatal screening and diagnosis.

Poor weight gain.

Failure to thrive.

Fever.

Diarrhea.

Increasing pallor.

Distended abdomen.

Signs

Pallor.

Heart failure.

Splenomegaly.

Jaundice.

Investigations

Blood tests: low hemoglobin, low mean corpuscular hemoglobin, low mean cell volume; absent or reduced hemoglobin A (β° or β+ thalassemia), variable hemoglobin F and A_2 (using electrophoresis).

Genetic analysis: defines specific mutations, may help to predict disease severity and prognosis and facilitate first-trimester diagnosis.

Complications

Splenomegaly leading to hypersplenism (neutropenia, thrombocytopenia, anemia).

Anemia causes severe bone changes, short stature, and heart failure.

Differential diagnosis

Iron deficiency.

Etiology

• Thalassemia is caused by defective synthesis of the α- or β-globin chain (α- and β-thalassemia, respectively). The disorder is inherited in autosomal-recessive fashion.

• It occurs in Mediterranean, Asian, Arabic, and Chinese groups because of a selective advantage against *Plasmodium falciparum*.

Epidemiology

• Thalassemia is one of the most common inherited disorders throughout the world.

• Among African Americans, approximately 30% of the population is either heterozygous or homozygous for the α-thalassemia-2 deletion.

• In southwest Europe, thalassemia is declining because of prevention programs; in consanguineous marriages, the birth rate of β-thalassemia increases by 30%.

Treatment

Diet and lifestyle
• Patients should avoid food with high iron content, such as red meat and liver, and they should be encouraged to lead a normal active lifestyle.

Pharmacologic treatment

For transfusional iron overload

Standard dosage	Desferrioxamine, infused s.c. over 8–12 hours from a portable syringe driver pump 5–6 nights per week. Chelation therapy is started when ferritin is 1 000 µg/L (after 12–24 transfusions).
Special points	*Desferrioxamine*: initial dose (20 mg/kg) is diluted in 5–10 mL water for injection; vitamin C, 100–200 mg orally (increases urinary iron excretion), is taken only when the patient is on desferrioxamine; in iron-overloaded patients, dose is 50 mg/kg/day; for cardiomyopathy, higher doses are given through an i.v. delivery device.

Complications of treatment
• Alloimmunization to blood group antigens (in 25% of patients), febrile and urticarial transfusion reactions (in 75% of patients), cytomegalovirus infection and immunosuppression, transfusion-transmitted hepatitis B and C viruses: caused by chronic transfusion (current risk of HIV estimated at 1:450 000 per unit transfused).

Cardiomyopathy (most common cause of death), reduced growth, hypoparathyroidism, diabetes, failure of puberty: due to transfusional iron overload.

Short stature, bone changes (metaphyseal dysplasia), visual disturbances, hypersensitivity, hearing problems, pulmonary hypersensitivity reaction: due to desferrioxamine toxicity (overchelation).

Treatment aims
To provide good quality of life.
To provide a long life.

Other treatments
Bone marrow transplantation: 94% success rate if patient has been compliant with desferrioxamine and has no liver fibrosis or enlargement.
Splenectomy for hypersplenism.

Prognosis
• Maintenance transfusion and regular iron chelation preserve excellent health, and the prognosis is now open-ended.
• Early death is generally the result of intractable heart failure secondary to iron overload and infections.

Follow-up and management
• The patient's ferritin, liver function, and bone metabolism must be monitored 3–4 times yearly, with annual anti-hepatitis C virus, anti-HIV, and hepatitis B surface antigen surveillance.
• Other endocrine and cardiac investigations should be made if clinically indicated.
• Patients should have routine audiometry and ophthalmologic evaluation.
• Splenectomized patients have higher risk of infection due to encapsulated organisms; they require vaccine against *Streptococcus pneumococcus, Haemophilus influenzae, Neisseria meningitidis* before splenectomy; penicillin prophylaxis is recommended indefinitely.

General references
1. Olivieri NF, Brittenham GM: Iron-chelating therapy and the treatment of thalassemia. *Blood* 1997, **89:**739–761.
2. Piomelli S: The management of patient's with Cooley's anemia: transfusion and splenectomy. *Seminars in Hematology* 1995, **32:**262–268.
3. Kattamis CA, Kattamis AC: Management of thalassemias: growth and development, hormone substitution, vitamin supplementation, and vaccination. *Seminars in Hematology* 1995, **32:**269–279.
4. Lucarelli G, Galimberti M, Polchi P, et al.: Bone marrow transplantation in patients with thalassemia. *N Engl J Med* 1990, **322:**417–421.

Tic disorders

Diagnosis

Symptoms

Brief, stereotyped, nonrhythmic movements or vocalizations that are essentially involuntary but are often transiently suppressible with voluntary effort and exacerbated by tension or anxiety; they reflect coordinated activation of a group of muscles.

Simple motor tics: eye blinking, upward or lateral eye deviation, grimacing, neck jerking, shoulder shrugging.

Complex motor tics: grooming behaviors (*eg*, sweeping one's hair back), gestures, jumping, touching.

Simple vocal tics: throat clearing, sniffing, grunting, barking, squeaking, or cooing.

Complex vocal tics: verbalizations, including obscenities (coprolalia), inappropriate repetition of one's own words or phrases (palilalia), or of the last sound, word, or phrase of another (echolalia).

Tic disorders: classified according to the chronicity and heterogeneity of the component tics. In practice, there is a continuous spectrum of chronicity and multiplicity of tics ranging from simple, transient motor tics to Tourette syndrome:

Transient tic disorder: single or multiple motor or vocal tics occurring frequently (*i.e.*, many times a day nearly every day) for at least 4 weeks but for less than 12 months.

Chronic tic disorder: single or multiple motor tics (but not both) occurring frequently for at least a year.

Tourette syndrome: multiple motor tics, and one or more vocal tics occurring frequently for at least a year.

Comorbidity: obsessions (recurrent, intrusive, and distressing thoughts or ideas) and compulsions (recurrent, ritualistic behaviors or mental acts such as hand washing or counting that are suppressed with difficulty) are common. In addition, many patients with tic disorders also have symptoms of attention deficit/hyperactivity disorder.

Family history: tics, obsessive–compulsive traits, or both may be present in one or more relatives, but most cases are sporadic.

Signs

• Except for tics, signs are usually absent. Occasionally, compulsive behaviors are directly observed, or may be inferred from signs such as erythema of the hands (from frequent washing) or around the mouth (from lip licking).

Investigations

• Investigation is generally not indicated. In exceptional instances, the following studies may be helpful in the exclusion of alternative diagnoses:

Electroencephalography: for epilepsy. In particular, eye blinking or eye rolling tics may mimic absence epilepsy, and facial grimace and jerking of the neck or trunk may mimic myoclonic epilepsy.

Neuroimaging (cranial CT, MRI, or MRA): for tumor, vascular malformation, other focal brain lesion, or basal ganglia abnormality.

Complications

Social isolation, poor self-esteem, depression.

Differential diagnosis

Other movement disorders: Sydenham's chorea, myoclonus.
Myoclonic or absence epilepsy.
• Stimulant drugs (methylphenidate, dexedrine, pemoline) may precipitate tics in individuals who have not previously suffered from them, or may exacerbate preexisting tic disorders. Generally, withdrawal of the stimulant results in amelioration within a few days (but occasionally not for several weeks). Rarely, the appearance or exacerbation of tics in association with stimulant use appears to be permanent. However, a causal relationship has not been established.

Etiology

• There is substantial evidence that most tic disorders are genetically determined, although the evidence for a single, autosomal dominant gene is debated.
• Because tics are often suppressed by neuroleptics (which are dopaminergic antagonists) and precipitated by stimulants such as amphetamines, it is speculated that they represent a developmental imbalance in neurotransmitter systems.

Epidemiology

• Tourette syndrome as currently defined is relatively common, affecting roughly 1:2000 individuals.
Mild, transient tic syndromes are relatively common, affecting 5%–10% of individuals at some point during childhood.

Treatment

Pharmacologic treatment

• Pharmacologic treatment is indicated only in the minority of patients who have severe, disabling tics.

• Clonidine is less toxic than neuroleptic drugs, but has limited efficacy (for dosage, see "Attention deficit–hyperactivity disorder").

• Neuroleptic agents, including haloperidol and pimozide, provide substantial benefit in up to 80% of patients. Newer agents may prove to be equally effective or less toxic; pediatric experience is limited. The following doses are for children.

Standard dosage	Haloperidol (Haldol), 0.5 mg daily in two divided doses, with weekly increases of 0.5 mg until significant benefit or unacceptable toxicity occurs. Usual maintenance dosage is 1–3 mg daily in two divided doses.
	Pimozide (Orap), 1 mg nightly for several days, then 1 mg twice daily. Weekly increases of 1–2 are made until significant benefit or unacceptable toxicity occurs. Usual maintenance dose is the lesser of 0.2 mg/kg/d or 10 mg/d.
Contraindications	*Pimozide*: long QT syndrome, drugs that prolong the QT interval.
Main side effects	*Haloperidol and pimozide*: tardive dyskinesia, akathisia (severe motor restlessness), acute dystonia, oculogyric crisis. Pimozide may prolong the QT interval and is suspected of causing sudden, fatal cardiac arrhythmia in rare instances.
Special points	Baseline and periodic EKG monitoring of QT interval is recommended by the manufacturer for patients on pimozide.
	The risk of tardive dyskinesia is probably increased in patients receiving prolonged therapy at high doses. Risperidone may prove to be preferable to other neuroleptics.
	Symptoms of obsessive compulsive disorder typically do not respond well to neuroleptic therapy; clomipramine (Anafranil) or fluoxetine (Prozac) may help suppress these symptoms.

Nonpharmacologic treatment

• Tics may be exacerbated by anxiety, which in some cases may be relieved by biofeedback or other relaxation techniques. However, insisting that a child simply exercise self-control may be ineffective or even counterproductive.

Treatment aims

To minimize anxiety.

To adjust pharmacologic treatment to the severity of the disorder.

To recognize and treat disabling obsessions and compulsions.

Prognosis

• Tourette syndrome most often persists for years or indefinitely. However, dramatic fluctuations in severity are common, and long-term spontaneous remissions occur in a significant minority of patients.

• Simple tic disorders most commonly remit spontaneously.

Follow-up and management

• Periodic follow-up is indicated to ensure optimal school and social function, to detect and manage long-term exacerbations, and to recognize and treat comorbidity.

General references

Singer HS: Tic disorders. *Pediatr Ann* 1993, **22**:22–29.

Diagnosis

Symptoms

Extremity pain.

Abnormal appearance: deformity, swelling, discoloration (bruising, cyanosis, pallor).

Altered motor function: extremity weakness, decreased range of motion, refusal or inability to move the extremity, weight bear, or ambulate.

Altered sensory function: numbness, tingling, paresthesias.

Signs

Tachycardia: blood loss from a closed femur fracture can be up to 30% of blood volume; blood loss from pelvic or open fractures can be even greater; hypotension is rare.

Pallor, cyanosis, delayed capillary refill, weak or absent pulses, extremity coolness: from vascular disruption, hematoma, or compartment syndrome.

Extremity deformity: angulation, shortening, malposition at rest, swelling, wounds.

Tenderness or crepitance: tenderness over a physis strongly suggests a growth plate injury.

Absent or decreased sensation.

Absent or decreased motor strength.

Abnormal range of motion: for example, inability to supinate or pronate the forearm is suggestive of a radial or ulnar injury.

Limp or inability to weight bear: very sensitive for a lower extremity fracture.

Investigations

Extremity radiographs: when indicated, to assess for fractures or dislocations. Unstable or significantly deformed fractures should be immobilized first, for patient comfort and to decrease further injury.

Doppler ultrasound: when indicated, to assess nonpalpable or weak pulses.

Computed tomography: for suspected pelvic fractures with significant abdominal bleeding.

Magnetic resonance imaging: rarely indicated.

Complications

• Permanent limb deformity or dysfunction.
• Altered limb growth (Salter–Harris fractures).

Differential Diagnosis

Fractures.

Contusions.

"Sprains" (ligamentous injury).

"Strains" (muscle-tendon unit injury).

Dislocations.

Injury to another joint (eg, an occult hip injury presenting with knee pain).

Child abuse.

Chondral injuries (eg, osteochondritis dessicans).

Disorders of bone or collagen formation.

Etiology

• Children's bones and joints are different than adults. The cartilaginous growth plate is the weakest part of their joints. Consequently, ligamentous sprains are rare in children who have open growth plates, ie, those who have not completed puberty; growth plate injuries (Salter–Harris fractures; see figure) are much more common.

• Children's bones are softer and more porous. The periosteum is thicker, which tends to reduce the amount of fracture displacement. Hence greenstick, buckle, and bow fractures are unique to children (see Fig. 2).

• Metaphyseal spiral fractures, except in toddlers, are considered the result of child abuse until proven otherwise.

• The etiology of extremity trauma in children includes:

Direct extremity trauma.

Occult extremity trauma (common in toddlers).

Excessive repetitive motion ("overuse" syndromes).

Epidemiology

• Childhood musculoskeletal trauma accounts for approximately 175,000 hospital admissions and 7.5 million emergency department visits annually in the U.S.

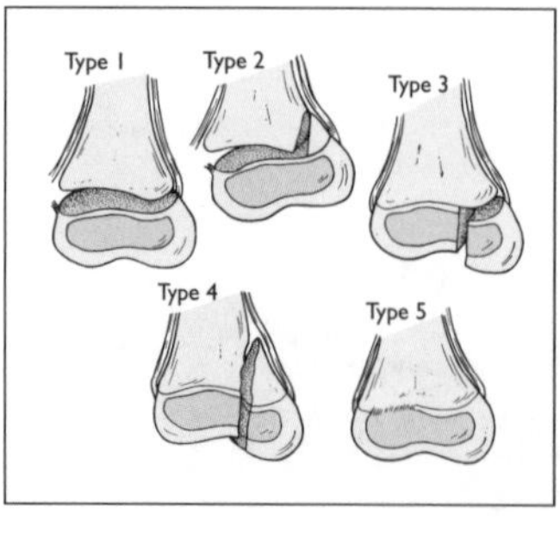

Figure 1. Salter-Harris physeal injury classification.
Type 1: epiphyseal separation through the physis only.
Type 2: epiphyseal separation with metaphyseal fracture.
Type 3: epiphyseal separation and fracture.
Type 4: fracture through the metaphysis, growth plate, and epiphysis.
Type 5: physis compression injury.

Treatment

Diet and lifestyle

• Prevention strategies, such as proper safety equipment, and appropriate strength, conditioning, and stretching regimens for athletes, are recommended.

Pharmacologic treatment

Nonsteroidal anti-inflammatory drugs

Standard dosage	Acetaminophen, 15 mg/kg every 4 h. Ibuprofen, 10 mg/kg every 6 h.
Contraindications	Hypersensitivity.
Main drug interactions	None.
Main side effects	Gastrointestinal distress (ibuprofen).

Other analgesic agents

Standard dosage	Morphine sulfate, 0.1–0.2 mg/kg/dose. Fentanyl, 1–2 µg/kg/dose.
Contraindications	Hypersensitivity, hypotension, shock, respiratory depression.
Main drug interactions	Other sedatives and analgesics.
Main side effects	Central nervous system and respiratory depression.

Nerve blocks

Standard dosage	Lidocaine, 5 mg/kg (maximum infiltration dose).

Nonpharmacologic treatment

"RICE": *R*est, *I*ce, *C*ompression (*eg*, ace wrap), and *E*levation, where indicated.

Immobilization: fiberglass, plaster, or air splints, casts, knee immobilizers, arm slings, ace wraps, and "figure-of-eight" bandages (for clavicle fractures), "buddy-taping" (of digits), and crutches to assist with ambulation in children able to use them (usually over age 6), where indicated.

Dislocation reduction: where indicated.

Orthopedic referral: mandatory in the following conditions: significant growth plate injury, open or severely displaced fractures, neurovascular compromise, suspected or severe ligament injury, dislocations (other than of the shoulder or digits).

Treatment aims

To ensure proper healing and normal subsequent growth and function.

To relieve discomfort.

To detect and report child abuse, where applicable.

Prognosis

• The main determinant of outcome is the type and degree of injury. Neurovascular compromise or growth plate injury can be very significant. Minor extremity trauma has an excellent overall prognosis.

Follow-up and management

• The focus of follow-up care is neurovascular and functional assessment of the injured extremity. Patients who are placed in casts should be checked the following day, as subsequent swelling inside the cast may cause neurovascular compromise. Those with persistent symptoms or poor return of function should be referred to an orthopedist.

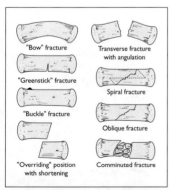

Figure 2. Fracture patterns.

"Bow" fracture

Transverse fracture with angulation

"Greenstick" fracture

Spiral fracture

"Buckle" fracture

Oblique fracture

"Overriding" position with shortening

Comminuted fracture

General references

Rosenthal RE: Office evaluation and management of acute orthopedic trauma. *Orthop Clin North Am* 1988, **19**:675–688.

Stanitski CL: Management of sports injuries in children and adolescents. *Orthop Clin North Am* 1988, **19**:689–698.

England SP, Sundberg S: Management of common pediatric fractures. *Pediatr Clin North Am* 1996, **43**:991–1012.

Saperstein AL, Nicholas SJ: Pediatric and adolescent sports medicine. *Pediatr Clin North Am* 1996, **43**:1013–1033.

Cramer KE: The pediatric polytrauma patient. *Clin Orthop* 1995, **318**:125–135.

Trauma, head and neck

Diagnosis

Symptoms

• Patients may initially be asymptomatic. Symptoms may be masked by preexisting conditions (intoxication, medication use) or acute medical issues (hypovolemia, postictal state, hypoglycemia, other dramatic or painful injuries).

Head trauma: headache, nausea, weakness, amnesia.

Neck injury: headache, neck pain, stiff neck, paresthesias, weakness, dyspnea.

Signs

Head injury

• Minimal to significantly altered level of consciousness, neurologic compromise, seizures, herniation, Cushing's triad (hypertension, bradycardia, respiratory irregularity), retinal hemorrhages, visual abnormalities [1]. Hypovolemic shock from an isolated intracranial bleed is rare, but is occasionally seen in neonates, those with acute blood extravasation to the subgaleal space through a communicating fracture, and children with large preexisting cerebrospinal fluid (CSF) spaces.

Neck injury

Blunt trauma: minimal to complete motor–sensory changes, altered mental status, hyporeflexia, paralysis, respiratory insufficiency, torticollis, midline neck tenderness, ataxia, spinal shock.

Penetrating trauma: subcutaneous emphysema, asymmetric neck contour, airway obstruction, vocal changes, bleeding, bruit, neurologic or vascular compromise.

Investigations

Head injury

History of injury mechanism.

Frequent reevaluations.

Skull radiography if concerned about bony injury in stable child <2 years of age, depressed fracture, foreign body, child abuse.

CT scan (noncontrast) [2]: to investigate for acute space occupying lesion or one amenable to surgical intervention (epidural, subdural, or parenchymal hematoma, depressed skull fracture), cerebral edema, intracranial projectile.

MRI: not necessary in acute patient; quite helpful in identifying extent of trauma with subacute injury.

Neck injury

Complete neurologic examination, including history of transient numbness, tingling, weakness, paralysis or other paresthesias [5].

Radiographs: need at least three view series (anteroposterior [AP] view C3-C7, odontoid view [AP C1-C2], and lateral view through C7/T1). Many authors recommend addition of oblique films to complete five-view trauma series. Flexion and extension films may be useful in an awake patient to investigate ligamentous stability [3–5].

CT scan: useful to augment radiographic findings or when radiographs are inadequate.

MRI: useful for parenchymal, ligamentous, vascular information.

Complications

Head injury: inadequate evaluation or recognition of intracranial injury can lead to severe neurologic compromise or death.

Neck injury: inadequate evaluation or recognition of cervical spine or cord injury can lead to permanent neurologic compromise. Airway and vascular compromise can be severe if not recognized and managed appropriately.

Differential diagnosis

• Altered mental status may be due to other causes than head and neck injury (eg, hypotension, inebriation, medications). If hypotension is evident with an apparent isolated closed head injury, suspect other injury as the cause.

Etiology

• Etiology can be categorized as blunt (majority), penetrating, or perforating. Specific signs and symptoms will often relate to the category of injury, although there is significant overlap. Head and neck trauma may be obvious (usual) or require a high index of suspicion for diagnosis. Seemingly minor trauma such as falls from short distances, walker injuries, localized blunt trauma (rock, baseball bat, golf club) can lead to severe intracranial (epidural, subdural hematoma) or cranial (depressed fractures) problems. Small penetrating injuries may be missed without radiographic assistance.

Prevalence

• 60%–70% of severe trauma in children will involve head trauma.

Concussions are seen in up to 20% of high school football players per year.

• Cervical spine injury occurs in approximately 1%–2% of severely xtraumatized children.

• Up to two thirds of pediatric spinal cord injuries may present without obvious bony cervical spine injury [5].

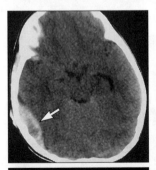

Computed tomographic scan of acute epidural hematoma (*arrow*) resulting from a short fall.

Treatment

Lifestyle management

Injury prevention is most effective treatment.

Use of protective gear (helmets) when appropriate.

Avoidance of high-risk activities.

Change in activity (*eg*, trampoline avoidance) and activity rules ("spearing") in football.

Pharmacologic treatment [2]

For acute seizure management in head injury

Standard dosage	Lorazepam, 0.05–1.0 mg/kg i.v.
Main side effects	Respiratory depression and hypotension.

For seizure prophylaxis and prolonged seizure management in head injury

Standard dosage	Phenytoin, 18 mg/kg slowly.
Special points	Advantage is no change in neurologic examination.
Main side effects	Cardiac dysrhythmias with rapid administration.

For sedation in head injury

Standard dosage	Midazolam, 0.1 mg/kg i.v.
	Sodium pentothal, 3–5 mg/kg i.v. (anesthetic for intubation).
Main side effects	*Midazolam*: respiratory depression and hypotension.
	Sodium pentothal: respiratory depression, hyperexcitability phase, hypotension.

Prevention of intracranial pressure increase with intubation in head injury

Standard dosage	Sodium pentothal, 3–5 mg/kg i.v.
	Midazolam, 0.1 mg/kg i.v.
	Lidocaine, 1–1.5 mg/kg i.v.
Main side effects	*Sodium pentothal*: respiratory depression, hyperexcitability phase, hypotension.
	Midazolam: respiratory depression and hypotension.

For paralysis in head injury

Standard dosage	Norcuron, 0.1–0.3 mg/kg.
Special points	Onset of action decreased and duration increased with increasing dosage.

Osmotic diuretic for head injury

Standard dosage	Mannitol, 0.5–1 g/kg.
Special points	Use only in cases of extremis when other basic modalities are exhausted, or to temporize a preoperative patient.
Main side effects	Hypovolemia, potential increased free water content in injured area (with disrupted blood–brain barrier), bladder rupture if urinary catheter not in place, and hyperosmolarity.

To decrease injury severity in neck injury

Standard dosage	Methylprednisolone, 30 mg/kg over 15 minutes in first hour followed by 5.4 mg/kg/h for 23 hours.
Special points	Best if started within 8 hours of injury; may not be useful in penetrating injuries.

Treatment aims

Strict adherence to the "ABCs":

Airway assistance or intervention.

Maintenance of the neck in the midline and elevation, as able, of the head to 30°.

Adequate oxygenation and ventilation with Po_2 of >100 torr and Pco_2 30–35 torr.

• Avoid overaggressive hyperventilation.

• Rapid sequence intubation will help stabilize the airway quickly and avoid secondary injuries.

• Avoiding ICP spikes by the use of sedation, pharmacologic paralysis, and seizure prevention should be considered.

• Recognition of a potential surgical lesion with appropriate neurosurgical referral is mandatory.

• Potential cervical spine injury involves total body immobilization:

• Use a long spine board with spacer under the torso (~1-in high) to accommodate the large occiput in children <8 y of age.

• Use hard cervical collar.

• Straps should be placed across the bony prominences of shoulders, pelvis and forehead, as well as over the chin area of hard collar [9].

• Frequently reassess immobilization.

• Tongs or other immobilization devices *should be directed by a neurosurgeon.*

Key references

1. Bruce D: Head trauma. In *Textbook of Pediatric Emergency Medicine*, ed 3. Edited by Fleisher G, Ludwig S. Baltimore: Williams & Wilkins; 1993:1102–1112.

2. Bullock R, Chesnut RM, Clifton C, *et al.*: Guidelines for the Management of Severe Head Injury. New York: Brain Trauma Foundation; 1995.

3. Bonadio W: Cervical spine trauma in children: part I. General concepts, normal anatomy, radiographic evaluation. *Am J Emerg Med* 1993, 11:158–165.

4. Bonadio W: Cervical spine trauma in children: part II. Mechanisms and manifestations of injury, therapeutic considerations. *Am J Emerg Med* 1993, 11:256–277.

5. Woodward G: Neck trauma. In *Textbook of Pediatric Emergency Medicine*, ed 3. Edited by Fleisher G, Ludwig S. Baltimore: Williams & Wilkins; 1993:1113–1142.

Diagnosis

Symptoms
- Most children are asymptomatic.

Cough: productive or nonproductive.

Fever.

Weight loss.

Malaise.

Night sweats.

Chills.

Hemoptysis.

Signs
- Examination may be normal.

Erythema nodosum.

Adenopathy: especially in the hilum, mediastinum, and neck

Rhonchi or rales over the affected lobe.

Decreased breath sounds over an atelectatic lobe.

Wheezing: if a bronchus is obstructed.

Investigations

Multiple puncture tests: (*eg*, Tine test) are not as useful for mass tuberculosis (TB) screenings as originally thought.

Tuberculin (Mantoux) skin test (purified protein derivative [PPD]): best test for confirming infection in children at risk or symptomatic for disease (*see* table).

Intradermal injection of 5 tuberculin units of PPD.

Read after 48– 72 h.

In healthy children >4 y old with no risk factors, positive test is <15 mm induration.

In healthy children <4 y old or children with risk factors for TB, positive test is = 10 mm induration.

In immunocompromised hosts or children suspected of having active TB, positive test is >5 mm induration.

A control (*ie*, tetanus toxoid, mumps, *Candida*) should be performed to rule out anergy as a cause for a false-negative TB test in immunocompromised patients.

A positive PPD only tests for exposure to TB; a chest radiograph is needed to assess the extent of the disease.

Chest radiograph: if PPD is positive; may be normal; suggests only exposure to TB (TB converter), not active disease; if active disease, findings include hilar adenopathy, lobar infiltrate, cavitation; must obtain both posteroanterior and lateral views (hilar adenopathy sometimes not visualized on the posteroanterior view).

Computer tomography chest scan: useful for assessing hilar and mediastinal adenopathy.

Sputum evaluation: acid-fast bacteria (AFB) stain to determine the presence of bacteria; culture to determine sensitivity of organism; may be collected by 1) productive cough, 2) early morning gastric aspirates (done on 3 consecutive mornings), 3) bronchoscopic lavage, or 4) biopsy (of the pleura, a lymph node, bone marrow aspirate, or other affected organ); polymerase chain reaction tests are useful if the AFB stain is positive.

Differential diagnosis
Pneumonia from other bacteria.

Congenital cyst.

Intrathoracic tumors (eg, lymphoma).

Systemic malignancy.

Sarcoidosis.

Etiology
Infection with *Mycobacterium tuberculosis*.
- Patients may be infected with TB but not have active disease (TB converters: positive PPD with no clinical evidence of disease and a normal chest radiograph).

Epidemiology
- Overall incidence in the US was decreasing until the mid-1980s; since then there has been an epidemic increase in newly diagnosed cases.
- Incidence is 9.4:100,000 (7% of which are children).
- Highest incidence occurs in immigrants from Southeast Asia, patients infected with HIV, other immunocompromised hosts, and i.v. drug abusers.
- Primary route of infection is through inhalation of viable tubercle bacilli.
- Easily spread in situations where health care is not easily accessible, hygiene is poor, and many people are in closed situations (eg, inner-city housing).
- A positive skin test usually develops within 2–12 wk of exposure (median, 3–4 wk).
- The risk for developing active disease is highest 6–24 mo after developing a positive skin test.
- The risk for developing disseminated disease (ie, miliary TB, meningitis) is highest in the first 3–12 mo after infection.
- Infants with active TB will rarely have a positive skin test before 6 mo of age.

Complications
Lobar atelectasis: especially if an endobronchial lesion or an encroaching hilar node is obstructing a major bronchus.

Pleural effusion.

Respiratory distress.

Pericardial effusion.

Hemoptysis.

Miliary TB.

TB meningitis.

Bone or joint involvement.

Treatment

Diet and lifestyle

Patients should be given vitamin B_6 (pyridoxine) supplements if their diet is limited or they are being breast fed (isoniazid can interfere with vitamin B_6 metabolism, leading to neuropathies and seizures).

• Compliance with therapy is essential, given the duration of treatment and the ramifications of incomplete therapy (*eg*, progression of disease, infecting others, increased risk for the development of drug resistant organisms). Directly observed therapy is sometimes indicated to assure compliance.

• Children who are not sputum producers are not considered infectious.

• Children who do produce sputum are infectious up to several weeks after therapy has started.

Pharmacologic treatment

For drug-susceptible organisms

Standard dosage Isoniazid, 10 mg/kg/d (maximum, 300 mg/d) may be given as daily dosage or divided twice daily for 9 mo if patient is a TB converter, or for 6 mo in cases of active TB and part of a multidrug regimen (may be given twice weekly during last 4 mo of therapy if under direct observation of a healthcare worker).

Rifampin, 10 mg/kg/d (maximum, 600 mg/d) for 6 mo in cases of active TB and part of a multi-drug regimen (may be given twice weekly during last 4 mo of therapy if under direct observation of a healthcare worker).

Pyrazinamide, 30 mg/kg/day (maximum, 2 g/d) for first 2 mo of a 6-mo multidrug regimen.

For drug-resistant organisms

• Administer isoniazid, rifampin, pyrazinamide at above doses *plus*:

Standard dosage Ethambutol, 15–25 mg/kg/d (maximum, 2.5 g/d), or Streptomycin, 30 mg/kg/d (maximum, 1 g/d).

Special points Duration is controversial and dependent on the underlying organism(s) and the host's situation; between 6 and 24 mo has been advocated.

Corticosteroids

Corticosteroids are used in cases of pleural and pericardial effusions, endobronchial disease, miliary TB and TB meningitis.

Standard dosage Prednisone, 1–2 mg/kg/d for 6–8 wk.

Bacille Calmette–Guerin (BCG)

Vaccine is frequently used where TB is endemic. It is useful in conferring partial immunity in this population. In patients who have received the BCG vaccine, they will have PPD tests that are borderline positive (<10 mm). If they have a true positive result, they should be considered infected with TB.

Treatment aims

To treat active disease.
To prevent progression of TB infection to active disease.

Prognosis

• If compliant with therapy: excellent prognosis.

Follow-up and management

• Liver function tests (transaminases) should be monitored to assess for isoniazid hepatotoxicity in patients at high risk or if higher than usual doses are used. Monitoring in otherwise healthy or low risk children is controversial.
• Follow-up chest radiographs should be obtained if the initial study is abnormal.
• Close follow-up is required to assure compliance with treatment plan.

Other information

• All new cases need to be reported to the local public health agency.
• All close contacts of the patient should be tested for TB.
• Isolation of the infected child is not required if they are at low risk for dissemination. If they have a productive cough, isolation is indicated until therapy has started. Newborns should be separated from mothers who have active disease until the mother has initiated anti-TB therapy.
• Tuberculin skin test will usually remain positive throughout life.

General references

Abernahy RS: Tuberculosis: An update. *Pediatr Rev* 1997, **18**:50–58.

American Academy of Pediatrics: *1997 Red Book: Report of the Committee on Infectious Diseases.* 1997:541–562.

American Thoracic Society: Treatment of tuberculosis and tuberculosis infection in adults and children. *Am J Respir Crit Care Med* 1994, **149**:1359–1374.

Correa AG: Unique aspects of tuberculosis in the pediatric population. *Clin Chest Med* 1997, **18**:89–98.

Hillman BC: *Pediatric Respiratory Disease: Diagnosis and Treatment.* Philadelphia: WB Saunders; 1993:311–320.

Inselman LS: Tuberculosis in children: an update. *Pediatr Pulmonol* 1996, **21**:101–120.

Diagnosis

Symptoms

Short stature: the birth height and weight are usually in the low–normal range; growth slows after age 3 years; mean adult height, 143 cm; short stature is present in virtually all affected individuals.

Delayed puberty/infertility: due to ovarian dysgenesis.

• Significantly, a substantial number of individuals with Turner syndrome have short stature and/or pubertal delay as the major presenting symptom, and the diagnosis must be considered in females who present with either feature, even in the absence of other associated dysmorphism.

Signs

Dysmorphic features: inverted triangular facies with narrow mandible, protuberant and simple ears, broad chest with nipples appearing widely spaced, prominent ears, low posterior hairline, short neck (present in 80%), webbed posterior neck (present in 50%), cubitus valgus, short 4th metacarpal, and hyperconvex nails; it is important to note that no single dysmorphism is required or pathognomonic for the diagnosis of Turner syndrome.

Lymphatic abnormalities: can present as edema of the hands, feet, and digits in the neonatal period; the webbed neck, low posterior hair line, and appearance of the ears may also be related to fetal lymphatic obstruction.

Investigations

Karyotype: required to confirm the diagnosis and to determine if Y chromosome material is present.

Cardiac evaluation.

Renal evaluation.

Complications

Cardiac defects: most commonly bicuspid aortic valve, coarctation of the aorta. Aortic stenosis and anomalous pulmonary venous return may also occur.

Hearing loss: often sensorineural, although chronic otitis media frequently occurs and may cause a conductive loss.

Renal anomalies: often asymptomatic, most commonly horseshoe kidney or pelvic kidney. Duplicated collecting system and ureteropelvic junction obstruction have been noted and may require treatment.

Infertility: initial ovarian development *in utero* is normal; however, stromal fibrosis occurs at an accelerated rate and the ovaries become "streak," usually during childhood, and some patients will develop some pubertal development and a few may have transient menses; retention of some ovarian function is more common in mosaic Turner syndrome; fertility has been reported but is extremely uncommon; women with Turner syndrome are able to bear children through egg donation if the uterus is normal.

Autoimmune disease: an increased frequency of autoimmune thyroid disease (most frequently Hashimoto's thyroiditis) has been noted, and hypothyroidism may result; inflammatory bowel disease also occurs at an increased frequency.

Gastrointestinal bleeding: may be due to telangiectasias or hemangiomas, and can be severe.

Differential diagnosis

• Noonan syndrome is an autosomal dominant condition that affects males and females. It shares with Turner syndrome the features of short stature; low posterior hairline; short, wide or webbed neck; cubitus valgus; widely spaced nipples; and lymphatic abnormalities. Facial features include downslanting palpebral fissures, ptosis, and ears with thick overturned helices. Congenital heart disease is present in approximately 40% of individuals (often pulmonary valve stenosis, occasionally generalized hypertrophic cardiomyopathy); Cryptorchidism, and sternal abnormalities may also be present. The karyotype is normal. The gene has been mapped to 12q but has not yet been identified. Cognitive development ranges from mental retardation (25%) to normal.

Etiology

• Most commonly due to monosomy of the entire X chromosome (karyotype 45,XO). Some individuals can be mosaic (XX/XO, or XY/XO), or have a structural abnormality of the X chromosome (eg, a ring or isochromosome) resulting in a deletion of a portion of the X chromosome. There is no association with advanced maternal age. It is generally sporadic with a low recurrence risk.

Epidemiology

• One in 2000 live-born females are affected.

Treatment

Pharmacologic treatment

Growth hormone therapy: short-term improvement of growth velocity, although the effect on final adult height is variable.

Estrogen replacement therapy: the timing of therapy should be individualized and psychological readiness is an important factor.

Nonpharmacologic treatment

Risk of gonadoblastoma: a dysgenetic gonad has not fully differentiated into either a normal ovary or a normal testis. If the dysgenetic gonad has some Y chromosome material, there is an increased risk for gonadoblastoma, which may be as high as 15%–30%. Some individuals with clinical Turner syndrome have a mosaic karyotype of XO/XY. The presence of the Y chromosome in some of the cells does not cause any consistent clinical effect, although virilization can occur. Individuals with Turner syndrome and Y chromosome material should undergo removal of the streak gonads to avoid the risk of gonadoblastoma.

Neuropsychologic function: individuals should be assessed for specific cognitive deficits such as nonverbal processing and visual–spatial difficulties. There is an increased incidence of low self-esteem and recognition of social cues, although the factors causing these features have not been delineated. Awareness of these potential neuropsychological difficulties should lead to appropriate support and intervention if needed. Psychological readiness is important for deciding on the timing of supplemental sex hormone therapy.

Prognosis/natural history

• Early motor milestones may be delayed, although overall intelligence is generally in the normal range. Verbal performance is relatively good, but visual–spatial organization and nonverbal problem-solving are frequently abnormal.

General references

American Academy of Pediatrics, Committee on Genetics: Health supervision for children with Turner syndrome. *Pediatrics* 1995, 96:1166–1173.

Chu CE, Paterson WF, Kelnar CJ, *et al.*: Variable effects of growth hormone on growth and final adult height in Scottish patients with Turner syndrome. *Acta Pediatrica* 1987, **86**:160–164.

Taback SP, Collin R, Deal CL, *et al.*: Does growth-hormone supplementation affect adult height in Turner syndrome? *Lancet* 1996, 384:25–27.

Lippe B: Turner syndrome. *Endocrinol Metab Clin North Am* 1991, 20:121–152.

Urinary tract infection

Diagnosis

Symptoms

• In infants, symptoms are nonspecific and include vomiting, poor feeding, and irritability.

• The symptoms in toddlers may be nonspecific as well.

• Older children develop dysuria, urgency, frequency, incontinence, hesitancy, and retention; fever, chills, back pain are symptoms that suggest an upper tract infection (pyelonephritis).

Signs

• Fever is the most common finding in infants; jaundice may be seen in neonates.

• Older children can demonstrate suprapubic or costovertebral angle tenderness. Other findings may suggest an anatomic or neuropathic cause of the infection.

• Uncircumcised males have 10 times the risk of infection compared with circumcised males.

Abdominal or flank mass: suggestive of obstructive uropathy.

Sacral dimple, hairy patch over the sacrum, abnormal gluteal cleft, decreased rectal tone, lipoma: suggest spinal cord anomalies.

Labial adhesion, trauma, and irritation: may increase the risk of infection.

Investigations

Urine culture: considered positive if any organisms are present on a suprapubic collection; > 10^4 colony forming units (CFU)/mL of a urinary pathogen from a catheterized specimen; > 10^5 CFU/mL of a urinary pathogen from a clean catch.

Bag specimens: should be avoided.

Urinalysis with dipstick: demonstrating positive leukocyte esterase and nitrite test with microscopic examination demonstrating more than five leukocytes per hpf, bacteria is highly suggestive of a urinary tract infection (UTI); this is not reliable in infants in whom the urine is dilute; 10% may have a negative urinalysis result despite a positive culture.

Radiographic imaging: indicated in every boy with an infection and girls with pyelonephritis; girls with recurrent lower tract infections or those who are younger than 5 years of age with their first infection should be studied as well.

Renal and bladder ultrasound: a noninvasive aid to look for hydroureteronephrosis, duplex kidneys, and ureteroceles, which may be a sign of obstruction.

Voiding cystourethrography: might demonstrate vesicoureteral reflux and is especially important in the male to exclude posterior urethral valves.

99mTc-DMSA scan: controversial; it is an excellent study to identify pyelonephritis as the cause of fever when the source is not known; it is the most sensitive study to determine the presence of scars; however, it may not ultimately change the course of treatment.

Complications

Septicemia: more likely to be present in neonates or in children with abnormal urinary tracts.

Renal scarring: can develop years after infections that occurred in infancy or early childhood; it is associated with hypertension, toxemia, and the risk of chronic renal failure leading to end-stage renal disease.

Staghorn calculi: can form in the presence of repeated infections.

Differential diagnosis

Urethritis (chemical; from irritants such as soap), vaginitis, trauma, and hypercalciuria can cause dysuria.

Detrusor/sphincter dysfunction can cause incontinence.

Pneumonia, gastroenteritis, appendicitis, and pelvic inflammatory disease can be associated with symptoms similar to acute pyelonephritis.

Etiology

• *Escherichia coli* is the most common cause of bacterial UTI; other organisms include *Klebsiella* spp, *Enterococcus*, *Staphylococcus saprophyticus*, and *Proteus mirabilis; Pseudomonas, Streptococcus*, and *Candida albicans* infections are usually associated with complicated UTIs or chronic antibiotic treatment.

• Risk factors in all children include indwelling catheters, urologic abnormalities, and neurogenic bladders; risk factors specific to girls include chemical irritants, sexual activity, sexual abuse, constipation, and pinworms.

• Uncircumcised boys have an incidence of infection 10 times that of circumcised boys.

Epidemiology

• Bacteriuria is present in 1%–2% of prepubertal children.

• In the first year of life, the risk of infection is equal among boys and girls; the risk in girls is considerably higher in toddlers and older children.

• The incidence of UTI was 3.0% in a large urban emergency department when all febrile infants younger than 12 mo and girls older than 24 mo of age without an obvious cause for fever were screened.

• Vesicoureteral reflux is present in 18%–50% of children with UTI; reflux is seen in 40% of siblings of index cases; it is also seen in 66% of offspring.

Treatment

Diet and lifestyle
• Increased water intake offers several benefits; it dilutes urine, increases voiding frequency, and reduces constipation. Stool softeners should be considered if the latter problem persists.
• Irritants, particularly soap, should be avoided near the perineum in prepubertal girls.
• Sexually active women may benefit from postcoital voiding.

Pharmacologic treatment
Complicated febrile urinary tract infections
• Complicated infections are defined as those seen in infants younger than 6 months of age and any child who is clinically ill, persistently vomiting, moderately dehydrated, or poorly compliant; these cases warrant intravenous antibiotics and hospitalization.

Standard dosage	Ampicillin, 50–100 mg/kg/d in four divided doses.
	Gentamicin, 2–2.5 mg/kg/dose every 8 h.
	Ceftriaxone, 75 mg/kg/dose every 12 h (does not cover *Enterococcus*, which is more frequently encountered in children with recurrent infection and should be avoided in neonates).
Special points	An oral agent can be used after the child improves clinically (>24 h afebrile) pending the results of the culture and sensitivities; total treatment should last 14 d or longer if there is a renal abscess or an abnormal urinary tract.

Uncomplicated febrile urinary tract infections
• These children do not appear clinically ill, can take oral antibiotics, and are only mildly dehydrated (if at all) and compliant. Treatment can start with one dose of a parenteral agent (ceftriaxone, 75 mg/kg i.v. or i.m.; gentamicin, 2.5 mg/kg i.v. or i.m.) followed by oral therapy or with oral therapy alone. Good follow-up is essential to ensure the child has responded appropriately, with treatment lasting 10–14 d.

Standard dosage	Cotrimoxazole, 6–12 mg/kg/d; trimethoprim divided twice daily.
	Amoxicillin, 20–40 mg/kg/d divided 3 times daily (many strains of *E. coli* are resistant to amoxicillin).
	Cephalexin, 25–50 mg/kg/d divided 4 times daily.
	Cefprozil, 15–30 mg/kg/d divided 2 times daily.

Afebrile urinary tract infections (acute cystitis)
• Oral therapy with the agents listed above for a total of 5–7 d assuming clinical improvement is seen; in addition, nitrofurantoin 5–7 mg/kg/d divided 4 times daily can be considered; the liquid form of nitrofurantoin is not well tolerated.

Covert (asymptomatic) bacteriuria
• The treatment of this subgroup is controversial even in the presence of reflux; treatment may lead to the emergence of resistant organisms.

Prophylaxis
Standard dosage	*Cotrimoxazole*: 1–2 mg/kg trimethoprim daily.
	Nitrofurantoin, 1–2 mg/kg/d.

• Both of the above medications should be avoided in infants younger than 6 months of age.
• Amoxicillin (10 mg/kg/d) or cephalexin (10 mg/kg/d) can be used instead.

General references
Dairiki Shortliffe LM: The management of urinary tract infections in children without urinary tract abnormalities. *Urol Clin North Am* 1995, 22:67–73.

Hellerstein S: Urinary tract infections: old and new concepts. *Pediatr Clin North Am* 1995, 42:1433–1457.

Sheldon CA: Vesicoureteral reflux. *Pediatr Rev* 1995, 16:22–27.

Urologic obstructive disorders

Diagnosis

Symptoms
• The introduction of antenatal ultrasonography has dramatically altered the presentation of urologic obstruction disorders; in contrast to 15 years ago, most infants now are asymptomatic when they come to the attention of the pediatrician and pediatric urologist.

Abdominal mass: primarily seen in neonates.

Vomiting, failure to thrive, and urinary tract infection: often noted as early as the first year of life.

Recurrent abdominal or flank pain: often seen in older children with uretero-pelvic junction obstruction (UPJ); Dietl's crisis (severe abdominal pain and vomiting) occurs in high flow states when the renal pelvis decompensates.

Gross hematuria: can occur either isolated or after mild abdominal trauma.

Abnormal urinary stream: can be indicative of posterior urethral valves (PUV) but may not be seen in all cases.

Daytime incontinence, nocturnal enuresis, and increased urinary frequency: may occur in older boys with mild obstruction secondary to PUV.

Signs
Abdominal mass on palpation in a neonate: most commonly associated with a genitourinary anomaly or obstruction.

Suprapubic mass: suggests PUV.

Abdominal distention secondary to urinary ascites: also seen in PUV with associated high pressure vesicoureteral reflux rupturing the renal fornices.

Respiratory distress and other features of oligohydramnios (contractures, "squashed facies"): can be seen in severe obstruction secondary to PUV.

Fever: may be the only sign indicating the presence of a urinary tract infection.

Failure to thrive, rickets, and irritability: signs of renal failure, can suggest the presence of PUV or, rarely, UPJ obstruction in a child with a single kidney.

Investigations
Renal ultrasonography: can help differentiate the forms of obstruction; hydronephrosis without ureteral dilitation suggests UPJ obstruction; if ureteral dilitation is present, either primary obstructed megaureter (POM) or vesicoureteral reflux must be considered; a thick-walled bladder with bilateral hydroureteronephrosis is seen in PUV.

Voiding cystourethrography: necessary to confirm PUV; a thick trabeculated bladder with dilitation of the posterior urethra and valve leaflets are seen; the study also demonstrates the presence of vesicoureteral reflux, which can be either isolated or in association with UPJ or PUV.

Diuretic renography (DPTA or MAG-3): helps differentiate the site of obstruction in UPJ versus POM, the latter remarkable for tracer present in the ureter; more importantly, it offers an opportunity to judge the degree of obstruction and differential renal function.

Intravenous pyelogram: is currently used less frequently but may be necessary if anatomic detail is required; its use is discouraged in infants younger than 6 months of age because the dye is not well concentrated.

Renal function studies, electrolytes: in cases of bilateral disease.

Complications
Urinary tract obstruction, pyelonephritis, urosepsis.

Renal failure: when PUV are present; UPJ obstruction and POM, if severe, may cause loss of function of the affected kidney.

Hypertension.

Nephrolithiasis.

Differential diagnosis
Vesicoureteral reflux must be considered in cases of antenatal hydronephrosis. Multicystic-dysplastic kidneys can mimic UPJ obstruction but show no function on nuclear renograms. Ureteoceles can obstruct the ureter and associated renal segment or act like a "valve" if it prolapses in the urethra. Ectopic ureters are usually associated with double collecting systems and obstruction of the upper pole moiety.

Etiology
• UPJ obstruction is most commonly congenital, caused by an intrinsic defect of abnormal muscle bundles that produce an adynamic segment at the junction. Extrinsic compression secondary to crossing vessels can also cause obstruction.
• POM is usually caused by a disruption in the normal ureteral musculature at the distal end that does not conduct a peristaltic wave to pass urine into the bladder.
• PUV form when the ventrolateral folds of the urogenital sinus fail to regress; these valves form a portion of the hymenal ring in females; thus, PUV may be likened to an "imperforate hymen" in males.

Epidemiology
UPJ obstruction is the most common obstruction in the urinary tract and is seen in 1:500 births, with male-to-female ratio of 3–4:1; bilateral lesions occur in 10%–40% of cases.
POM is seen in 1:10,000 births, with males affected 3:1.
PUV is seen in 1:8000 male births; familial cases have been reported.

Treatment

Diet and lifestyle

No specific modifications are necessary unless there is decreased renal function (*see* Renal failure, chronic).

There may be poor urinary concentrating ability and polyuria; there should be sufficient water available to avoid dehydration especially in infants.

Pharmacologic treatment

• Antibiotic prophylaxis is recommended in infants with urinary tract dilitation until a diagnosis is confirmed; children with reflux usually remain on prophylaxis until the reflux resolves.

Standard dosage	Cotrimoxazole, 1–2 mg/kg trimethoprim per day.
	Nitrofurantoin, 1–2 mg/kg/d.
Special points	*Cotrimoxazole* and *nitrofurantoin* should be avoided in infants younger than 6 wk.
	Amoxicillin (10 mg/kg/d) or cephalexin (10 mg/kg/d) can be used instead.
	In chronic renal failure, secondary to obstruction, various medications may be indicated (*see* Renal failure, chronic).

Other treatments

• Pyeloplasty is indicated in children with UPJ obstruction and compromised renal function or in instances in which the patient is experiencing painful crises.

• Reimplantation surgery is indicated in children with POM and deteriorating renal function or with symptomatology.

• Infants diagnosed with PUV usually undergo ablation of the valve; in some cases a vesicostomy is required.

• Nephrectomy is indicated in rare cases in which the affected renal unit has no function and symptoms are present.

Treatment aims

To preserve renal function in cases in which obstruction is significant.

To relieve symptoms of pain when present.

To decrease risk of infection.

Prognosis

Depends on the degree of renal damage at the time of diagnosis; because UPJ obstruction and POM are usually unilateral, a poorly or nonfunctioning kidney should not significantly affect overall renal function as the unaffected kidney will hypertrophy.

Because PUV affect both kidneys in most cases, the prognosis can vary from poor, if there is oligohydramnios, to good if the obstruction is mild.

Follow-up and management

Infants and children with UPJ obstruction and POM should be followed closely by a pediatric urologist until it is believed that renal function is stable; a pediatric nephrologist should also follow children with PUV because they may develop chronic renal failure.

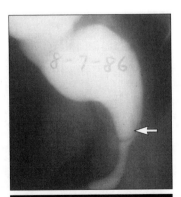

Posterior urethral valves. Arrow represents valves with dilated posterior urethra proximally.

General references

Denes ED, Barthold JS, Gonzalez R: Early prognostic value of serum creatinine levels in children with posterior urethral valves. *J Urol* 1997, 157:1441–1443.

Dinneen MD, Duffy PG: Posterior urethral valves. *Br J Urol* 1997, 78:275–281.

King LR: Hydronephrosis: when is obstruction not obstruction? *Urol Clin North Am* 1995, 22:31–42.

Noe HN: The wide ureter. In *Adult and Pediatric Urology.* Edited by Gillenwater JY, Grayhack JT, Howards SS, Duckett JW. St. Louis: Mosby; 1996:2233–2257.

Reznick VM, Budorick NE: Prenatal detection of congenital renal disease. *Urol Clin North Am* 1995, 22:21–30.

Diagnosis

Symptoms

Itching (pruritus) and swelling of the skin.

Arthralgia in severe urticaria (and urticarial vasculitis).

Painful or burning sensation of the skin: can reflect severe pruritus but more commonly found in urticarial vasculitis.

Abdominal cramping and symptoms of laryngeal edema (hoarseness, dyspnea): may appear in hereditary/acquired angioedema.

Signs

Urticaria: red, elevated, nonpitting papules or plaques usually associated with blanched, edematous centers; may be annular in appearance; usually pruritic; usually show at least transient response to antihistamine; individual lesions are transient (2 hours or less) and resolve without residuum.

Angioedema: especially of the lips and periorbital areas; usually nonpruritic and frequently not painful; as a manifestation of hereditary or acquired angioedema, lesions may involve both skin (face, neck limbs, trunk) and mucosa of upper respiratory and gastrointestinal tracts.

Investigations

Acute urticaria

Thorough history and physical examination: often uncovers trigger.

Examine for dermatographism.

Determine presence of allergen-specific immunoglobulin E (IgE): skin test most sensitive; RAST.

Challenge procedures: may be appropriate (*eg*, atopic, drug, physical triggers).

Evaluation for infection as appropriate.

General screening: may include complete blood count with differential, urinalysis, and ESR.

Chronic urticaria

Evaluation: should exclude presence of systemic illness (especially collagen-vascular, malignancy).

Consider skin biopsy with immunofluorescence studies: rule out vasculitis.

Consider baseline complement assays: (C1, C4 components; total serum hemolytic complement [CH_{50}]) to detect consumption.

Angioedema syndromes

Assay of C1 esterase function: quantitative and functional assays.

Assess complement component consumption in baseline state and during flare: (C1, C4, CH_{50}).

Complications

Anaphylactic shock: in acute, IgE-mediated reactions.

Asphyxiation (laryngospasm) or shock: in hereditary angioedema syndrome.

• Life-threatening systemic illness can exist in some cases of chronic urticaria.

Differential diagnoses

Urticarial vasculitis, erythema multiforme, erythema chronicum migrans, erythema marginatum, erythema infectiosum (fifth disease), dermal contact dermatitis, urticarial component of bullous pemphigoid, urticaria pigmentosa, systemic mastocytosis, papular urticaria (insect bites), erythropoietic protoporphyria, other drug hypersensitivity reactions, pityriasis rosea, atopic dermatitis (eczema), scabies, and psychogenic.

Etiology

Acute urticaria (<6 wk)

Immediate hypersensitivity (IgE-mediated): most common mechanism (eg, food, drug, stinging insect, or animal dander triggers).

Infection (viruses [respiratory, herpes, hepatitis] and bacterial [eg, *Streptococcus*]): common in childhood (idiopathic urticaria); fungal, helminthic possible.

Cytotoxic antibodies.

Antigen–antibody complexes (eg, serum sickness).

Direct histamine release.

Interference with arachidonic acid metabolism (aspirin, nonsteroidal anti-inflammatory drugs [NSAIDs]).

Physical factors (eg, cold, heat exercise).

Chronic urticaria (> 6 wk)

Etiology remains obscure in 80%–90% of cases.

• Intolerance to food additives, aspirin, NSAIDs, and foods is frequently suspected but uncommonly the final diagnosis.

• Underlying systemic disease is possible: collagen vascular disease, malignancy, endocrine disturbances (eg, hyperthyroidism, pregnancy), amyloidosis, hypereosinophilic syndromes, and most rarely, deficiency of C3b inactivator (factor I).

• Some cases are due to autoimmune phenomena.

Angioedema syndromes

• Absence of normal C1 esterase inhibitor (most commonly reduced production, but also nonfunctional protein); autosomal dominant transmission.

• Acquired forms of C1 esterase dysfunction occur rarely, mainly in association with malignancy or collagen-vascular disorders (heterogenous group; multiple pathogenic mechanisms).

Epidemiology

• Affects 10%–20% of population.

• Allergen-induced and infection-associated are most common etiologies in childhood.

Treatment

Diet and Lifestyle

- Avoidance of known triggers is essential.
- Chronic medication administration: compliance and side effects.
- Interference of social function: appearance; ability to work, attend school.
- Counseling for hereditary disorders (angioedema).

Pharmacologic treatment

Acute and chronic urticaria (standard dosages, adjusted for age/weight)

H1 antagonists: first-line modality.

Cetirizine: nonsedating.

Loratadine: nonsedating.

Fexofenidine: nonsedating.

Terfenadine: nonsedating.

Hydroxyzine.

Cyproheptadine: especially cold-, heat-induced urticaria.

Doxepin: tricyclic with H1 and H2 activity; optimize daily dose, avoid sedation unless sleep disrupted.

H2 antagonists: added to H1 regimen if control not achieved.

Ranitadine.

Cimetidine.

Contraindications	Porphyrias.
Main drug interactions	*Terfenadine*: associated with ventricular arrhythmias (with concurrent macrolides, antifungals, liver disease)
	Cimetidene and *ranitadine*: associated with increased theophylline levels.
Main side effects	Sedation, anticholinergic effects.

- Systemic corticosteroids often used as brief (3- to 5-day) course in acute urticaria but otherwise reserved for severe, difficult-to-control cases.

- For chronic administration, use minimize dose and attempt alternate-day regimen; plan periodic interruption to assess remission.

For hereditary angioedema

Acute attacks: Epinephrine can provide some benefit; corticosteroids and antihistamines not helpful; mild analgesia and intravenous fluids may suffice for mild attacks; meperidine useful to reduce severe pain; infusion of purified C1 inhibitor (experimental drug) or fresh frozen plasma (may worsen symptoms) to abort acute attacks.

Perioperative prophylaxis: fresh-frozen plasma or purified C1 inhibitor as above.

Long-term prophylaxis: antifibrinolytic agents (epsilon-aminocaproic acid and tranexamic acid [utility of each limited by toxicity and availability]); attenuated androgens (increase C1 inhibitor synthesis) can improve control but have residual androgenic side effects; acquired forms may have variable response to androgens; autoimmune forms may require fibrinolytic inhibitors, plasmapheresis, and/or immunosuppressive agents.

Treatment aims

Urticaria

To relieve symptoms, avoid treatment complications, detect underlying conditions.

Hereditary angioedema

To prevent recurrences, recommend family counseling, prepare for life-threatening episodes.

Prognosis

- Excellent for acute urticaria and idiopathic urticaria of childhood.
- Most children with chronic urticaria do well.
- Severity of hereditary angioedema varies.

Follow-up and management

Individualized for each patient.

General references

Horan R, Schneider LC, Sheffer AL: Allergic skin disorders and mastocytosis. *JAMA* 1992, **268:**2858–2868.

Huston DP, Bressler RB: Urticaria and angioedema. *Med Clin North Am* 1992, **76:**805–840.

Kaplan AP: Urticaria and angioedema. In *Allergy*. Edited by Kaplan AP. Philadelphia: WB Saunders Co.; 1997.

Soter NA: Urticaria: current therapy. *J Allergy Clin Immunol* 1990, **86:**1009–1014.

Diagnosis

• Vaginal complaints, either vaginal discharge or bleeding, in a preadolescent girl must be taken seriously. The differential diagnosis contains elements of serious medical problems. These complaints also raise the possibility of sexual abuse.

Symptoms

• The symptom of vaginal discharge and bleeding in the post-newborn period is not worrisome as it probably represents physiologic leukorrhea and/or withdrawal bleeding, both produced by the influence of maternal estrogen.

• After the newborn period, vaginal discharge may be noted by the child or parent as a stain on the underpants. The same is true for vaginal bleeding.

• Obtain history about the duration of the symptom and the nature of the discharge. Is there foul odor that might go along with a vaginal foreign body? What is the color and consistency of the discharge?

• Is there unusual behavior that might signal a child sexual abuse encounter? Is there a upper respiratory infection, sore throat, or skin infection that might point to a streptococcal infection? Does the child toilet themselves and what techniques are used for normal perineal care?

• Is there vaginal pain or dysuria? Is there itching? Have medications been administered? Does the child masturbate often? Has bubble bath been used or any other additives to the bath water?

• It is always appropriate to ask the child about any uncomfortable or unusual contacts that might elicit a history of possible sexual abuse.

Signs

• Examine the child to determine the nature and amount of vaginal discharge or bleeding.

• If there is steady blood flow and the child is clearly prepubertal, then gynocologic or pediatric surgical consultation should be obtained in order to perform an examination under anesthesia.

• Examine the child for their stage of pubertal development. Are their any other signs of developing secondary sexual characteristics such as increased body odor, breast development, hair growth in the pubic or axillary area? Has there been any recent change in growth?

• Perform a careful neurological examination.

• If the complaint is bleeding, try to localize the site of bleeding and attempt to quantitate the amount. Examine the child in both the frog leg and knee chest position to get an adequate view of the genitalia. Is there evidence of urethral prolapse?

Investigations

• For girls with vaginal discharge it is important to obtain a bacteriologic culture. Be certain that you can harvest both standard bacteria as well as *Neisseria gonorrhoeae* and *Chlamydia trachomatis*.

• If bleeding is of acute onset and sudden, consider the work-up of the child who has been sexually abused. This would include looking for sperm, semen, and evidence of sexual contact, *eg*, pubic hair.

Complications

• The main complications come in missing the primary diagnosis and the opportunity to correctly manage it.

Differential diagnosis

For vaginal bleeding

Trauma, including sexual abuse.

Foreign body.

Organisms associated with vaginitis: group A *Streptococcus, Shigella*.

Urethral prolapse.

Lichen sclerosis.

Precocious puberty.

Tumor.

Hemangioma.

For vaginal discharge

Vaginitis (nonspecific or specific organisms such as group A *Streptococcus, N. gonorrhoeae, C. trachomatis, Giardinerella, Candida, Trichomonas*, pinworms, and others.

Foreign body.

Anatomic abnormality, eg, ectopic ureter.

Physiologic leukorrhea.

Chemical irritant.

Allergic reaction.

Etiology

• The child's vaginal mucosa is thin and has no estrogenization. The pH is neutral and there is no glycogen in the vaginal lining, thus making it a perfect culture medium.

• Most children have perineal hygiene that is lacking. In addition, it is a site for exploration and masturbation with unclean hands.

Epidemiology

• Virtually every girl will have some vaginal irritation and scant amount of discharge sometime during childhood.

• Nonspecific vulvovaginitis accounts for 25%–75% of cases diagnosed.

Treatment

• Treatment depends on the underlying cause.

Pharmacologic therapy

• The following agents may be needed for corresponding infection:

Group A *Streptococcus*: penicillin V, 125–250 mg 4 times daily.

***Neisseria gonorrhoeae*:** cephtriaxone, 125 mg i.m. for older children > 8 years of age; also give doxycycline, 100 mg twice daily for 7 days.

***Candida*:** topical nystatin or clotrimazole cream.

Trichomonas: metronidazole, 125 mg 3 times daily for 7–10 days.

Pinworms: mebendazole, 1 chewable 100-mg tablet repeat in 2 weeks.

***Chlamydia trachomatis*:** children < 8 years of age: erythromycin, 50 mg/kg/d for 10 days; children > 8 years of age, deoxycycline 100-mg twice daily for 7 days.

Nonpharmacologic therapy

• Use of regular sitz baths with plain water is soothing and helps cleanse the area.

• The child should be encouraged to use good hygiene techniques.

• Also recommended is the avoidance of tight-fitting underpants, nylon or other synthetic nonabsorbent fibers, and chemical additives to bath water.

Treatment aimss

To identify a cause of vaginal bleeding or discharge.
To treat specific cause.
To rule out any child sexual abuse.
To reassure family.
To teach proper perineal care.

Prognosis

• Prognosis should be excellent if proper diagnosis has been ascertained and treatment provided.
• Child sexual abuse may be difficult to diagnose due to reluctance of the victim to identify the perpetrator. The prognosis in cases of child sexual abuse is more guarded.

Follow-up and management

• There is no need for any special follow-up.

Other information

• Consultation with a pediatric gynecologist, urologist, or child sexual abuse specialist may be indicated.

General references

Altchek A: Vaginal discharges. In *Difficult Diagnosis in Pediatrics.* Edited by Stockman J. Philadelphia: W.B. Saunders; 1990: 383–389 .

Berkowitz CD: Child sexual abuse. *Pediatr Rev* 1992, 13:443–452.

Paradise J: Vaginal bleeding and vaginal discharge. In *Textbook of Pediatric Emergency Medicine,* edn 3. Edited by Fleisher GR, Ludwig S. Baltimore: Williams & Wilkins; 1993: 494–505.

Vandeven AM, Emans SJ: Vulvovaginitis in the child and adolescent. *Pediatr Rev* 1993, 14:141–147.

Diagnosis

Symptoms

Wetting: occurring during the day, at night, or both; there may be overt episodes of soaking or underwear that is slightly damp; the pattern may be diurnal or nocturnal or both; primary (since toilet training) or secondary (at least 6 months dry).

Recurrent urinary tract infections (UTIs).

Urinary symptoms: such as increased urinary frequency, urgency, and hold maneuvers such as squatting to prevent leakage.

Interrupted urinary stream: or voiding associated with straining.

Constipation, encopresis, and other bowel complaints.

Signs

• Physical findings are usually rare; however, emphasis should be placed on abnormalities associated with anatomic or neuropathic causes of wetting.

Suprapubic mass: distended bladder, which can arise secondary to neuropathic, anatomic, or functional causes.

Labial adhesion: associated with postvoid leakage.

Sacral dimple or hairy tuft: suggestive of an occult spinal dysraphism.

Decreased rectal tone, perineal sensation, or severe constipation.

Neurological examination of the lower extremity.

Investigations

Urinalysis and urine culture: are the only studies necessary for children with isolated primary nocturnal enuresis; check for the presence of infection or occult renal disease (hematuria, proteinuria, poor concentrating ability).

Renal and bladder ultrasonography: should be considered in every patient with daytime wetting to exclude structural abnormalities and to determine the effect of pressure on the urinary tract (hydronephrosis, bladder wall thickening).

Voiding cystourethrography: in males with decreased urinary flow or UTI and in all children with febrile UTI to identify vesicoureteral reflux; girls may demonstrate a "spinning top" urethra, which suggests bladder or sphincter dysfunction.

Urodynamic studies: should be considered in older children not responding to initial treatment.

Spinal MRI: to exclude tethered cord when history, physical examination, and radiographic studies suggest a neuropathic bladder.

Complications

Hinman's syndrome: an uncommon complication associated with renal damage, hydroureteronephrosis, and a trabeculated bladder. Encopresis is seen in about one third of cases.

• **Poor self-esteem:** children are embarrassed and many refuse to participate in activities that might expose them to potential ridicule; many behavioral studies show improvement after treatment; the long-term effects are less clear.

Differential diagnosis

Anatomic causes of wetting: posterior urethral valves, ectopic ureter, ureterocele.

Neurological causes of wetting: occult spinal dysraphism, tumor, sacral agenesis.

UTI, chemical urethritis, pinworms, sexual abuse.

Any condition causing polyuria can cause enuresis.

Etiology

• Daytime wetting most likely represents an inability of the cortex to inhibited detrusor contractions and usually represents a maturational delay; other coinciding conditions such as recurrent UTIs and constipation may cause poor relaxation of the external sphincter.

• Nocturnal enuresis is familial in about 70% of cases; some children may have decreased functional capacity for the reasons cited above, and some children lack a nocturnal surge of antidiuretic hormone, which causes them to urinate inappropriately high volumes while sleeping.

• Sleep abnormalities, allergies, and primary behavioral disturbances have been implicated but not well substantiated as causes for wetting.

Epidemiology

• A Swedish study found 8.4% of girls and 1.7% of boys have voiding dysfunction manifest by wetting or recurrent UTIs.

• Nocturnal enuresis affects 20% of 5-year-old children; each year 15% recover spontaneously; about 1% of adults continue wetting at night; boys are affected more frequently than girls.

Treatment

Diet and lifestyle

• The age at which treatment should begin depends on several factors, including maturity, risk and type of infection, social pressures, and motivation; negative reinforcement should be strongly discouraged.

• A high fluid (water) intake can be beneficial in diluting urine and decreasing dysuria, thus decreasing future infections; it can also be used to treat constipation.

• Patients are encouraged to void regularly, prior to the sensation of urge; diaries can be used to increase compliance.

• A nocturnal enuresis alarm is a valuable tool for children with isolated night wetting. The alarm is inexpensive ($30–$50) and, if used properly, has a success rate approaching 80%.

• A high-fiber diet, stool softeners, and enemas may be recommended in children with associated symptoms of constipation.

Pharmacological treatment

• Children with severe urge and uninhibited detrusor contractions may benefit from an anticholinergic medication such as oxybutynin and hyoscyamine, which is available in a long-acting preparation.

Standard dosage	Oxybutynin, 2.5–5 mg 2 or 3 times daily.
	Hyoscyamine (LevBid), one half to 2 tablets 2 times daily.
Contraindications	Glaucoma, partial or complete intestinal obstruction, genitourinary obstruction.
Main side effects	Dry mouth, flushing, decreased sweating, constipation, drowsiness, blurry vision.

• Antibiotic prophylaxis in children with recurrent UTIs secondary to voiding dysfunction can break the cycle of discomfort, poor relaxation, incomplete emptying, infection, and discomfort; examples include cotrimoxazole and nitrofurantoin.

For isolated nocturnal enuresis

• Imipramine is effective in up to 50% of cases; over 60% relapse after the medication is discontinued.

• Desmopressin acetate (DDAVP) is an analogue of antidiuretic hormone; its use causes a 30%–60% reduction in wetting and, in some reports, a 50% cure rate; relapses are high when the medication is stopped.

Standard dosage	Imipramine, 25–50 mg at night for younger children; 75 mg nightly is maximum dose in older children (> 12 years); wean medication slowly when considering discontinuation.
	Desmopressin acetate, 20–40 µg (2–4 sprays) intranasally 1 hour before bedtime; an oral formulation is pending approval from the FDA for this indication.
Contraindications	*Imipramine:* concomitant use of monoamine oxidase inhibitors.
Special points	*Imipramine:* warn parents to keep out of reach of younger children as an overdose can be lethal.
	Desmopressin acetate: children should be advised to limit their intake of fluids near and after then time of administration to decrease the potential occurrence of water intoxication; the medication's absorption is impaired when the nasal mucosa is edematous.
Main side effects	*Imipramine:* personality changes, insomnia, nausea, nervousness.
	Desmopressin acetate: epistaxis, headache, nausea.

Treatment aims

To reduce the frequency of wetting episodes and UTIs.

To prevent the development of renal damage.

To improve self-esteem.

Other treatments

• Biofeedback has been shown to be helpful in older children with an inability to relax the external sphincter who develop recurrent UTIs; sessions are performed with repeated voiding using urine flows as a guide to relaxation.

• Rarely, some children with severe hydronephrosis and poor emptying require clean intermittent catheterization.

Prognosis

• Most children improve spontaneously, especially those with isolated nocturnal enuresis.

• A few children develop renal impairment in the form of renal scarring or insufficiency.

Follow-up and management

• Patients with enuresis and normal urinary tracts need not be followed up after resolution of the symptoms.

• Patients with abnormal urinary tracts should be followed up until improvement is seen.

• Those with renal scarring should have blood pressure monitoring and urinalysis on a yearly basis to look for proteinuria.

General references

Alon U: Nocturnal enuresis. *Pediatr Nephrol* 1995, **9:**94–103.

van Gool JD: Non-neuropathic and neuropathic bladder-sphincter dysfunction in children. *Pediatric Adolescent Medicine* 1994, **5:**178–192.

Rushton HG: Wetting and functional voiding disorders. *Urol Clin North Am* 1995, **22:**75–93.

Diagnosis

Symptoms

Fever: usually signifies infectious etiology.

Frequent, effortless regurgitation, heartburn: gastroesophageal reflux.

Persistent bilious vomiting, decreased stool output: intestinal obstruction.

Dysphagia, odynophagia, globus: esophageal abnormality.

Nausea, epigastric pain, water brash: origin of vomiting is typically gastric or motility disorder.

Early-morning vomiting, headaches, lethargy: neurologic etiology.

Pain radiating to back or abdominal trauma: pancreatitis.

Mental retardation, history of pica: foreign body ingestion.

Right upper quadrant pain: gallbladder disease or hepatitis.

Right lower quadrant pain: appendicitis, ectopic pregnancy.

Signs

Newborn with palpable "olive-sized" mass in right upper quadrant: hypertrophic pyloric stenosis [1].

Infant with unusual odor: metabolic disease.

Papilledema: increased intracranial pressure.

Heme-positive stools: gastrointestinal etiology (ulcer, esophagitis, intussusception, duplication).

Visible bowel loops (peristalsis), borborygmi: intestinal obstruction.

Enlarged parotid glands: bulimia.

Investigations

Complete blood count: anemia may suggest chronic gastrointestinal blood loss.

Electrolytes: indicates dehydration; hypochloremic alkalosis in an infant suggests pyloric stenosis; chronic acidosis may indicate metabolic disease or renal tubular acidosis.

Chemistry panel: hyperbilirubinemia, gamma-glutamyl transpherase, and elevated liver enzymes (biliary or liver disease); hypoalbuminemia may denote intestinal or renal disease; elevated blood urea nitrogen or creatinine suggests kidney disease.

Urinalysis, urine culture: abnormalities may prompt renal evaluation.

Elevated amylase/lipase: suggests pancreatic dysfunction.

Abdominal obstruction series: useful in determining intestinal obstruction (air/fluid levels); some gallstones or renal stones; appendicolith.

Abdominal ultrasound: noninvasive test, rapidly evaluates abdominal organs; test of choice for pyloric stenosis, gallbladder, pancreatic, renal, and ovarian disease.

Upper gastrointestinal contrast series: useful in determining anatomic and mucosal intestinal diseases.

Endoscopy: most reliable test for determining esophageal, gastric, and duodenal causes of vomiting.

Abdominal CT: only when increased anatomic detail required (abscess, tumor).

Head MRI: indicated for the evaluation of neurologic causes of vomiting.

Ophthalmologic examination: may indicate increased intracranial pressure (papilledema) or metabolic abnormality.

Complications

Mallory–Weiss tear, hemetemesis: linear mucosal tear in the distal esophagus causing hemetemesis, which occurs secondary to forceful vomiting or retching; diagnosed endoscopically; usually requires no treatment [2].

Esophageal stricture, Barrett's esophagus: esophageal abnormalities that develop subsequent to disorders causing poor esophageal acid clearance.

Differential diagnosis [3]

Infections: otitis media, meningitis, viral or bacterial enteritis, *Giardia lamblia*, urinary tract infection.

Motility: gastroesophageal reflux, pseudoobstruction, achalasia.

Esophagus: stricture or web.

Gastric: bezoar, pyloric stenosis, *Helicobacter pylori*, ulcer disease.

Intestine: malrotation or atresia, duplication, volvulus, appendicitis, foreign body.

Gallbladder/liver: cholecystitis or cholelithiasis, hepatitis.

Other gastrointestinal: pancreatitis, celiac disease, inflammatory bowel disease, cyclic vomiting syndrome.

Neurologic: cerebral edema, tumor, hydrocephalus, pseudotumor cerebri, migraine, seizure.

Renal: ureteropelvic junction obstruction (UPJ), nephrolithiasis, glomerulonephritis.

Allergic: environmental or food allergies.

Other: drugs, pregnancy (ectopic), anorexia/bulimia, pneumonia, sepsis, diabetes, superior mesenteric artery (SMA) syndrome.

Definitions

Vomiting: forceful expulsion of stomach or intestinal contents.

Regurgitation: effortless ejection of stomach fluids or foods.

Nausea: offensive esophageal or stomach sensation of impending vomitus without emesis occurring.

Rumination: voluntary, pleasurable act of regurgitation.

Retching: serial, forceful, straining vomiting episodes that may be associated with petechiae or gastrointestinal bleeding.

Cyclic vomiting: episodes of extreme vomiting episodes of unknown etiology interspersed with long periods of normal activity and health.

Metabolic causes of vomiting

Galactosemia, tyrosinemia, hereditary fructose intolerance.

Urea cycle disorders.

Hyperglycemia.

Renal tubular acidosis.

Methylmalonic acidemia, phenylketonuria, maple syrup urine disease.

Leigh disease.

Congenital adrenal hyperplasia.

Treatment

Diet and lifestyle

• The provision of adequate oral fluids and nutrition is essential in preventing dehydration and malnutrition. In severe cases of vomiting, the intake of fluids should be stressed. Patients with dysphagia may require soft or pureed foods. Infants with gastroesophageal reflux improve with the addition of thickened liquids and solid foods and should be positioned in a prone position with their head elevated 30°. Motility disorders may be exacerbated by foods containing caffeine, spicy foods and peppermint. Cigarette smoking should be avoided.

• Special lifetime diets may be required for specific allergic or metabolic disorders.

Pharmacologic treatment

• Medical therapy for vomiting depends on its etiology.

Phenothiazines

Prochlorperazine, chlorpromazine: these medications should not be routinely used to control vomiting; they should only be used in cases of severe vomiting with impending dehydration.

Motility-enhancing agents

Standard dosage:	Cisapride, 0.2–0.3 mg/kg/dose 3 or 4 times daily (maximum, 15 to 20 mg/dose).
	Metoclopromide, 0.1–0.5 mg/kg/d in three to four divided doses.
Contraindications:	*Cisapride*: hypersensitivity, bowel obstruction, gastrointestinal hemorrhage, or perforation.
	Metoclopromide: hypersensitivity, gastrointestinal obstruction, pheochromocytoma, seizure disorder.
Main drug interactions:	*Cisapride*: should not be given with erythromycin compounds, antifungal agents.
	Metoclopramide: anticholinergic or opioid drugs interfere with action.
Main side effects:	*Cisapride*:diarrhea, headache, rash, arrhythmia.
	Metoclopramide: extrapyramidal reactions, drowsiness, restlessness, rash, diarrhea, gynecomastia.

For *H. pylori* infection [4]

Standard dosage:	Omeprazole: 5 to 20 mg daily or twice daily.
	Clarithromycin: 7.5 mg/kg twice daily (maximum, 500 mg/kg twice daily).
	Metronidazole: 35 to 50 mg/kg/d 3 times daily (maximum, 500 mg/kg 3 times daily).
Contraindications:	*Omeprazole*: hypersensitivity.
	Clarithromycin: hypersensitivity.
	Metronidazole: hypersensitivity, first trimester of pregnancy.
Main drug interactions:	*Omeprazole:* delays the elimination of phenytoin, warfarin, diazepam.
Clarithromycin:	*Cisapride*: decreases elimination of digoxin and theophylline.
	Metronidazole: alcohol, phenytoin, warfarin, phenobarbitol.
Main side effects:	*Omeprazole*: headache, rash, diarrhea, abdominal pain.
	Clarithromycin: diarrhea, nausea, abdominal pain.
	Metronidazole: thrombophlebitis, peripheral neuropathy, rash, headache, dizziness, metallic taste, leukopenia, diarrhea, dry mouth.

Treatment aims

To relieve vomiting and prevent dehydration and malnutrition.

Prognosis

Depends on the cause of vomiting.

Follow-up and management

• The majority of disorders causing vomiting require long-term management of the underlying disorder and nutritional evaluation. Treated infectious causes typically do not need follow-up.

Nonpharmacologic treatment

Surgery: indicated for appendicitis, biliary and anatomic gastrointestinal disorders, tumors, UPJ obstruction.

Endoscopy: indicated for dilatation of esophageal strictures and webs and for removal of foreign bodies.

Key references

1. Benson CD: Infantile hypertrophic pyloric stenosis. In *Pediatric Surgery*, edn 4. Edited by Welsh KJ. Chicago: Yearbook Medical Publishers; 1986: 811–815.

2. Knauer CM: Mallory-Weiss syndrome. *Gastroenterology* 1976, **71**:5–8.

3. Orenstein SR: Dysphagia and vomiting. In *Pediatric Gastrointestinal Disease.* Edited by Hyams JS, Wyllie R. Philadelphia: WB Saunders; 1993:135–150.

4. Dohil R, Israel DM, Hassall E: Effective 2-wk therapy for Helicobacter pylori disease in children. *Am J Gastroenterology* 1997, **92**:244–247.

Diagnosis

Symptoms
• Frequent vomiting starts soon after birth. Often the infant screams most of the day and refuses feedings. Irritability may persist for most of the first year. These symptoms may be due to gastroesophageal reflux causing esophagitis, hypercalcemia, or both.

Signs
• Gestation is usually approximately 42 weeks, with birth weight and length in the lower half or below the normal growth curves. Infant facies may be coarse or fine, with periorbital fullness, medial flare to the eyebrows, blue irises (frequently) with a stellate pattern, epicanthic folds, chubby "low-set" cheeks, flat nose bridge with full nasal tip and anteverted nares, long or undefined philtrum, thick lips at birth or later, diminished or absent "cupid's bow," small chin and large ears, dolicocephalic head (increased anteroposterior diameter) and curly hair. Face and body may become gaunt in childhood or adolescence.

• Supravalvular aortic stenosis (SVAS) or peripheral pulmonic stenosis (PPS) (>50%) may manifest in the newborn period or infancy; rarely, coarctation of the aorta; occasionally, mitral valve prolapse, atrial or ventricular septal defects. Narrowing (stenosis or coarctation) of other vessels, including the aorta, renal, and cerebral arteries may occur.

• Mild hypotonia is common. Moderate global developmental delay with a specific pattern of strengths and weaknesses is usual, with rare individuals having normal IQ or severe retardation. Strengths include good expressive language, good recognition of faces, (indiscriminate) friendliness, empathy, musicality, and sometimes short-term memory. Difficulties include poor visual motor abilities (eg, writing and drawing figures), mathematical reasoning, understanding money, and subtle social interactions. Hyperactivity is common and can be controlled with methylphenidate and similar drugs, improving learning and performance. Difficulties with falling and staying asleep, especially in young children.

• Skin is very soft; skin and hair age prematurely; the voice is deep or hoarse.

• Musculoskeletal signs include cervical kyphosis and lumbar lordosis in childhood, occasional scoliosis, disproportionately short limbs (may not be obvious in the newborn period), clinodactyly (incurving) of the fifth fingers, and an occasional inability to pronate and supinate the forearm.

Investigations

Blood
Fluorescent *in situ* hybridization (FISH): to confirm diagnosis.
Calcium: (ionized is more accurate) for hypercalcemia.
Renal function: 1–2 yearly.
Thyroid function:

Other studies
Urine: calcium/creatinine ratio (timed collection); urinalysis.
Renal ultrasound: for malformations, nephrocalcinosis, bladder diverticula.
Echocardiography and electrocardiography: for structural cardiac defects, SVAS and PPS.
MRI and angiography: for Chiari malformation, narrowing of blood vessels.
Developmental and psychometric testing: preferably by tester experienced with Williams syndrome).
Gastrointestinal endoscopy, upper gastrointestinal scan, milk scan: for reflux and esophagitis.
Urodynamic studies: for dysfunctional voiding, urinary frequency.
Sleep study (if relevant).

Differential diagnosis
• Lysosomal storage disease in neonate/infant, especially GM_1 gangliosidosis, or mucolipidosis II (I cell disease), may have coarse facial features, joint contractures, and cardiomyopathy but not arterial narrowing and other features.
• Noonan syndrome may have coarse features, valvar pulmonic stenosis, but not usually PPS.
• Coffin-Lowry syndrome (adolescent-adult) may have coarse features and mental retardation.
• Autosomal dominant SVAS is not associated with all the other features of Williams syndrome. Often there are other affected family members.

Etiology
• Contiguous gene deletion syndrome resulting from a partial deletion on one chromosome 7 (7q11.23). At least nine genes are deleted, including elastin (causing arterial narrowing, diverticula, skin and joint problems, some facial characteristics, and deep voice), replication factor C subunit 2 (may be important for cell growth), LIM kinase 1 (visual motor dysfunction).
• The deletion occurs equally in chromosomes of maternal and paternal origin; may be more severe growth retardation if maternal. Deletion can be demonstrated with FISH using a probe that includes the elastin gene and extends beyond it.

Complications
Hypertension: due to arterial stenosis or renal disease.
Lifespan may be shortened by cardiac or renal failure: cardiac failure is less common now, because of earlier diagnosis, rigorous routine monitoring, and intervention with cardiac medications or surgery; renal failure, associated with interstitial nephritis, is rare.
Cerebral artery stenosis: may cause strokes in first and second decades (rare).
Diverticulosis of bowel (associated with chronic constipation) and bladder (associated with chronic dyssynergia of bladder emptying): may develop in adolescence or adulthood. Bowel diverticulitis can cause "acute abdomen."
Enuresis, urinary frequency, or dysfunctional voiding.
Contractures can impair daily function: rare; caused by tethered spinal cord.

Treatment

General information

• It is recommended that continuous monitoring and treatment be given in a multispecialty clinic consisting of experienced physicians and therapists: geneticist, cardiologist, feeding specialist, developmental pediatrician, behavior specialist, sleep pulmonologist, ophthalmologist, nephrologist, urologist, speech therapist, occupational therapist, physical therapist .

Diet

• Low-calcium diet, including low-calcium infant formula, if hypercalcemic; do not restrict too severely.

Pharmacologic treatment

Acid antisecretory agents for gastroesophageal reflux and esophagitis: proton pump inhibitors (*eg*, omeprazole) and H_2 antagonists (*eg*, ranitidine).

Prevent constipation.

Antihypertensive agents for hypertension: use appropriate agent determined by normal or high renin secretion.

Optional: **acetylsalicylic acid if cerebral artery narrowing or stroke (usefulness has not yet been determined).**

Anticholinergic agents (*eg*, hyoscamine or oxybutynin): if dysfunctional voiding cannot be treated with functional bladder training alone.

Inheritance

• Most cases are sporadic occurrences in a family; however, we are aware of one affected sibling pair with unaffected parents (Scott, Personal communication), possibly due to germline mosaicism in one parent. The risk for recurrence in a sibling of a sporadic case is probably ~5%, (based on experience with osteogenesis imperfecta). Each child of a person with Williams syndrome has a 50% chance of inheriting the chromosome 7 with the deletion and manifesting the disorder
Prenatal diagnosis: FISH in chorionic villous cells and amniocytes.

Support group

Williams Syndrome Association, PO Box 297, Clawson, MI 48017-0297. Tel:810-541-3630; e-mail:WSAoffice@aol.com.

General references

Byers PH, Tsipouras P, Bonadio JF, et al.: Perinatal lethal osteogenesis imperfecta (OI type II): a biochemically heterogeneous disorder usually due to new mutations in the genes for type I collagen. Am J Hum Genet 1988, 42:237–248.

Ewart AE, Morris CA, Atkinson D, et al.: Hemizygosity at the elastin locus in a developmental disorder: Williams syndrome. Nat Genet 1993, 5:11–16.

Kaplan P, Levinson M, Kaplan BS: Cerebral artery stenoses in Williams syndrome cause strokes in childhood. J Pediatr 1995, 126:943–945.

Morris CA, Demsey SA, Leonard CO, et al.: Natural history of Williams syndrome: physical characteristics. J Pediatr 1988, 113:318–326.

Perez Jurado LA, Peoples R, Kaplan P, et al.: Molecular definition of the chromosome 7 deletion in Williams syndrome and parent-of-origin effects on growth. Am J Hum Genet 1996, 59:781–792.

Power TJ, Blum NJ, Jones S, et al.: Response to methylphenidate in two children with Williams syndrome [brief report]. J Autism Dev Dis 1997, 27:79–87.

Schulman SL, Zderic S, Kaplan P: Increased prevalence of urinary symptoms and voiding dysfunction in Williams syndrome. J Pediatr 1996, 129:466–469.

Diagnosis

Symptoms

Abdominal mass or pain, constipation, weight loss, malaise, urinary tract infections, diarrhea.

Signs

Abdominal or flank mass (70%): may present with rupture and hemorrhage into the tumor mass mimicking an acute abdomen.

Hematuria (25%).

Hypertension (25%): due to excess renin production; may cause hypertensive cardiomyopathy as presenting sign.

Investigations

History and physical examination: fixed abdominal mass in or crossing the midline is likely a neuroblastoma, whereas a displaceable flank mass suggests Wilms' tumor.

Ascertain whether there is a family history of Wilms' tumor.

Assess for stigmata of associated diseases: *see* Epidemiology.

Abdominal imaging: with flat plate, ultrasound, and/or CT.

Complete blood count (anemia more commonly associated with intratumor hemorrhage than bone marrow involvement), chemistry panel, and urine analysis.

Tissue: is necessary for the diagnosis, and should be obtained from the time of resection of the mass when possible (including nephrectomy) or as a diagnostic biopsy.

Histology: as defined by the National Wilms' Tumor Study group, is crucial to planning appropriate therapy.

Metastatic evaluation: liver evaluation with abdominal imaging (CT), lung evaluation with chest radiography (CT may be too sensitive in this setting).

• Because Wilms' tumor may extend through the great vessels of the abdomen (and even into the heart), vascular imaging with echocardiography may be appropriate.

• In special circumstances: bone scan and bone marrow evaluation (clear cell sarcoma) or neuroimaging (clear cell sarcoma or rhabdoid renal tumor).

Complications

• Therapy for Wilms' tumor is generally well tolerated with infrequent long-term side effects. However, tumor may extend through the great vessels (*eg*, the inferior vena cava), causing complications.

Metastatic spread: primarily to the lungs and liver.

Therapy-related toxicities: will depend on the specific treatment. Cardiac toxicity is a complication of anthrocycline use and/or chest radiotherapy; liver dysfunction is related to the use of actinomycin D and/or abdominal radiotherapy. There is a life-long potential for second malignant neoplasms.

Differential diagnosis

Nonneoplastic renal masses (multicystic and polycystic kidney disease, renal hematoma, congenital mesoblastic nephroma).

Other renal neoplasms (clear-cell sarcoma, rhabdoid renal tumor, renal cell carcinoma).

Neuroblastoma (tends to displace the kidney rather than distort it or arise within it); less commonly lymphoma, adrenal carcinoma, hepatoblastoma.

Staging

Stage I: limited to kidney; can be completely resected with negative margins.

Stage II: tumor extends beyond kidney, but can be completely resected.

Stage III: Residual tumor is present but confined locally (including nodes and peritoneal spread), tumors are unresectable..

Stage IV: Hematologic metastases or lymphatic metastases are beyond the abdominopelvic region.

Stage V: Bilateral renal disease at diagnosis.

Etiology

• Wilms' tumor is a primary malignant renal neoplasm causing enlargement of the kidney with distortion and invasion of surrounding tissues (also referred to as a nephroblastoma).

• The majority of spontaneously arising Wilms' tumors are of unknown cause,

Epidemiology

Most common renal tumor of childhood; accounting for 5%–6% of childhood cancers.

Incidence: 1:14 000 children.

Male to female ratio: 1:1.

Most present between 1–5 y of age (peak is 2–3 y).

• Approximately 10% are bilateral at diagnosis, and approximately 10% are metastatic at diagnosis.

• 15% are hereditary in origin (often occur bilaterally and in younger children).

• Wilms' tumor is associated with congenital anomalies in 10%–15% of cases (genitourinary, musculoskeletal, reproductive anomalies; neurofibromatosis; Beckwith-Wiedemann syndrome; aniridia; mental retardation; hemihypertrophy).

Treatment

Diet and lifestyle
• There are no particular dietary restrictions.
• The current Wilms' tumor therapies are very well tolerated by children, often delivered exclusively in the outpatient setting.
• Children receiving more intensive therapies for advanced disease sometimes require nutritional supplementation via the enteral or parenteral route.
• Those on more intensive regimens with poor-prognosis disease may require supportive hospital care.
• Children should wear a kidney guard to protect the remaining unaffected kidney when playing certain sports.

Treatment aims
• The goal of therapy is disease cure, with preservation of as much renal panenchyma and renal function as possible.
• Due to the outstanding success of the collaborative Wilms' protocols in disease cure, current strategies are addressing less-aggressive therapies to diminish therapy-related toxicities in good-risk groups.

Prognosis
• Prognosis depends on two factors: extent of primary lesion at diagnosis and its pathology (favorable, unfavorable, or variant renal neoplasm). Over 90% of low-stage disease patients are long-term survivors.
• Even in advanced stages of disease, current multidrug protocols, with or without abdominal or pulmonary radiotherapy, cure the majority of patients.

Follow-up and management
• Post-therapy management is designed for two purposes: to evaluate for disease recurrence and to assess for toxicities incurred by the therapy.
• Patients are routinely assessed for recurrence by radiographic studies of the primary disease site (ie, renal ultrasound every 3–6 mo for 3 y). Urinalysis and chest radiography to evaluate for pulmonary spread are also routinely performed during this period.
• Specific follow-up recommendations for toxicity are dependent on the therapy received, and children receiving chemoradiotherapy will require long-term follow-up for side effects.
• Immunizations to prevent childhood diseases may be resumed after immunocompetence is restored following therapy.

General references

White KS, Grossman H: Wilms' and associated renal tumors of childhood. *Pediatr Radiol* 1991, 21:81–88.

Kobrinsky NL, Talgoy M, Shuckett B, et al.: Solid tumors in children: Wilms' tumor. *Hematol Oncol Ann* 1993, 1:173–185.

Paulino AC: Current issues in the diagnosis and management of Wilms' tumor. *Oncology* 1996, 10:1553–1571.

Principles and Practice of Pediatric Oncology, ed 3. Edited by Pizzo PA, Poplack DG. Philadelphia: JB Lippincott; 1997:733–759.

Index

Page ranges in **bold type** indicate major discussion.

Index

Arthritis
  with celiac disease, 60
  with chronic granulomatous, 134
  with chronic hepatitis, 148
  with dermatomyositis/polymyositis, 86
  with hemophilia, 142
  infectious, 260
  with inflammatory bowel disease, 176
  juvenile rheumatoid, 8, 24, 34, 34–35, 182, 196, 260, 266
  with Lyme disease, 196
  with microscopic hematuria, 204
  nonerosive symmetric, 288
  nonsuppurative, 174
  poststreptococcal, 260
  reactive, 34, 196
  with rheumatic fever, 260
  rheumatoid, 288
  septic, 34, 36–37, 40, 120, 224
  with sexually transmitted diseases, 270
  viral, 34
Arthrodesis
  for juvenile rheumatoid arthritis, 35
Arthropathy
  with infectious diarrhea, 174
Arthroplasty
  for juvenile rheumatoid arthritis, 35
Ascaris spp.
  and infectious diarrhea, 174
Ascites, 2
  with chronic hepatitis, 148
  with Gaucher disease, 130
  with glomerulonephritis, 132
  with hepatosplenomegaly, 150
  with minimal-change nephrotic syndrome, 208
Asperger's syndrome, 48
Aspergillosis, 246
Aspergillus
  and endocarditis, 110
Asphyxiation, 164
  anaphylactic, 310
Aspiration, 20
  with dermatomyositis/polymyositis, 86
  with esophagitis, 114
Aspiration pneumonia, 82
  and cardiopulmonary resuscitation, 58
  with gastrointestinal foreign body, 124
  with hypotonia, 170
Aspirin
  for Kawasaki disease, 183
  for murmurs, 213
  for pericarditis/tamponade, 227
  for rheumatic fever, 261
Astemizole
  for allergic rhinoconjunctivitis, 17
  effects of, 192
Asterixis
  with acute viral hepatitis, 146
Asthma, 20, 38–39, 52, 82, 122, 158
  and cardiopulmonary resuscitation, 58
Ataxia
  acute, 40–41
  with encephalitis, 106
  with Gaucher disease, 130
  with head and neck trauma, 300
Ataxia-telangiectasia, 88, 268
Atelectasis, 228, 230
  lobar, 302
Atenolol
  for cardiomyopathies, 57
  for supraventricular tachycardia, 291
  for syncope, 287
  for ventricular tachycardia, 293
Atherosclerosis
  with insulin-dependent diabetes mellitus, 94
Atresia, 178, 316

Atrial flutter
  with acyanotic congenital heart disease, 6
Atrial septal defect, 212
  with acyanotic heart disease, 6
  and atrioventricular block, 42
Atrioventricular block, **42**
  with endocarditis, 110
  with Lyme disease, 196
Atrioventricular canal defect, 212
  with acyanotic heart disease, 6
  and atrioventricular block, 42
Atrophic glossitis
  with inflammatory bowel disease, 176
Atropine
  for atrioventricular block, 43
  for cardiopulmonary resuscitation, 59
  for poisoning, 237
Attempted suicide, **44–45**
Attention deficit–hyperactivity disorder, **46–47**, 162
Autistic disorder, 48
Autistic spectrum disorders, **48–49**
  with fragile X syndrome, 126
Autoimmune adrenalitis
  and adrenal insufficiency, 12
Autoimmune diseases, 186
  with Di George syndrome, 88
  with Turner syndrome, 304
Avascular necrosis, 36
Azathioprine
  for dermatomyositis/polymyositis, 87
  effects of, 30
  for inflammatory bowel disease, 177
Azithromax
  for sexually transmitted diseases, 271
Azithromycin
  for bacterial pneumonia, 231
  for endocarditis prophylaxis, 111
  for epididymitis, 5
Azotemia
  with glomerulonephritis, 132

Babinski sign
  with cerebral palsy, 62
Bacille Calmette–Guerin
  for tuberculosis, 303
Baclofen
  for cerebral palsy, 63
Bacteremia, **120–121**
  with bacterial pneumonia, 230
  and cervical lymphadenitis, 64
  with HIV, 152
Bacterial conjunctivitis, 16
Bacterial endocarditis
  and atrioventricular block, 42
  and septic arthritis, 36
Bacterial infections, 176, 184
  with HIV, 152
Bacterial overgrowth syndrome, 174
Bacterial peritonitis
  with chronic hepatitis, 148
Bacterial tracheitis, 76
Bactrim
  for Di George syndrome, 89
  effects of, 192
Bag-valve mask ventilation
  and cardiopulmonary resuscitation, 59
Balloon tamponade
  for bleeding varices, 129
Bare lymphocyte syndrome, 88
Barium
  for congenital airway disorders, 14
  for constipation, 74
Barotrauma
  with asthma, 38

Barrel-chest deformity of thorax
  with cystic fibrosis, 82
Barrett's esophagus
  with esophagitis, 114
  with vomiting, 316
Bartonella henselae
  and cervical lymphadenitis, 65
Bartter's syndrome, 258–259
Beals congenital contractural arachnodactyly syndrome, 198
Becker's muscular dystrophy, **214–215**
Beckwith–Wiedemann syndrome, 150
Beclomethasone
  for allergic rhinoconjunctivitis, 17
Behavior abnormalities
  with adenopathy, 8
  with attention deficit–hyperactivity disorder, 46
  with celiac disease, 60
  with cerebral palsy, 62
  with encephalitis, 106
  with hypoglycemia, 164
Behavioral therapy
  for attention deficit–hyperactivity disorder, 47
  for autistic spectrum disorders, 49
  for encopresis, 109
Bell clapper deformity, 4
Bell's palsy
  with hypertension, 160
Benign juvenile myoclonic epilepsy, 130
Benzathine penicillin
  for sore throat, 281
Benzathine
  for rheumatic fever, 261
  for sexually transmitted diseases, 271
Benzodiazepines
  and attempted suicide, 45
  for autistic spectrum disorders, 49
  for cerebral palsy, 63
  for insomnia, 279
Bezoar, 2, 316
Bicarbonate
  for diabetic ketoacidosis, 99
  for Fanconi's syndrome, 259
Biguanide
  for non–insulin-independent diabetes mellitus, 97
Bilateral conjunctival injection
  with Kawasaki disease, 182
Bilateral disease
  with acute scrotum, 4
Bile acid synthetic disorders, 148
Biliary abnormality
  and abdominal masses, 2
Biliary atresia, 150
Biliary disease
  and abdominal masses, 2
Bilirubin levels
  with jaundice, 180
Biofeedback
  for voiding dysfunction, 316
Bitolterol
  for asthma, 39
Bladder dysfunction
  with neuroblastoma, 218
Blastomycosis, 246
Bleeding
  with acute lymphoblastic leukemia, 186
  with acute myeloid leukemia, 188
  with esophagitis, 114
  with head and neck trauma, 300
  with hemophilia, 142
  with immune thrombocytopenic purpura, 172
Bleeding varices, 129
Blindness
  with brain tumors, 50
  with poisoning, 236

Index

Index